Joint Stiffness of the Upper Limb

ALSO AVAILABLE

Wrist Instability
Edited by Ueli Büchler

Joint Stiffness of the Upper Limb

Edited by

Stephen A Copeland, FRCS
Royal Berkshire Hospital
Reading, UK

Norbert Gschwend, MD
Schulthess Klinik
Zurich, Switzerland

Antonio Landi, MD
Clinica Ortopedica e Traumatologica
University of Modena
Modena, Italy

Philippe Saffar, MD
Institut Français de Chirurgie de la Main
Paris, France

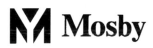

St. Louis Baltimore Boston Carlsbad Chicago Naples New York Philadelphia Portland
London Madrid Mexico City Singapore Sydney Tokyo Toronto Wiesbaden

MARTIN DUNITZ

© **Martin Dunitz Ltd 1997**

First published in the United Kingdom in 1997
by Martin Dunitz Ltd, The Livery House, 7–9 Pratt Street, London NW1 0AE

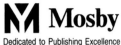
Dedicated to Publishing Excellence

A Times Mirror
Company

Distributed in the U.S.A and Canada by

Mosby–Year Book
11830 Westline Industrial Drive
St. Louis, Missouri 63146

Times Mirror Professional Publishing Ltd.
130 Flaska Drive
Markham, Ontario L6G 1B8

A CIP record for this book is available from the British Library.

ISBN 1 85317 414 9

Composition by Wearset, Boldon, Tyne and Wear, UK
Printed and bound in Spain by Grafos, S.A. Arte sobre papel

Contents

List of contributors   ix
Preface   xiii

I   SHOULDER STIFFNESS

1   Introduction   3
Stephen A Copeland

2   Anatomy   7
Herbert Resch and Herbert Maurer

3   Fibrosis and adhesion formation   15
James Crossan, Dominic Meek and Homa Darmani

4   Medical management   25
Brian Hazleman

5   Assessment   33
Christopher Constant

6   Post-traumatic stiffness   37
Herbert Resch and Herbert Maurer

7   Rehabilitation of the stiff and postoperative shoulder   41
Didier Mailhe and Veronique Aurand

8   The frozen shoulder   47
Brian Hazleman

9   Arthroscopic management   55
Philippe Beaufils, Thierry Boyer and Gilles Walch

10   Arthrodesis   63
Stephen A Copeland

11   Arthroplasty   67
Stephen A Copeland

II   ELBOW STIFFNESS

12   Aetiology and incidence   73
Jens Ole Søjbjerg

13   Classification and assessment   77
Francesco Catalano, Francesco Fanfani, Giuseppe Taccardo, Antonio Pagliei and Antonio Tulli

14   The contribution of the elbow joint to upper limb function   81
       William A Souter

15   Arthroscopic arthrolysis   85
       Franklin Chen and A Lee Osterman

16   Open arthrolysis with distraction   91
       Thierry Judet, Philippe Piriou, Christian Garreau, Godfrey Charnley and †Robert Judet

17   Open arthrolysis and rehabilitation   95
       Joachim Hassenpflug

18   Arthrolysis: our experience   99
       Francesco Catalano, Francesco Fanfani, Antonio Tulli, Antonio Pagliei and Giuseppe Taccardo

19   Elbow replacement arthroplasty: long-term results   103
       Allan E Inglis

20   Total replacement arthroplasty in the management of the ankylosed elbow   111
       William A Souter

21   The GSB III elbow prosthesis   119
       Norbert Gschwend, Hans-Kasper Schwyzer, Beat R Simmen and Jochen F Loehr

III   WRIST STIFFNESS

22   Radiocarpal stiffness: introduction   133
       Philippe Saffar

23   Radiocarpal joint: anatomy and biomechanics   135
       Marc Garcia-Elias

24   Congenital radiocarpal stiffness   143
       Ann Nachemson

25   Extrinsic and intrinsic causes of radiocarpal stiffness   149
       Philippe Saffar

26   General causes of radiocarpal stiffness   169
       Marc Garcia-Elias

27   Flaps and tenolysis for radiocarpal joint stiffness   179
       Guy Foucher

28   Limited arthrodesis and scapholunate advanced collapse treatment for radiocarpal joint stiffness   185
       Philippe Saffar

29   Arthroscopic wrist joint arthrolysis and proximal row carpectomy   193
       John Stanley

30   Rehabilitation for radiocarpal joint stiffness   197
       Jean-Luc Roux, Jean-Claude Rouzaud, Jean Goubau and Yves Allieu

31   Causes of stiffness of the distal radioulnar joint   203
       John Stanley

32   Treatment of stiffness of the distal radioulnar joint   221
       Philippe Saffar

33   Rehabilitation of the distal radioulnar joint   227
       Lynda Gwilliam

IV FINGER STIFFNESS

34 Causes of post-traumatic metacarpophalangeal joint stiffness — 231
Jean-Yves Alnot and Emmanuel H Masmejean

35 Flaps and tenolysis for metacarpophalangeal joint stiffness — 237
Guy Foucher

36 Treatment of metacarpophalangeal joint stiffness — 243
Philippe Saffar

37 Rehabilitation of metacarpophalangeal joint stiffness — 247
Patrice Morla

38 Extrinsic causes of stiffness of the proximal interphalangeal joint — 251
Constantin Sokolow

39 Intrinsic causes of stiffness of the interphalangeal joints — 259
Alberto Lluch

40 Treatment of stiffness of the proximal interphalangeal joint — 265
Philippe Saffar

41 Rehabilitation of the proximal interphalangeal joint — 273
Patrice Morla

42 Stiffness of the thumb — 277
Antonio Landi, Giuseppe Caserta, Antonio Saracino and Maria Cristina Facchini

43 Stiffness of the base of the thumb — 289
Giorgio A Brunelli and Giovanni R Brunelli

44 Rehabilitation of the stiff thumb — 299
Jacques Otthiers

V INTERRELATED STIFFNESS

45 Clinical and neurophysiological aspects of the spastic upper limb — 307
Rudolf Schoenhuber and Francesco Teatini

46 Hyponeurotization in spastic palsy — 315
Giorgio A Brunelli and Giovanni R Brunelli

47 Spasticity after prolonged coma — 319
Antonio Landi, Giuseppe Caserta, Lidia Buscaroli, Marco Esposito and Antonio Saracino

48 Surgical rehabilitation of the spastic upper limb — 331
Eduardo A Zancolli

49 Neuro-rehabilitation of the spastic upper limb — 349
M Antonietta Vannini

50 Arthrogryposis multiplex congenita of the elbow — 355
Loris Valdiserri, Stefano Stilli and Raffaele Pascarella

51 Arthrogryposis multiplex congenita of the hand and wrist — 361
Paul J Smith and Adriaan O Grobbelaar

52 Atypical compartment syndromes of the upper limb — 365
Antonio Landi, Giuseppe Caserta, Antonio Saracino and Marco Esposito

53   Reflex sympathetic dystrophy: an overview   381
      Christopher B Wynn Parry

Index   391

List of contributors

Yves Allieu
Chirurgie Orthopédique et Traumatologique II
Hôpital Lapeyronie
555, route de Ganges
F-34295 Montpellier Cedex 5, France

Jean-Yves Alnot
Hand Surgery
Centre de Chirurgie
Orthopédique et Traumatologique
Hôpital Bichat
46, rue Henri Huchard
F-75877 Paris Cedex 18, France

Veronique Aurand
UTAM
26, cours Gambetta
F-34000 Montpellier, France

Philippe Beaufils
Centre Hospitalier de Versailles
F-78157 Le Chesnay Cedex, France

Thierry Boyer
Clinique Nollet
21, rue Brochant
F-75017 Paris, France

Giorgio A Brunelli
Clinica Ortopedica dell'Università
Spedali Civili
Piazzale Ospedale Civile, 2
I-25124 Brescia, Italy

Giovanni R Brunnelli
Clinica Ortopedica dell'Università
Spedali Civili
Piazzale Ospedale Civile, 2
I-25124 Brescia, Italy

Lidia Buscaroli
Ospedale di Rieducazione Funzionale
Via Monte Cantone, 37
Monte Catone
I-40026 Inola, Italy

Giuseppe Caserta
Clinica Ortopedica e Traumatologica
Università di Modena
Policlinico
Largo del Pozzo, 71
I-41100 Modena, Italy

Francesco Catalano
Istituto di Clinica Ortopedica
Università Cattolica del Sacro Cuore
Largo F Vito, 1
I-00168 Rome, Italy

Franklin Chen
Department of Orthopaedics, Northwestern
University
and Evanbrook Orthopaedic and Sports Medicine
Associates, Ltd
1144 Wilmette Avenue
Wilmette, Illinois 60091–1604, USA

Christopher Constant
Department of Orthopaedic Surgery
Addenbrooke's Hospital
Hills Road
Cambridge CB2 2QQ, UK

Stephen A Copeland
Department of Orthopaedic Surgery
Royal Berkshire Hospital
London Road
Reading RG1 5AN, UK

James Crossan
Department of Orthopaedic Surgery
Western Infirmary
Glasgow G11 6NT, UK

Homa Darmani
Laboratory of Cell Biology
Institute of Biomedical and Life Sciences
University of Glasgow
Glasgow, UK

Marco Esposito
Clinica Ortopedica a Traumatologica
Università di Modena
Policlinico
Largo del Pozzo, 71
I-41100 Modena, Italy

Maria Cristina Facchini
Clinica Ortopedica a Traumatologica
Università di Modena
Policlinico
Largo del Pozzo, 71
I-41100 Modena, Italy

Francesco Fanfani
Istituto di Clinica Ortopedica
Università Cattolica del Sacro Cuore
Largo F Vito, 1
I-00168 Rome, Italy

Guy Foucher
SOS Main/Clinique du Parc
4, boulevard du Président-Edwards
F-67000 Strasbourg, France

Marc Garcia-Elias
Institut Kaplan
Paseo Bonanova, 9
08022 Barcelona, Spain

C Garreau
Hôpital Tenon
4, rue de la Chine
F-75970 Paris Cedex 20, France

Jean Goubau
Chirurgie Orthopédique et Traumatologique II
Hôpital Lapeyronie
555, route de Ganges
F-34295 Montpellier Cedex 5, France

Adriaan O Grobbelaar
Plastic Surgery Unit
Mount Vernon Hospital
Rickmansworth Road
Northwood HA6 2RN, UK

Norbert Gschwend
Schulthess Klinik
Lengghalde 2
CH-8008 Zürich, Switzerland

Lynda Gwilliam
Upper Limb Unit
Wrightington Hospital for Joint Disease
Hall Lane, Appley Bridge
Wigan WN6 9EP, UK

Joachim Hassenpflug
Klinik für Orthopädie
Christian-Albrechts-Universität
Michaelisstraße 1
D-24105 Kiel, Germany

Brian Hazleman
Rheumatology Research Unit
Box 194, Unit E6
Addenbrooke's Hospital
Hills Road
Cambridge CB2 2QQ, UK

Allan E Inglis
Hospital for Special Surgery and
Center for Advanced Orthopaedic Surgery
Beth Israel Medical Center North Division
1725 York Avenue, 89th Street
New York, New York 10128, USA

Thierry Judet
Hôpital Tenon
4, rue de la Chine
F-75970 Paris Cedex 20, France

†Robert Judet

Antonio Landi
Microvascular Unit
Clinica Ortopedica e Traumatologica
Università di Modena
Policlinico
Largo del Pozzo, 71
I-41100 Modena, Italy

Alberto Lluch
Institut Kaplan
Paseo Bonanova, 9
08022 Barcelona, Spain

Jochen F Loehr
Schulthess Klinik
Lengghalde 2
CH-8008 Zürich, Switzerland

Didier Mailhe
Cabinet de Chirurgie Orthopédique
5, rue Gerhardt
F-34000 Montpellier, France

Emmanuel H Masmejean
Hand Surgery
Centre de Chirurgie
Orthopédique et Traumatologique
Hôpital Bichat
46, rue Henri Huchard
F-75877 Paris Cedex 18, France

Herbert Maurer
Anatomical Institute
Müllerstraße 59
A-5020 Innsbruck, Austria

Dominic Meek
Department of Orthopaedic Surgery
Western Infirmary
Glasgow G11 6NT, UK

Patrice Morla
Institut Français de Chirurgie de la Main
5, rue du Dôme
F-75116 Paris, France

Ann Nachemson
Department of Hand Surgery
Sahlgrenska University Hospital
S-413 45 Göteborg, Sweden

A Lee Osterman
Hand Surgery, Department of Orthopaedic Surgery
Thomas Jefferson University Hospital
Philadelphia
and The Philadelphia Hand Center
700 South Henderson Road, Suite 200
King of Prussia, Pennsylvania 19406, USA

Jacques Otthiers
Centre de Chirurgie de la Main
Clinique du Parc Léopold
Rue Froissart, 38
B-1040 Brussels, Belgium

Antonio Pagliei
Istituto di Clinica Ortopedica
Università Cattolica del Sacro Cuore
Largo F Vito, 1
I-00168 Rome, Italy

Raffaele Pascarella
Istituto Ortopedico Rizzoli, Div. III
Via GC Pupilli, 1
I-40136 Bologna, Italy

P Piriou
Hôpital Tenon
4, rue de la Chine
F-75970 Paris Cedex 20, France

Herbert Resch
Abteilung für Unfallchirurgie
Landeskrankenanstalten Salzburg
Müllnerhauptstraße 48
A-5020 Salzburg, Austria

Jean-Luc Roux
Chirurgie Orthopédique et Traumatologique II
Hôpital Lapeyronie
555, route de Ganges
F-34295 Montpellier Cedex 5, France

Jean-Claude Rouzaud
Hôpital Lapeyronie
555, route de Ganges
F-34295 Montpellier Cedex 5, France

Philippe Saffar
Institut Français de Chirurgie de la Main
5, rue du Dôme
F-75116 Paris, France

Antonio Saracino
Clinica Ortopedica e Traumatologica
Università di Modena
Policlinico
Largo del Pozzo, 71
I-41100 Modena, Italy

Rudolf Schoenhuber
Divisione Neurologica
Ospedale Regionale
Via Böhler, 127
I-39100 Bolzano, Italy

Hans-Kasper Schwyzer
Schulthess Klinik
Lengghalde 2
CH-8008 Zürich, Switzerland

Beat R Simmen
Schulthess Klinik
Lengghalde 2
CH-8008 Zürich, Switzerland

Paul J Smith
Plastic Surgery Unit
Mount Vernon Hospital
Rickmansworth Road
Northwood HA6 2RN, UK

Jens Ole Søjbjerg
Shoulder and Elbow Clinic
Department of Orthopaedic Surgery
University Hospital of Aarhus
Randersvej 1
DK-Aarhus, N, Denmark

Constantin Sokolow
Institut Français de Chirurgie de la Main
5, rue du Dôme
F-75116 Paris, France

William A Souter
Surgical Arthritis Unit
Princess Margaret Rose Orthopaedic Hospital
41–43 Frogston Road West
Edinburgh EH10 7ED, UK

John Stanley
Centre for Hand and Upper Limb Surgery
Wrightington Hospital for Joint Disease
Hall Lane, Appley Bridge
Wigan WN6 9EP, UK

Stefano Stilli
Paediatric Department
Istituto Ortopedico Rizzoli
Via GC Pupilli, 1
I-40136 Bologna, Italy

Giuseppe Taccardo
Istituto di Clinica Ortopedica
Università Cattolica del Sacro Cuore
Largo F Vito, 1
I-00168 Rome, Italy

Francesco Teatini
Divisione Neurologica
Ospedale Regionale
Via Böhler, 137
I-39100 Bolzano, Italy

Antonio Tulli
Istituto di Clinica Ortopedica
Università Cattolica del Sacro Cuore
Largo F Vito, 1
I-00168 Rome, Italy

Loris Valdiserri
Paediatric Department
Istituto Ortopedico Rizzoli
Via GC Pupilli, 1
I-40436 Bologna, Italy

M Antonietta Vannini
Studio Medico
Via S Stefano, 130
I-40125 Bologna, Italy

Gilles Walch
Clinique Orthopédique Émile de Vialar
116, rue Antoine Charial
F-69003 Lyon, France

Christopher B Wynn Parry
Devonshire Hospital
29–31 Devonshire Street
London W1N 1RF, UK

Eduardo A Zancolli
Avenida Alvear 1535
1014 Buenos Aires, Argentina

Preface

The choice of the topic 'Joint Stiffness of the Upper Limb' was entirely that of my friend Antonio Landi, President of the Fourth Congress of the Federation of European Societies for Surgery of the Hand, at Bologna. The title is beguilingly simplistic and when he asked me to run an instructional course for the Congress, I readily accepted.

From the beginning it was envisaged that a book should be published to accompany this course. It was only when I started to assemble the contributors and organize the topics to be discussed that I realized what a very complex task I had taken on: it cuts across all boundaries, scientific, anatomic and therapeutic. However, I think it is extremely timely that a very old problem be carefully examined in a multi-disciplinary approach. The function of the upper limb is much more of mobility and agility compared to the lower limb, where strength and stamina are of far greater importance; hence any loss of movement is a far greater problem in the upper limb than in the lower limb. There is no one cause of stiffness, and prevention is better than cure, but in order to prevent we have first to understand. Although we have become very divided in our surgical subspecialties, our problems are surprisingly similar when it comes to stiffness, and we can therefore all learn from each other. In this regard I am particularly grateful to my co-editors, Norbert Gschwend, Philippe Saffar and Antonio Landi, who were each responsible for their own sections of the book. They are well known and highly respected in their fields and have gathered together a magnificent and varied collection of contributors, all of whom illuminate some aspect of a problem that besets us all. The book therefore became very much a cooperative effort. The section on interrelated stiffness in particular draws together these disparate topics into a cohesive whole.

Compiling this book was made relatively easy by the inexhaustible efforts of Robert Peden of Martin Dunitz Publishers. He has an amazingly innate sense of timing, in combination with an 'elastic' deadline, and brought the book to fruition with remarkable good humour. Compiling this book was certainly a greatly enjoyable learning experience, and I hope reading it will be for you also.

Stephen A Copeland

Part I
Shoulder stiffness

1
Introduction

Stephen A Copeland

The term stiffness when applied to a joint can be defined as the loss of the normal active and passive range of motion for that joint. Obviously this is simplistic and begs the question of what is the normal range of motion. This varies as to age, ethnic background, familial laxity, training, custom and lifestyle. For example, the range of motion at the hip and knee is greater in people who customarily squat to eat, and any minor loss of movement is not well tolerated. Such movement loss may be easily accepted in westernized society.

The shoulder is the most mobile joint in the body with a combined motion of almost 360°. Stiffness at the shoulder may be particularly difficult to define as movement of the arm in relation to the trunk is a combination of movement taking place at the sternoclavicular joint, acromioclavicular joint, thoracoscapular joint and the true glenohumeral joint. Hence, loss of motion at any one of these links can put strain on to the next joint. For example, loss of movement at the glenohumeral joint may be accompanied by increased movement in the thoracoscapular articulation which causes added stress on the acromioclavicular joint and hence, the patient may present with acromioclavicular joint pain.

When clinically assessing patients, the range of motion is most often assessed by movement of the arm in relation to the trunk and therefore, known as combined shoulder movement. It is obviously this combined shoulder movement which is of importance to the patient and hence, function is dependent on this combined range. However, from a diagnostic point of view, an attempt may be made to define true thoracoscapular range and glenohumeral range. A joint may be described as stiff, when both active and passive range is lost secondary to pain, but if the patient is given an anaesthetic and pain abolished, there may be a full range of movement in the joint. Is this true stiffness or pseudo-stiffness?

The end result of stiffening of a joint is ankylosis where no true movement takes place at the joint interface. At the shoulder, this may be surprisingly difficult to diagnose as there is compensatory movement at the thoracoscapular joint.

Transient stiffness

Sometimes stiffness may be a purely temporary phenomenon. For example, if a loose body 'catches' in the shoulder joint, whilst the loose body is jammed in the shoulder joint there may be complete loss of active and passive motion. However, as soon as the joint is unlocked, motion is regained.

We are all aware of the stiff joint following overenthusiastic athletic pursuits. The next day the joints may be stiff and painful, but as soon as localized muscle swelling resolves, then joint motion returns. A good example of transient stiffness is in the inflammatory arthropathies when morning stiffness can be characteristic.

Congenital stiffness

Shoulder stiffness may be further defined on a pathological basis as congenital and acquired. Occasionally a patient may be born with a primary dysplasia of the shoulder which may not allow for any normal range of motion. Congenital loss of motion may be due to extrinsic or intrinsic factors which may be applied to any category of shoulder stiffness. For example, an extrinsic cause of congenital stiffness may be a brachial plexus palsy causing loss of muscle action around the shoulder and, hence, secondary shoulder stiffness. Whereas an intrinsic cause would be a congenital dislocation of shoulder which may be left unrecognized and so cause stiffness.

Acquired stiffness

One of the commonest causes for shoulder stiffness is trauma which may be due to direct fracture of joint surfaces causing incongruity or soft tissue destruction resulting in loss of the gliding motion around the joint. Recognition of both these factors at an early stage can make a significant difference to the outcome of the degree of stiffness around the shoulder. The role of rehabilitation following trauma is therefore of particular importance.

Inflammatory

The second commonest cause of shoulder stiffness after trauma are the effects of arthritis, particularly osteoarthritis and rheumatoid arthritis. The diagnosis and treatment of these will be discussed in a later chapter. Soft tissue inflammation may also cause secondary joint stiffness. For example, tendinitis of the rotator cuff with impingement and subacromial bursitis may result in permanent loss of movement. It is known that any immobilization of the shoulder may result in permanent loss of motion as the shoulder is particularly sensitive to this. The other inflammatory arthropathies need to be excluded, both monarticular and polyarticular, including crystalline arthropathy, haemophilic arthritis, osteochondromatosis, pigmented villonodular synovitis, etc. It is impossible to give an exhaustive list of causes of stiffness of the shoulder.

Bony disorders

These may be primary or secondary involving joints in general, or just specifically the shoulder joint, e.g. avascular necrosis, metastatic tumour, primary bone tumour, Paget's disease, osteomalacia, hyperparathyroidism and multiple myeloma.

Neurological stiff shoulder

Stiffness may be caused by primary central spasticity or stiffness due to nerve damage leading to loss of muscular action and secondary stiffness. A common cause of pain around the shoulder area may arise from primary pathology in the cervical spine, e.g. cervical spondylosis, cervical disc herniation, neoplasm or infection, and these must be excluded.

Shoulder stiffness from remote sites

It is well known that shoulder pain may result from a diaphragmatic irritation, but it also may result from a Pancoast's tumour, myocardial infarction, oesophagitis, subphrenic abscess, cholecystitis or gastric ulcer. Consequently, no history or examination of a stiff shoulder is complete without a general systemic enquiry or examination.

Finally, no differential diagnosis of a stiff shoulder is complete without considering a psychogenic aetiology. The more bizarre the presenting pattern of shoulder positioning or movement loss, the more likely a psychogenic cause.

Primary frozen shoulder: adhesive capsulitis

The one condition not discussed yet is the true primary frozen shoulder. This should always be the last consideration in the diagnosis as it is essentially a diagnosis of exclusion.

It presents with a characteristic history and runs a typical pattern, but this pattern may masquerade as any other stiff shoulder. Some believe that the true frozen shoulder does not exist, but is only a plain stiff shoulder for which we have not found the cause. This 'frozen' syndrome does not occur at any other joint. There is no such thing as a frozen knee or frozen ankle. Why should the shoulder have a separate aetiology? This is an area of great interest involving much controversy and discussion and would be a fruitful area for research. Frozen shoulder is discussed in detail in a later chapter.

Clinical evaluation of the stiff shoulder

It can be concluded from the above brief differential diagnosis, that history taking and examination of the patient must indeed be thorough, and this will be dealt with in each of the separate chapters. The more thorough the clinical examination and history, then usually the fewer specialist investigations are required.

Conventional radiography is considered to be the starting point for most shoulder evaluation following baseline blood tests.

By using standard projection, it is possible to detect most bony abnormalities such as fractures, calcification, osteonecrosis and arthritic change. However, more subtle changes can be appreciated in the impingement syndrome or rotator cuff disease such as hooked acromion, narrowing of the subacromial space, cysts and sclerosis of the greater tuberosity. Arthrography and sonography both have their place, but sonography particularly is operator dependent and great experience is required to gain valuable information. Magnetic resonance imaging (MRI) is the most reliable imaging technique for most pathological conditions around the shoulder. It is non-invasive and safe, but as it is

time consuming and expensive it can only be used very sparingly as clinical history and evaluation dictates. With obliques, sagittal and coronal planes, any impingement of the rotator cuff by degenerative change at the acromioclavicular joint can be appreciated and, hence, the size, degree and retraction of tendons can be seen, as well as possible fatty degeneration which may have an influence on the outcome of repair. MRI is the procedure of choice to delineate soft tissue or bone infection and also the extent of bony tumours. Computed tomography (CT) scanning is also useful for planning major bony surgery, e.g. if total shoulder replacement is considered, then the CT scan can be very helpful in assessing glenoid bone stock and, hence, planning glenoid replacement.

It can be seen from the above that stiffness is the final common pathway of many different aetiologies and there are many common factors in the development of stiffness despite the differences in the initiating causes. It is the purpose of this symposium to enumerate the different causes, discuss methods of investigation and treatment. One of the main requirements of the shoulder is a full range of motion. Any loss of this causes significant functional impairment. Early recognition and treatment of shoulder stiffness is therefore vital for our patients' welfare.

2
Anatomy

Herbert Resch and Herbert Maurer

When performing shoulder surgery, knowledge of the muscles, nerves and vessels is important to prevent unnecessary complications.

Shoulder joint

The shoulder joint is a typical ball-and-socket joint and is protected by enveloping muscles. These muscles must be crossed when introducing the arthroscope and the necessary instruments.

Articular surfaces

As a classic ball-and-socket joint, the shoulder has a ball which is formed by the head of the humerus and a socket which is formed by the glenoid (Figs 1 and 2). The socket is not exactly perpendicular to the blade of the scapula, but has a physiological retroversion of 5°. The head of the humerus is separated from the shaft of the humerus by the anatomical neck. At the level of the greater tuberosity, the cartilage covering of the articular surface has a recess which varies in size.

The bony socket is formed by the glenoid cavity, narrowing superiorly, and has an anterior recess, the glenoid notch. The glenoid labrum enlarges the contact surface between the socket and the humeral head, which is three to four times larger. This articular lip is attached at the rim of the bony socket.

In section the glenoid labrum is triangular, approximately 4–6 mm thick at its base, 4 mm high from the base to the margin. It consists of a ring of collagen fibre bundles interspersed with fibrous cartilage in the surface facing the joint and at the base.

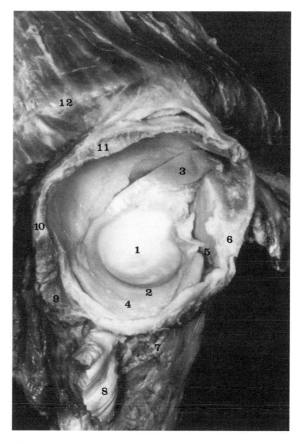

Figure 1

Lateral view of shoulder joint (with humerus removed). 1 Glenoid cavity, 2 glenoid labrum, 3 long head of biceps brachii muscle, 4 axillary recess, 5 subtendinous bursa of the subscapularis muscle, 6 tendon of subscapularis muscle, 7 subscapularis muscle, 8 long head of triceps brachii muscle, 9 teres minor muscle, 10 infraspinatus muscle, 11 supraspinatus muscle, 12 deltoid muscle.

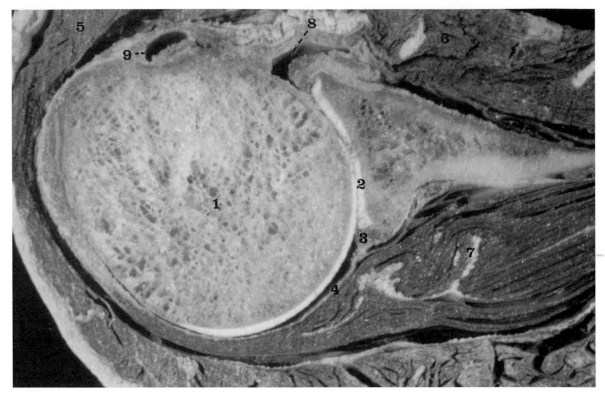

Figure 2

Transverse section through the shoulder joint. 1 Head of humerus, 2 glenoid cavity, 3 glenoid labrum, 4 articular capsule, 5 deltoid muscle, 6 subscapularis muscle, 7 subtendinous bursa of subscapularis muscle, 9 intertubercular synovial sac.

Except for one point at the anterior rim of the socket, the synovial layer of the joint capsule is attached to the glenoid labrum. This is the point where we may find the entrance to the subtendinous bursa of the subscapular muscle. Here, the articular lip is usually rather flat and protrudes freely into the joint cavity.

In the region of the supraglenoid tubercle, the origin of the long head of the biceps is in continuity with the glenoid labrum. In the region of the infraglenoid tubercle, the origin of the long head of the triceps is connected to the labrum.

Joint capsule

The capsule of the shoulder joint is slack with very weak ligaments, and is protected by a tendinous hood, the so-called rotator cuff. The synovial membrane arises from the scapula at the free border of the glenoid labrum, except for the site where the joint space communicates ventrally with the subtendinous bursa of the subscapular muscle and where the attachment recedes to the base of the labrum. The fibrous membrane fuses with the outer surface of the glenoid labrum and radiates into the bone at its base. At the supraglenoid tubercle the fibrous capsule encloses the origin of the long head of the biceps brachii muscle. The capsule is attached to the humerus at its anatomical neck and only extends distally within the intertubercular sulcus. This is where the fibrous membrane, reinforced by fibres of the subscapular tendon, form the roof of the osteofibrous synovial canal in which the tendon of the long head of the biceps extends, surrounded by a 2- to 5-cm long tubular sheath (vagina synovialis intertubercularis).

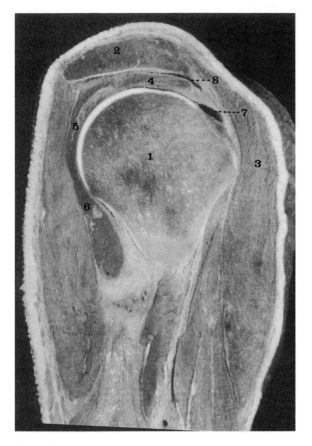

Figure 3

Sagittal section through the shoulder joint. 1 Head of humerus, 2 acromion, 3 deltoid muscle, 4 supraspinatus muscle, 5 infraspinatus muscle, 6 teres minor muscle, 7 intertubercular synovial sac, 8 subacromial bursa.

When the arm hangs in its normal anatomical position, the capsule is slack and forms the axillary recess, which disappears when lifting the arm.

Ligaments

The ligaments of the shoulder joint are very weak and consist of the glenohumeral ligaments, which are interwoven with the fibrous membrane, and the coracohumeral ligament. The ventrally located glenohumeral ligaments are divided into the supe-

rior, middle and inferior glenohumeral ligaments. The opening of the subtendinous bursa of the subscapularis muscle lies between the superior and the middle glenohumeral ligaments. There is a recess in the region of the glenoid notch between the middle glenohumeral ligament and the glenoid labrum. The opening of the bursa, the middle glenohumeral ligament, as well as the subscapularis tendon can be readily viewed arthroscopically.

The coracohumeral ligament arises from the base of the coracoid process, radiates into the capsule and extends to the greater and lesser tuberosities.

Fornix of the humerus

The roof of the shoulder indirectly secures the shoulder joint and prevents the dislocation of the humeral head in a cranial direction (Figs 3, 4 and 5).

The fornix of the humerus is formed by the acromion, the coracoid process and the coracoacromial ligament which extends between both. The latter serves as a reinforcement at the point where the subdeltoid fascia and the surpraspinatus fascia merge, and it generally has a triangular shape, the tip lying at the acromion. A lateral, stronger bundle of fibres extends from the undersurface of the acromion to the tip of the coracoid process and a medial, weaker bundle runs from the acromion to the base of the coracoid process. Occasionally this ligament is rectangular and then consists of parallel running fibre bundles.

Joint cavity

The joint cavity is very spacious and has several recesses. The largest recess is formed anteriorly, connecting with the subtendinous bursa of the subscapularis muscle. Often it communicates with the subcoracoid bursa, thus further enlarging the joint cavity.

The synovial intertubercular sac is also one of the recesses of the joint cavity. The axillary recess is only evident with the arm by the side.

The joint cavity may be expanded to its maximum extent by filling it with fluid, thus making arthroscopy of the shoulder joint easier. It is also advisable to perform the arthroscopy when the arm is in mid-position.

Movements

Movements in the shoulder joint are possible around three main axes. From the neutral position, anteversion (flexion) and retroversion (extension) are performed around a transverse axis, abduction and adduction around the sagittal axis of the scapula, and finally external and internal rotation on an axis running through the head and the capitulum of the humerus.

Elevation of the arm from the neutral position is referred to as vertical movement. In the shoulder joint, anteversion and abduction are limited to approximately 90°, and retroversion to 40–50°. When the arm is slightly anteverted, adduction of 45° is possible.

Forward and backward movement with a 90° abduction of the arm is termed horizontal movement.

The range of rotation depends on the position of the shoulder joint and may be examined when the elbow joint is flexed. Thereby, additional rotation in the elbow joint is prevented. With the arm hanging by the side, internal rotation of up to 90° and external rotation of up to 60° is possible.

Rotator cuff

The shoulder joint is largely stabilized by the tone of the surrounding muscles. The tendons of these muscles enclose the head of the humerus superiorly, anteriorly and posteriorly, thus forming a tendon hood which covers three-quarters of the joint capsule. The tendon hood is fused with the capsule, thereby preventing the formation of folds and incarceration of the capsule. Additional stability is provided by the overlying muscle belly of the deltoid and the long head of the biceps tendon, which runs through the joint cavity and passes over the humeral head.

The bursae of the subacromial and subdeltoid spaces are of considerable importance for rotator cuff function. In particular, they aid movement of the supraspinatus tendon, as it passes through a constriction between the fornix of the humerus and the proximal end of the humerus when leaving the osteofibrous space of the supraspinous fossa.

Pathological changes in this region can result in pain on abduction ('painful arc'). Ruptures of the tendon usually lead to tears in the joint capsule and the synovium.

Supraspinatus muscle

The supraspinatus muscle is completely covered by other muscles. Its origin in the supraspinous fossa and fascia lies deep to the trapezius muscle. Its tendon passes below the fornix of the humerus and the deltoid muscle, where it then becomes fused superiorly with the shoulder joint capsule, to reach the upper facet of the greater tuberosity of the humerus.

The supraspinatus muscle is an abductor, a capsule tensor and a guiding muscle in the shoulder joint. When abducting the arm, the deltoid muscle pulls the greater tuberosity under the fornix of the humerus. Rotation of the humerus displaces the supraspinatus tendon. External rotation positions it under the acromion and internal rotation positions it under the coracoacromial ligament (Fig. 4). The supraspinatus muscle is supplied by the suprascapular nerve.

Infraspinatus muscle

This muscle arises from the infraspinous fossa and fascia, leaving space for the neurovascular bundle of the suprascapular nerve and vessels at the neck of the scapula. Covered by the posterior part of the deltoid, which in part arises from the infraspinous fascia, the infraspinatus muscle, fuses dorsally with the joint capsule and inserts into the middle facet of the greater tuberosity. The upper surface of the tendon is covered by the subacromial bursa. The main function of the infraspinatus muscle is external rotation but its lower fibres also contribute to adduction. It is innervated by the suprascapular nerve.

Teres minor muscle

This muscle arises from the lateral margin of the scapula, superior to the origin of the teres major and inserts on the lower facet of the greater tuberosity. Its tendon strengthens the joint capsule posteriorly and inferiorly. The teres minor acts as an external rotator of the arm and contributes to adduction. It is innervated by the axillary nerve.

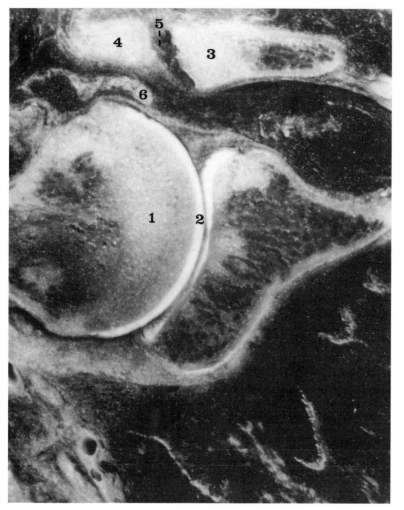

Figure 4

Frontal section through the shoulder joint with abducted arm. 1 Head of humerus, 2 glenoid cavity, 3 clavicle, 4 acromion, 5 acromioclavicular joint, 6 supraspinatus muscle in the subacromial space.

Subscapularis muscle

This muscle arises in the subscapular fossa. Its tendon passes anteriorly to the shoulder joint and inserts into the lesser tuberosity and the proximal part of its crest. Some of its fibres pass over the intertubercular sulcus and reach the crest of the greater tuberosity. The subscapularis tendon is fused with the anterior surface of the joint capsule, thereby strengthening it.

The subtendinous bursa of the subscapularis muscle lies between the subscapularis tendon and the neck of the scapula. It communicates with the glenohumeral joint and often also with the subcoracoid bursa. The upper margin of the tendon protrudes freely into the bursa.

The subscapularis is a strong internal rotator and its cranial fibres participate in abduction. It is supplied by the subscapularis nerve.

Deltoid muscle

The three sections of this muscle take origin from the lateral one-third of the clavicle (clavicular part), the acromion (acromial part) and the spine of the scapula (scapular part). All three parts insert into the deltoid tuberosity on the lateral aspect of the humeral shaft.

The three parts of the muscle differ in function depending on the relative position of the shoulder joint and the muscle fibres to the axes of movement. The acromial part of the deltoid muscle is the most important abductor of the shoulder joint. This function cannot be replaced by the other abductors. When abduction is over 60°, the action of the acromial part is assisted by the other two parts, which are normally active in adduction. The clavicular part effects anteversion and internal rotation. The spinal part helps with retroversion and external rotation. The deltoid muscle plays a major role in all movements of the shoulder joint, thus indirectly stabilizing the joint. Innervation is supplied by the axillary nerve.

Biceps brachii muscle

The long head of this muscle takes its origin from the supraglenoid tubercle and from the glenoid labrum which is intracapsular. At the level of the deltoid tuberosity it joins with the short head arising from the coracoid process. The biceps brachii muscle has two insertions. The deep insertion is into the radial tuberosity, whereas the superficial insertion is into the bicipital aponeurosis, passing medially into the antebrachial fascia. With its long head the biceps acts as an abductor and internal rotator, whilst the short head aids adduction and anteversion of the shoulder joint. At the elbow joint the function of the biceps is flexion and, in the flexed position, it also acts as a strong supinator of the forearm. Innervation is supplied by the musculocutaneous nerve.

The tendon of the long head plays an important role in arthroscopy of the shoulder joint because of its location within the joint space. Surrounded by a synovial membrane, the tendon passes over the humeral head to the intertubercular sulcus in which it continues distally, enclosed by the intertubercular synovial sac. When the arm is rotated internally, tension of the tendon decreases, whereas in external rotation, tension increases.

Subacromial space

The narrow osseofibrous space between the fornix of the humerus and the subdeltoid space on the one hand, and the proximal end of the humerus and the joint capsule on the other, contains the supraspinatus tendon and the cranial part of the infraspinatus tendon.

When abduction moves the arm from the neutral position, the greater tuberosity is pulled under the fornix of the humerus by the supraspinatus muscle, and the tendons mentioned above are protected by the subacromial and the subdeltoid bursae (Fig. 5). The two bursae are usually connected with each other (Fig. 6).

The roof of the two bursae is formed by the deltoid muscle, the coracoacromial ligament and the acromion. The upper surface of the supraspinatus tendon lies in the floor. Pathological changes in this region cause pain when abducting the arm up to 120°.

The subacromial space can be examined by bursoscopy. The arm should be abducted only slightly to avoid excessive constriction of the subacromial space. Pathological changes in this region may lead to the development of additional articular surfaces on the undersurface of the acromion.

Relationships to nerves and vessels

To protect the neurovascular structures of the axilla the arm should be only moderately abducted.

In marked abduction, the axillary vessels and the infraclavicular part of the brachial plexus are under tension and may be damaged if the anterior portal is made too far medially and/or inferiorly with the musculocutaneous nerve being especially vulnerable.

If the posterior portal is located too far inferiorly, the axillary nerve may be damaged. Lesions of nerves and vessels can be avoided if the portals are located correctly.

Innervation of the skin

Anteriorly, superiorly and laterally the skin of the shoulder is innervated by the supraclavicular nerves of the cervical plexus. The lateral superior cuta-

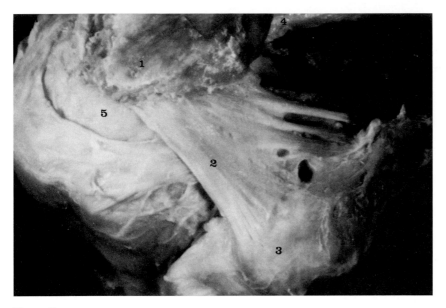

Figure 5

Cranial view of subacromial synovial space. 1 Acromion, 2 coracoacromial ligament, 3 coracoid process, 4 supraspinatus muscle, 5 subacromial bursa (opened cranially).

neous branch of the axillary nerve innervates the so-called 'badge area' laterally. Posteriorly, the region supplied by the dorsal branches of the spinal nerves may extend to the area of the posterior approach. This can be important during regional anaesthesia, as a brachial plexus block may not produce complete anaesthesia posteriorly.

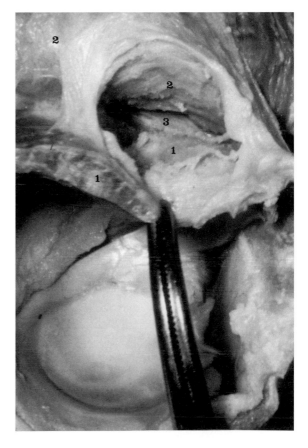

Figure 6

Lateral view of subdeltoid bursa and subacromial bursa (communicating). 1 Tendon of supraspinatus muscle (floor of bursa), 2 deltoid muscle (roof of bursa), 3 coracoacromial ligament (roof of bursa).

3
Fibrosis and adhesion formation

James Crossan, Dominic Meek, and Homa Darmani

The deposition of fibrous scar tissue can be the surgeon's friend or foe. It is clearly desirable that strong scar tissue forms in wounds following injury or surgery and that this process should be expedited rapidly and efficiently. On the other hand, mesothelial tissues which include the synovial cavity of the shoulder joint and its surrounding bursae, must reconstitute themselves fully following injury in order to maintain satisfactory shoulder function. Unfortunately fibrosis often occurs in structures such as the subacromial bursa leading to chronic pain and stiffness. At present, physiotherapy offers the only useful treatment for this complication, but it is likely that future developments in cellular and molecular biology will lead to the design of specific antifibrotic drugs.

The pathogenesis of fibrosis is similar throughout a whole range of tissues (Kovacs and DiPietro 1994). The sequence of events which leads to fibrosis commences when inflammatory cells infiltrate an injured area in response to chemotactic signals produced largely by endothelial cells. The influx of inflammatory cells leads to the elaboration of many cellular messengers called cytokines (or growth factors), and these induce proliferation of fibroblasts and endothelial cells to form granulation tissue. At a later stage a number of fibrogenic cytokines released from inflammatory cells induce the synthesis and deposition of extracellular matrix, initially in the form of fibronectin and later in the form of collagen. Under normal circumstances inhibitory signals bring this process to a halt within a few weeks of injury, but continued production of these mediators leads to progressive connective tissue accumulation and scarring. In the long term this causes permanent alteration to tissue structure and function.

The classical extra-articular manifestations of this process are best seen around the shoulder joint following burns when axillary fibrosis limits shoulder abduction. The threshold for involvement of bursae in fibrosis is much lower than it is for non-mesothelial soft tissues, and even a relatively small amount of bursal fibrosis can produce marked impairment of function. A good example of this complication occurs in patients who develop severe adhesions between the rotator cuff and the undersurface of the acromion as a result of trauma or in the chronic impingement syndrome.

Clinical causes of fibrosis and adhesions

On the basis that adhesions in the subacromial bursa are induced by inflammatory disorders one can classify the types of insult which lead to adhesion formation in the shoulder according to the type of inflammatory response which is elicited.

Soft tissue trauma and fracture

Soft tissue injuries around the shoulder often lead to adhesion formation between the rotator cuff and the undersurface of the acromion. Tuberosity fractures of the shoulder can induce additional adhesions between the deltoid muscle and the bony tragments, including the proximal shaft of the humerus. Both types of injury produce a similar wound healing response in the soft tissues (Cohen et al 1992). This response is characterized by a rapid accumulation of neutrophils in the injured tissues. The function of these cells is to release a number of enzymes which digest damaged tissue and facilitate its later phagocytosis by macrophages. Unless infection sets in, the neutrophil response subsides rapidly and disappears almost completely within 48 h of the injury.

Within 12 h circulating peripheral blood monocytes migrate across the injured endothelium and enter the tissues. Monocytes are the most important cell type in wound healing. Indeed if monocytes are rendered inert, wounds will not heal or do so very poorly (Liebovich and Ross 1975). Monocytes convert rapidly to tissue macrophages and these cells are the main scavengers within the healing wound. In addition to their scavenging function, they manufacture and release large quantities of cytokines. Cytokines can be regarded as hormones which are released by cells and which influence the behaviour of adjacent cells within a local environment. This mode of action contrasts with the more traditional concept of endocrine hormones which pass through the bloodstream and exert their influence on a large number of cells in many tissues throughout the body. Cytokines can transfer signals between adjacent cells, this is called paracrine action. In some circumstances they can also induce their own synthesis by the cells which manufacture them and this is known as an autocrine loop. Continued activation of macrophages through such loops can be engendered by foreign material, infection or inflammation and can lead to sustained and uncontrolled production of scar tissue with consequent loss of function.

Macrophages are assisted in their actions by lymphocytes which appear in the wound within 3 days of tendon injury and which disappear again within a week (Wojciak and Crossan 1993). Lymphocytes, like macrophages, can produce a large number of growth factors which can act in autocrine and paracrine fashions, thereby potentiating and perpetuating the actions of macrophages (Wojciak and Crossan 1994). Indeed, many chronic fibrotic conditions are characterized by the sustained presence of lymphocytes within the affected area.

Some 2 weeks following injury, the wound becomes much less cellular as many of the invading inflammatory cells disappear either by necrosis or by the process of apoptosis in which the individual cells appear to commit 'cell suicide' (Desmouliere et al 1995). This regression within the inflammatory cell population leads to an ordered repair of the wound with sufficient scar formation to achieve good healing, but without the problems of excessive scar formation. Operative intervention around the shoulder for elective purposes induces this sequence of events in the extra-articular and extra-bursal tissues, but often leads to proliferation of bursal fibroblasts and partial obliteration of bursae by adhesions.

Thermal burns

Burns are another source of chronic inflammation around the shoulder joint. A similar sequence of inflammatory cell infiltration occurs in thermal burns as in soft tissue trauma, but there is a much greater tendency for the macrophage and lymphocyte infiltration to be sustained for some considerable time following injury and this leads to excessive scar formation. This is most commonly seen in the extra-articular tissues beneath the shoulder joint. The bursae, because of their deeper anatomical location, are involved to much lesser extent, although the inferior capsule of the shoulder joint may be involved and this will produce a severely disabling adduction contracture.

Inflammation

The commonest pathological conditions involving the shoulder are inflammatory disorders. These are mainly of a non-specific nature and are thought to be caused by inflammation in the rotator cuff and subacromial bursa. Similar inflammatory changes can be induced by calcific deposits in the rotator cuff. The presence of acute inflammation of the bursal tissues in patients with a painful arc syndrome can be inferred from the rapid resolution of these symptoms following injection of anti-inflammatory agents, in the form of cortiocosteroids, into the subacromial bursa. In the case of the calcific tendonitis the acute episode is commonly more severe and can progress likewise to chronic inflammation mediated by macrophages, lymphocytes and multinuclear giant cells which produce fibrogenic cytokines for a long time.

Impingement syndrome

Neer (1983) has described the process of chronic inflammatory change in the subacromial bursa in relation to the subacromial impingement syndrome.

In the early stages of the disorder he records the presence of acute inflammatory change with inflammation and oedema. Subsequently, chronic minor trauma brought about by anterior spurs on the acromion (Neer 1972) will perpetuate this inflammatory response which is characterized by macrophage and lymphocyte invasion. The cytokines which these cells produce in a chronic fashion may induce scar formation across the bursa together with proliferation of cells lining the bursal walls. This may explain the features observed in subacromial bursography of patients with impingement syndrome in whom the volume of the bursa is reduced from the normal 5–10 ml down to 1–2 ml (Strizak et al 1982).

A small group of patients who undergo surgery for impingement syndrome develop severe adhesions between the rotator cuff and the undersurface of the acromion. Revision surgery in these patients is generally unsuccessful as a similarly severe inflammatory cell invasion generally ensues and causes further obliteration of the subacromial space by adhesions. This complication is often characterized by intractible pain and stiffness in the affected shoulder.

Irradiation

Irridation of the shoulder is undertaken less frequently in modern times following the severe problems which it caused by inducing soft tissue inflammation and limb oedema when it was used in a less controlled fashion in the 1970s. The early effects of irradiation are visible in the skin which demonstrates redness, oedema and new blood vessel formation. These changes extend into the deeper tissues, and the inflammatory response engendered, particularly around the inferior recess of the shoulder and the bursae, can lead to the sustained production of fibrogenic cytokines by monocytes and lymphocytes. Obliteration of the bursae or the inferior recess of the shoulder causes severe shoulder stiffness and is often painful.

Rheumatoid arthritis

Although rheumatoid arthritis can cause clinically obvious effusions in the shoulder joint and espe-

cially in the subacromial bursa, a group of rheumatoid patients have been described by Neer (1981) as having 'dry disease', and develop a form of arthropathy in which a great deal of fibrous tissue is deposited within the subacromial bursa and the glenohumeral joint. Such patients require extensive freeing of adhesions between the rotator cuff and the undersurface of the acromion and acromioclavicular joint at the time of arthroplasty. In addition, it is often difficult to dislocate the glenohumeral joint easily and safely when undertaking arthroplasty because of extensive fibrous adhesion within the synovial cavity of the joint. The pathology of rheumatoid arthritis is marked by the continuing presence of large numbers of lymphocytes and macrophages in the tissues. It is likely that the lymphocytes amplify and perpetuate the inflammatory response by their interactions with macrophages, and this leads to sustained production of fibrogenic cytokines over months or years.

Infection

Fortunately, infection, both acute and chronic is now a rarity in and around the shoulder. When it does occur, it is generally diagnosed at an early stage and settles well with prompt and vigorous antibiotic treatment. An exception is seen in the patient who suffers from recurrent axillary abscess formation, often secondary to hyperhidrosis. Repeated episodes of infection and surgical drainage can be followed by the development of scarring in the extra-articular tissues beneath the glenohumeral joint and can cause painful adduction contracture of the shoulder. Tuberculosis still occurs within the shoulder joint and its bursae and produces fibrous contracture. The presence of soft tissue contractures may be disguised by intra-articular bony and cartilaginous destruction which can produce intrinsic stiffness of the joint.

Abduction contractures due to fibrosis of deltoid

Abduction contractures of the deltoid can be congenital or acquired. The acquired form of the disorder is rare and occurs as a result of multiple injections of therapeutic agents into the deltoid muscle. The agents most commonly involved are pentazocine and antibiotics which are administered in high volume injections on several occasions (Groves and Goldner 1974). The explanation for the development of contracture may lie in the genesis of inflammatory cell infiltration either as a result of haematoma or as a reaction to the injection of foreign material. It is likely that multiple injections of irritant substances will produce a chronic low grade inflammatory response leading to the release of fibrogenic cytokines over weeks or months. The fibrous tissue produced by these cytokines will subsequently contract by mechanisms which remain obscure and produce a deltoid contracture which requires surgical correction.

Biological molecules implicated in fibrosis and adhesion

Future prevention of fibrosis and adhesion formation by biological means demands an understanding of the cellular and molecular events which induce these changes. At present there is evidence that at least two groups of substances play a major role in this process. It has been recognized for some time that free radicals can induce fibrosis and this has been highlighted recently in the orthopaedic literature by the demonstration that the level of reactive oxygen species is increased sixfold in Dupuytren's disease, a disorder characterized by fibrosis and contracture (Murrel 1992). More recently, growth factors such as TGF-β (transforming growth factor) and PDGF (platelet derived growth factor), have also been implicated in this process (Kovacs and DiPietro 1994).

Free radicals – key players in fibrosis

Man cannot exist without oxygen, yet oxygen in the form of its free radicals has long been recognized as being inherently dangerous to his existence. Superoxide anion radical, hydrogen peroxide and the extremely reactive hydroxyl radical are common products of life in an aerobic environment, and these agents are known to play a role in the aetiology of fibrosis (Cerutti et al 1992). The superoxide anion is a molecule which is continuously produced and released by metabolically active cells such as

those which invade tissue following injury or inflammation and it acts as an important mediator of tissue damage. Mast cells which appear in large numbers close to injured tendon (Broadley et al 1997), are triggered by oxidative events (Qu et al 1995). Superoxide anion induces mast cells to degranulate and release mediators which may promote the development of fibrosis. These agents include TGF-β and TNF-(tumour necrosis factor) α (Gordon and Galli 1994).

Nitric oxide is another free radical which is produced by activated inflammatory cells. Its role in wound healing has not been established, but will be important to define, as both its production and inhibition can be controlled by pharmacological agents. It is a scavenger of superoxide anion (Midorikawa and Ogata 1996) and in this role it could serve a defensive function by protecting tissues from superoxide-induced mast cell release of fibrogenic mediators. However, in theory this molecule could contribute to tissue damage by producing peroxynitrite anion through its interaction with superoxide. Peroxynitrite is a powerful long-lived oxidant which is known to cause acute inflammation and oedema (Salvemini et al 1996).

TGF-β – another key player in fibrosis

Transforming growth factor-β is a small polypeptide molecule which was characterized a little over 10 years ago. It is an important cytokine in embryological development and its central role in the control of wound healing is undisputed (Border and Noble 1994). Its relevance in the production of scarring and fibrosis was highlighted when it was discovered that foetal wounds, which heal without scar, have little or no TGF-β in the healing tissues, but can be induced to produce scar tissue if exogenous TGF-β is administered to the wound (Krummel et al 1988). Adult wounds on the other hand contain large amounts of this peptide in the infiltrating inflammatory cells and in the extracellular matrix. The expression of TGF-β in a variety of tissues correlates well with areas of fibrosis (reviewed by Border and Ruoslahti 1992). Thus it is overexpressed in fibrotic conditions of kidney, lung and liver. It also occurs in increased levels in proliferative vitreoretinopathy and is associated with a variety of fibrotic skin diseases such as systemic sclerosis.

Of direct relevance to adhesion formation around

the tendon is the fact that injection of TGF-β into another mesothelial tissue, namely peritoneum, in unwounded animals, causes adhesions to form (Williams et al 1992). In addition, injection of TGF-β following experimental intraperitoneal surgery increases the number and severity of the adhesions which form within the peritoneal cavity.

Although many cytokines and growth factors are produced within healing wounds, TGF-β above all others appears to control the level of tissue fibrosis (Wahl 1992). Its central role in these processes is due, firstly, to the enormous number of effects that it exerts on a variety of cell types and its ability to cause differing effects at different stages of matura-

tion in inflammatory cells. Secondly, as a result of its ability to autoinduce its own production (Kim et al 1990), it can induce a vicious circle of events leading to its chronic overproduction.

Mechanisms of action of TGF-β in wound healing

The events leading to fibrosis originate during the final stages of the blood clotting cascade when platelets are deposited into the wound (Fig. 1). Platelets are a rich source of TGF-β (Assoian and

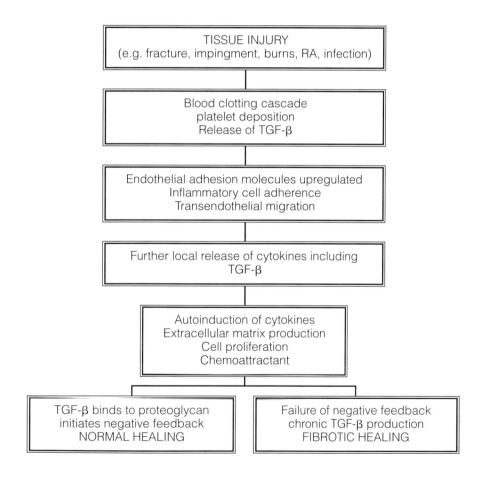

Figure 1

The cascade of events which leads to fibrosis and scar formation is initiated by deposition of blood clot in the wound. These events can terminate in sound wound healing with deposition of normal amounts of scar tissue and restoration of function. However, if control mechanisms fail, hypertrophic scarring occurs, causing scar contracture in the extra-articular tissues and adhesion formation in the bursae and the synovial cavity of the shoulder joint.

Sporn 1986) and the low concentrations of the peptide which are released into the wound exert a strong chemotactic effect on circulating inflammatory cells (Adams et al 1991) and fibroblasts (Postlethwaite et al 1987).

Lymphocytes, monocytes and macrophages

Low concentrations of TGF-β are chemotactic for circulating monocytes and lymphocytes which are thus drawn into the wound. As these activated inflammatory cells enter the injured tissues they begin to manufacture cytokines and growth factors independently. Among these growth factors, TGF-β is of primary importance as it is released by inflammatory cells and induces those very cells to produce more of itself by an autocrine loop (Kim et al 1990). This autoinduction of TGF-β amplifies its biological effects and leads to chronic inflammatory cell activation. TGF-β activates monocytes and lymphocytes to produce a variety of other growth factors which play important roles in wound healing (McCartney-Francis et al 1990; Ahuja et al 1993) and it promotes peak inflammatory cell infiltration for 3 days following injury. After 3 days, its tissue concentration rises to levels at which it begins to downregulate activity in mature lymphocytes and macrophages by complex mechanisms of negative-feedback loops (Tsunawaki et al 1988).

Fibroblasts

As the inflammatory response is downregulated, TGF-β begins to exert major effects on the metabolism of wound-healing fibroblasts and causes them to deposit large amounts of extracellular matrix within 7 days of injury (reviewed by Border and Noble 1994). At first this matrix consists of the sticky extracellular matrix protein, fibronectin, which forms a scaffold for the later deposition of collagen. TGF-β induces wound-healing fibroblasts to produce large amounts of collagen and proteoglycans which form scar tissue in the extrasynovial tissues and adhesions within synovial structures such as the glenohumeral joint and the subacromial bursa. Its potent fibrotic effect is magnified by its ability to inhibit the action of tissue proteases which would normally break down much of the newly formed extracellular matrix.

Under normal circumstances this fibrotic reaction is gradually downregulated when active TGF-β assumes a latent form by binding to certain proteoglycans in the matrix. When this negative feedback loop fails to become activated, chronic overproduction of TGF-β ensues and leads to hypertrophic scarring. It is self-evident that mesothelial tissues such as bursae and the synovial cavity of the shoulder joint itself will be much more susceptible to malfunction than the extra-articular soft tissues, as even small fibrous adhesions can impair their delicate gliding function. It is not surprising, therefore, that fibrous adhesion formation within bursae is such a common and disabling complication of surgical practice.

Experimental prevention of adhesions between tendon and synovium by inhibiting TGF-β

The hypothesis that inhibition of TGF-β reduces adhesions between tendon and synovium has been tested in a rat model in which a crush injury was applied to the flexor tendon and its synovial sheath (Crossan et al 1996). Normal tendon has a superficial layer of epitenon cells which are separated from the synovial lining by a layer of synovial fluid (Fig. 2). Following injury there is a rapid but transient influx of polymorphs over the first 24 h (Fig. 3). This infiltrate is replaced by a predominantly monocyte/macrophage and mast cell infiltration which is maximal at 3 days but which persists for more than 3 weeks (Fig. 4). Lymphocytes appear transiently between 3 and 10 days following injury. The inflammatory cells accumulate in their highest concentrations in the subsynovial tissues and also infiltrate the superficial layer of tendon. In contrast, the numbers of infiltrating inflammatory cells are greatly reduced in the wounds of animals treated by antibody neutralization of TGF-β at the time of the injury and on the following 2 days. Three weeks following injury, extensive adhesion formation between tendon and synovium occurs in untreated animals (Fig. 5), whilst animals treated with neutralizing antibodies to TGF-β form few adhesions (Fig. 6). Peritendinous deposition of collagen is reduced greatly in treated animals from 7 days onwards, and biomechanical measurements at 3 weeks demonstrate that neutralization of TGF-β results in a greater than four-fold reduction in the strength of adhesions.

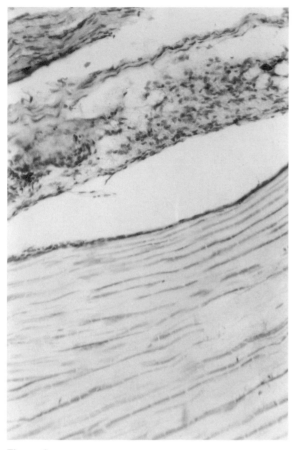

Figure 2

Uninjured flexor tendon and synovial sheath in rat (×10, Toluidine blue). The normal synovial and subsynovial tissues (top) contain modest numbers of fibroblasts and macrophages. Tendon (below) is covered by a single layer of epitenon cells, which, like the synovial lining cells, secretes synovial fluid into the synovial canal.

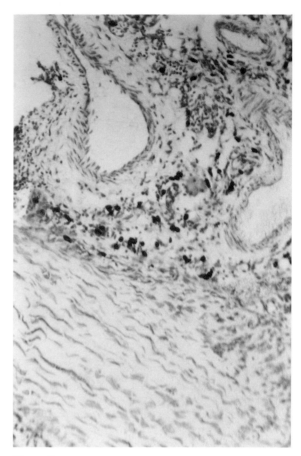

Figure 3

Twenty-four hours after tendon injury in untreated wound in rat (×10, Toluidine blue). The synovium (top) is oedematous and is invaded by polymorphs, some monocytes and mast cells which are large and darkly staining. The synovial space is obliterated in this specimen and some inflammatory cells are beginning to invade the superficial layer of tendon (below).

Thus, experimental adhesion formation between tendon and synovium can be reduced by inhibiting TGF-β over the first 2–3 days following injury. These observations infer that the cellular and molecular events which occur during the earliest phase of wound healing are crucial in determining the development of adhesions. This experimental work gives hope that, in future, biological manipulation of inflammatory cell migration and growth factor production may reduce adhesion formation in synovial tissues following injury, surgery, inflammation and infection in man and may therefore have a large impact on rehabilitation after shoulder trauma and surgery. Progress in pharmacology is likely to lead to the introduction of TGF-β antagonists and antioxidants which may be effective in controlling excessive fibrosis and adhesion formation. The introduction of such agents into clinical practice may transform the management of surgical conditions of the shoulder joint leading to swift rehabilitation and restoration of function.

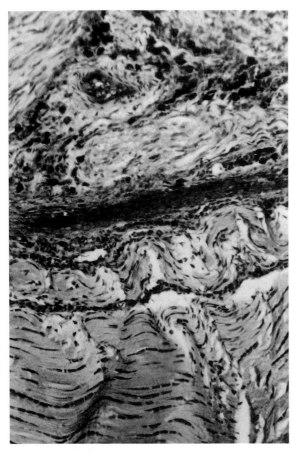

Figure 4

Seventy-two hours after tendon injury in untreated wound in rat (×10, Toluidine blue). The synovium (top) is invaded by numerous cells of monocyte/macrophage lineage, some lymphocytes and mast cells. The intense central band of staining, which separates synovium from tendon (below), represents newly formed proteoglycan matrix containing a high density of inflammatory cells. This marks the peak phase of inflammatory cell infiltration.

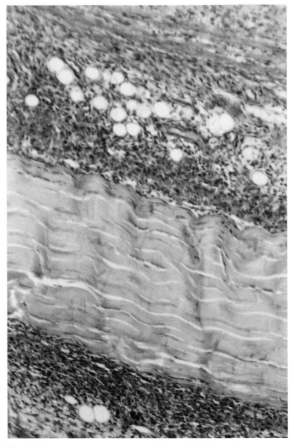

Figure 5

Twenty-one days after tendon injury in untreated wound in rat (×10, Toluidine blue). A particularly pronounced inflammatory cell accumulation is present in the subsynovial tissues surrounding tendon (centre). The synovial space is completely obliterated by adhesion formation. Some of the dark staining is caused by proteoglycan deposition in the peritendinous tissues.

References

Adams DH, Hathaway M, Shaw J, Burnett D, Elias E, Strain AJ (1991) Transforming growth factor-β induces human T lymphocyte migration in vitro, *J Immunol* **147**:609–15.

Ahuja SS, Paliogianni F, Yamada H, Balow JE, Boumpas DT (1993) Effect of transforming growth factor-β on early and late activation events in human T cells, *J Immunol* **150**:3109–18.

Assoian RK, Sporn MB (1986) Type β transforming growth factor in human platelets: release during platelet degranulation and action on vascular smooth muscle cells, *J Cell Biol* **102**:1217–23.

Border WA, Noble NA (1994) Transforming growth factor β in tissue fibrosis, *New Engl J Med* **331**:1286–92.

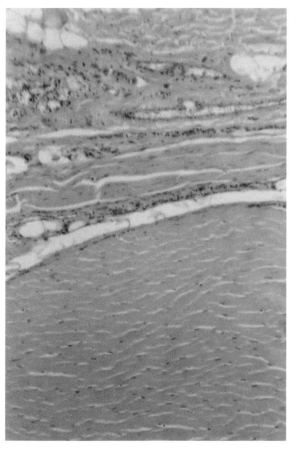

Figure 6

Twenty-one days after tendon injury in rat wound treated with neutralizing antibodies to TGF-β 1 and 2 on days 0, 1 and 2 (×10, Toluidine blue). The synovial space remains well preserved with no more than wisps of acellular fibrous tissue transgressing the synovial canal. There are no substantial adhesions. Synovium (top) shows slight thickening of the lining cell layer and only a mild subsynovial infiltrate of inflammatory cells. There are no inflammatory cells in the tendon (below).

Border WA, Ruoslahti E (1992) Transforming growth factor-β in disease: the dark side of tissue repair, *J Clin Invest* **90**:1–7.

Broadley C, Crossan JF, Reid S, McLay ALC (1997) Pathogenesis of adhesion formation between injured tendon and synovium and its inhibition by antibodies to TGF-β 1 and 2 (submitted).

Cerutti P, Shah G, Peskin A, Amstad P (1992) Oxidant carcinogenesis and antioxidant defence, *Ann NY Acad Sci* **663**:158–66.

Cohen IK, Diegelmann N RF, Lindblad WJ (1992) *Wound Healing – Biochemical and Clinical Aspects*. WB Saunders: Philadelphia.

Crossan JF, Craen J, Broadley C, Nicol AS, Barbanel J (1996) Antibodies to transforming growth factor-β inhibit adhesion between injured tendon and synovium in the rat. In: *Abstracts of the 9th Congress of European Society for Surgery of Shoulder and Elbow*: 146.

Desmouliere A, Redard M, Darby I, Gabbiani G (1995) Apoptosis mediates the decrease in cellularity during the transition between granulation tissue and scar, *Am J Path* **146**:56–66.

Gordon JR, Galli SJ (1994) Promotion of mouse fibroblast collagen gene expression by mast cells stimulated via the Fc (epsilon) RI. Role for mast cell-derived TGF-β and TNF-α, *J Exp Med* **180**:2027–37.

Groves J, Goldner JL (1974) Contracture of the deltoid muscle in the adult after intramuscular injections, *J Bone Joint Surg* **56A**:817–20.

Kim S-J, Angel P, Lafyatis R (1990) Autoinduction of transforming growth factor β1 is mediate by the AP-1 complex, *Mol Cell Biol* **10**:1492–7.

Kovacs EJ, DiPietro LA (1994) Fibrogenic cytokines and connective tissue production, *FASEB J* **8**:854–61.

Krummel TM, Michna BA, Thomas BL (1988) Transforming growth factor-β induces fibrosis in a fetal wound model, *J Paediatr Surg* **23**:647–52.

Leibovich SJ, Ross R (1975) The role of the macrophage in wound repair: a study with hydrocortisone and anti-macrophage serum, *Am J Pathol* **78**:71–91.

McCartney-Francis N, Mizel D, Wong H, Wahl L, Wahl S (1990) TGF-β regulates production of growth factors and TGF-β by human peripheral blood monocytes, *Growth Factors* **4**:27–35.

Midorikawa Y, Ogata H (1996) Influence of nitric oxide on superoxide anion radical generation in vivo, *Jap J Anaesth* **45**:1088–95.

Murrell GAC (1992) An insight into Dupuytren's contracture, *Ann Royal Coll Eng* **74**:156–61.

Neer CS (1972) Anterior acromioplasty for the chronic impingement syndrome in the shoulder. A preliminary report, *J Bone Joint Surg* **54A**:41–50.

Neer CS (1981) Reconstructive surgery and rehabilitation of the shoulder. In: Kelley WN, Harris ED, Ruddy S, Sledge CB, eds. *Textbook of Rheumatology*. WB Saunders: Philadelphia: 1944–59.

Neer CS (1983) Impingement lesions, *Clin Orthop* **173**:70–7.

Postlethwaite AE, Keski-Oja J, Moses HL, Kang HL (1987) Stimulation of the chemotactic migration of human fibroblasts by transforming growth factor-β, *J Exp Med* **165**:251–6.

Qu Z, Liebler JM, Powers MR, Galey T, Ahmadi P, Huang XL, Ansell JC, Butterfield JH, Planck SR, Rosenbaum JT (1995) Mast cells are a major source of basic fibroblast growth factor in chronic inflammation and cutaneous haemangioma, *Am J Pathol* **147**:564–73.

Salvemini D, Wang ZQ, Bourdon DM, Stern MK, Currie MG, Manning PT (1996) Evidence of peroxynitrite involvement in carrageenan-induced rat paw oedema, *Eur J Pharmacol* **303**:217–20.

Strizak AM, Danzig LA, Jackson DW, Greenway G, Resnick D, Staple T (1982) Subacromial bursography: an anatomical and clinical study, *J Bone Joint Surg* **64A**:196–201.

Tsunawaki S, Sporn M, Ding A, Nathan C (1988) Deactivation of macrophages by transforming growth factor-β, *Nature (Lond)* **334**:260.

Wahl SM (1992) Transforming growth factor beta in inflammation. A cause and a cure, *J Clin Immunol* **12**:61.

Wahl SM, Hunt DA, Wakefield LM, McCartney-Francis N, Wahl LM, Roberts AB, Sporn MB (1987) Transforming growth factor type-β induces monocyte chemotaxis and growth factor production, *Proc Natl Acad Sci USA* **84**:5788–92.

Williams RS, Rossi AM, Chegini N, Schultz G (1992) Effect of transforming growth factor-β on postoperative adhesion formation and intact peritoneum, *J Surg Res* **52**:65–70.

Wojciak B, Crossan JF (1993) The accumulation of inflammatory cells in synovial sheath and epitenon during adhesion formation in healing rat flexor tendons, *Clin Exp Immunol* **93**:108–14.

Wojciak B, Crossan JF (1994) The effects of T cells and their products on in vitro healing of epitenon cell microwounds, *Immunology* **83**:93–8.

4

Medical management

Brian Hazleman

Introduction

Arthritis of the glenohumeral joint is a common problem. Whilst crystal arthritis, rheumatoid arthritis (RA) and other inflammatory joint disease account for most cases of arthritis at this site, several other diseases may also affect the joint (Table 1). Recently it has been recognized that the glenohumeral joint is frequently affected in the elderly (Chard and Hazleman 1987).

Table 1 Causes of glenohumeral arthritis

Crystal arthropathies
    Calcium pyrophosphate dihydrate
    Gout (very rare)
    Hydroxyapatite (basic calcium phosphate crystals)
    Cholesterol
Inflammatory joint disease
    Rheumatoid arthritis
    Juvenile chronic arthritis
    Ankylosing spondylitis
    Seronegative spondarthropathies
    Systemic lupus erythematosus
Septic arthritis
Osteoarthritis
Destructive arthritis of the elderly
Neuropathic (Charcot's) arthritis

Crystal arthropathies

Crystal deposition occurs frequently in and around joints. Calcium pyrophosphate dihydrate and basic calcium phosphate (mostly hydroxyapatite) are the crystals most commonly deposited in the shoulder.

Involvement of the glenohumeral joint is one of the features that distinguishes chronic pyrophosphate arthropathy from primary osteoarthritis. In a series of 105 patients with pyrophosphate arthropa-

thy, shoulder involvement occurred in more than one-third of patients, was the first joint involved in 8% of females and 3.6% of males, and was the most troublesome joint in 4% of females and 7% of males (Dieppe et al 1982).

Clinically, chronic pyrophosphate arthropathy of the glenohumeral joint may cause pain, restriction of movement and functional impairment. Some patients may have a history of previous attacks of pseudogout in the shoulder or elsewhere. The joint may be worn, with restricted movement and with an effusion. Some patients will have clinical signs of a rotator cuff rupture.

A small number of patients with pyrophosphate arthropathy develop a destructive arthritis (Menkes et al 1976) which most commonly involves the shoulder, knee or hip. These destructive changes may involve one or both shoulders and occasionally affect multiple sites in the same patient.

No specific treatment is available for pyrophosphate arthropathy. Treatment should be similar to that of osteoarthritis, with analgesia, non-steroidal anti-inflammatory drugs and physiotherapy. Persistent synovitis may respond to intra-articular steroid. Promising results with intra-articular radiocolloid (yttrium-90) has been reported in pyrophosphate arthropathy of the knee (Doherty and Dieppe 1981) but studies on the shoulder joint are not available.

Inflammatory polyarthritis

Involvement of the glenohumeral joint may occur in any inflammatory arthritis, especially RA. Of patients with RA, 99% suffer shoulder pain at some time (Petersson 1986). In a study of 105 patients with rheumatoid arthritis (average duration 17 years) he found that 33 had severe shoulder problems with pain, restriction and functional impairment in at least one shoulder (bilateral in 18 of 33). A further 48 patients had shoulder pain; 42 of these had restricted movement.

Clinically, rheumatoid involvement of the shoulder presents usually as a painful restriction of movement. Severe involvement will cause severe functional impairment, with difficulty dressing and with personal toilet. There is usually restriction in all directions with a joint effusion. With more severe involvement there may be signs of rotator cuff rupture and there may be involvement of other joints and bursae around the shoulder with particular involvement of the acromioclavicular joint and the subacromial bursa.

Treatment of rheumatoid involvement of the glenohumeral joint is the same as for other joints in RA, including the use of analgesics, anti-inflammatory drugs and the use of slow-acting antirheumatoid drugs when necessary. Local corticosteroid injections into the glenohumeral joint may be useful, often with good short-term benefit.

The glenohumeral joint may be involved at some time in most of the other types of inflammatory arthritis. The seronegative spondarthropathies usually involve lower limbs rather than upper limb joints, but glenohumeral joint involvement is relatively common and may be the presenting feature in ankylosing spondylitis.

At the time of diagnosis of systemic lupus erythematosus, up to 45% of patients have arthralgias or arthritis involving the shoulder joints (Rothfield 1985). This involvement usually occurs as part of a symmetrical polyarthritis; when there is severe involvement of the shoulder in systemic lupus erythematosus, it is usually due to avascular necrosis rather than synovitis.

Principles of management in inflammatory arthritis

The progressive destructive inflammatory process in RA may cause not only crippling deformity, but also systemic illness and changes outside the joints that may prove fatal. In its early stages, before joint destruction and deformity have occurred, it can be a reversible disease.

It is important to remember that drug treatment is just one component in the total management of arthritic patients. Management must also include advice about rest and exercises, splintage, the provision of appliances designed to reduce dependence upon others, and advice about employment.

The general principle of drug therapy is to use the least number of agents in the lowest effective dosage. Drug regimens must be tailored to the needs of the individual patients.

RA is often badly treated; patients are kept on anti-inflammatory drugs alone for long periods, in the face of obvious deterioration, or corticosteroids are given early with considerable immediate effect but at the cost of complications later on. There is an understandable tendency to increase gradually the dose of drugs to alleviate the patient's symptoms. This is dangerous, however, and often unnecessary.

The inflammatory process can usually be suppressed, with symptomatic improvement, better function, less stiffness and considerable pain relief, but the disease cannot be cured. Hence, adequate patient education is required from the outset, stressing the importance of controlling the disease, to help give the patient realistic expectations.

The aims of treatment are to reduce inflammation, maintain function and prevent deformities. Adequate suppression of chronic inflammation allows secondary manifestations, such as anaemia, to revert to normal.

Improving the outcome with early treatment

Improving the outcome can be achieved in three ways: developing new and better drugs; more effective use of current drugs; or starting therapy with current drugs earlier in the disease. There is now good evidence that early intervention represents the maximum long-term benefit for the minimum risk. The use of suppressive drugs within 6 months of disease onset improves function; at this stage there is inflammation present but little joint destruction.

At an early stage RA usually involves the small joints of the hands and the feet; large joints such as the knee are less frequently involved. Destructive arthritis is best indicated at the onset of the inflammation; synovitis by the presence of rheumatoid factor, prolonged morning stiffness, rheumatoid nodules, a high erythrocyte sedimentation rate (ESR) and early erosive arthritis. There is little advantage in using human leucocyte antigen (HLA) typing to predict outcome, although some subtypes such as DRB1*0401 may be more closely related to progression.

Drug therapy

Alteration in disease activity in response to a drug treatment can be assessed by a number of subjective and objective parameters, as follows:

- Assessment of pain
- Measurement of joint tenderness
- Measurement of grip strength
- Measurement of joint size
- Assessment of joint stiffness
- Functional evaluation
- Aspirin or paracetamol consumption
- Patient's drug preference
- Radioactive technetium bone scans
- Laboratory correlates (ESR, acute phase proteins)

Pain remains the parameter that correlates best with the overall assessment of a change in disease activity.

Analgesics

Most patients with RA see pain relief as their most desirable objective. Simple analgesics, such as paracetamol with or without dextropropoxyphene, are usually considered to be best because of their lack of central nervous system side-effects. Codeine-containing preparations can be associated with constipation, particularly in the elderly.

Non-steroidal anti-inflammatory drugs (NSAIDs)

The class of NSAIDs encompasses both aspirin and its derivative, indomethacin, the more recently introduced propionic acid derivatives, oxicams and phenylacetic acids. These drugs must be given in full dosage to achieve a continuing anti-inflammatory effect, lower dosage merely producing analgesia. Many NSAIDs are available, which indicates that no single drug is perfect.

There is little to choose between the non-steroidal anti-inflammatory analgesics in terms of

pain relief, nor is it likely that using them in combination will provide any more relief than using them singly. Because of the increasing evidence of pharmacokinetic interaction between these drugs, pain should, whenever possible, be controlled with a single drug.

There is a large variation in an individual's response to NSAIDs. It is often necessary to try several drugs for a particular patient before finding one that provides adequate relief of symptoms. Each drug should be given for 2 weeks to assess its efficacy. Aspirin has now been replaced by newer NSAIDs as first-line treatment since these can be given in a convenient dosage schedule and have a lower incidence of side-effects.

Guidelines for prescribing an NSAID include:

- use a drug you are familiar with
- prescribe cheaper, established drugs
- prescribe only one drug at a time
- prescribe an adequate dose
- encourage compliance by flexible dosing
- prescribe for 2 weeks and review.

Non-steroidal drugs

The major advantage of these compounds is a reduction in adverse effects rather than an improvement in efficacy. They also have advantages over aspirin in the smaller number of tablets required and often, using drugs such as benorylate and naproxen, less frequent administration is needed. When NSAIDs have been compared in controlled studies, no significant differences have been found in terms of pain relief or the patient's assessment of efficacy.

NSAIDs can be divided broadly into those with a short half-life (ibuprofen) or those with a long half-life (piroxicam). Many of the short half-life NSAIDs can be effective in a twice-daily dosing regimen. Long half-life NSAIDs remain in the body for longer once administration has ceased; adverse effects may persist for many days. Also a steady-state level is not reached for 2 weeks and the onset of action is slow.

All anti-inflammatory drugs can cause gastrointestinal bleeding, partly by a local action on the stomach and partly by a systemic effect. About 20% of all cases of ulceration, haemorrhage and small bowel perforation are directly attributable to the use of NSAIDs. The risk is increased in elderly females. If patients develop severe indigestion of peptic ulceration it is best to discontinue the NSAID. If this is not possible, an H2-antagonist may allow healing to occur; this is less likely with a gastric ulcer. There is increasing evidence that prophylactic use of prostaglandin analogues (e.g. misoprostol) may reduce the incidence of side-effects of NSAIDs. Other side-effects may be renal, hepatic, of the skin, pulmonary, CNS, or haematological.

More specific antirheumatic drugs

The theory that selective inhibition of cyclo-oxygenase (COX) might solve the problem of gastrointestinal and renal side-effects is now being put to the test with new drugs. Inhibition of the so-called 'housekeeping' COX-1 is thought to result in NSAID side-effects, whereas inhibition of inflammatory COX-2 gives rise to therapeutic benefits. Drugs are therefore being developed that selectively inhibit COX-2.

If an adequate trial of treatment with a combination of physical therapy and anti-inflammatory drugs fails to reduce inflammation after 2 or 3 months, then treatment with gold salts, chloroquine, sulphasalazine or methotrexate should be considered. The aim is to initiate disease-suppressing treatment before irreversible joint destruction has occurred. Of the three, gold salts are particularly popular and effective, although their adverse effects have led to periods when their use has fallen into disfavour. None of these drugs has a short-term effect in relieving symptoms; however, they suppress the underlying disease process in a proportion of patients when given over a period of months. The characteristics of these drugs are as follows:

• Slow action; begin working after 4–6 weeks and may take 6 months to produce full benefit
• Improvement in joint symptoms accompanied by fall in ESR and RF
• May retard progression of erosive change seen on X-ray
• Patients feel much improved in general health

Major side-effects include renal hepatic and haematological toxicity.

A pyramidal stepwise approach has been widely adopted, moving from the least toxic to the more aggressive therapies (Fig. 1). Recently, Yocum (1994) argued for an inversion of this pyramid on the basis that aggressive disease modifying anti-rheumatic drugs (DMARDs) should be used early in inflammatory disease before most of the joint damage occurs. While there is evidence that some DMARDs have a beneficial effect, long-term data are needed to show that this early benefit is maintained. Unfortunately, because of toxicity or lack of response, after a 1-year period only about 50% of patients will still be on a given agent.

Some DMARDs act slowly, improve symptoms and suppress clinical and serological markers of RA activity. Markers of inflammation include duration of morning stiffness and the number of swollen or painful joints. The ESR is usually elevated as is the C-reactive protein (CRP) and there may be anaemia.

Patients used not to start these drugs until there was radiological evidence of erosive disease, but it is now thought illogical to wait since damage will already have taken place. Patients who have failed to improve after at least 6 months treatment with one drug or who stop responding may still gain benefit with a different DMARD.

Osteoarthritis

Osteoarthritis is thought to be relatively uncommon in the shoulder. It may be idiopathic or secondary to numerous other conditions such as trauma (which includes recurrent dislocation or previous fracture), pyrophosphate arthropathy, rheumatoid and inflammatory joint disease, avascular necrosis, neuropathic arthropathy, ochronosis, acromegaly and haemophilia.

Chard and Hazleman (1987) found secondary osteoarthritis in two of a 100 subjects over the age of 70 years. Kerr et al (1985) showed moderate to severe osteophyte formation in 24% of cadaveric humeri and 25% of cadaveric scapulae. They also described moderate to severe osteoarthritis of the glenohumeral joint in 14% of 50 men (over 60 years old) with shoulder pain.

Pain from glenohumeral osteoarthritis is managed with analgesics, NSAIDs and physiotherapy. Intra-articular corticosteroids may be used and may provide symptomatic improvement. Most consider that they should not be repeated more frequently than every 3–4 months (Wilde 1984). Suprascapular nerve blocks may provide significant improvement in patients with intractable pain.

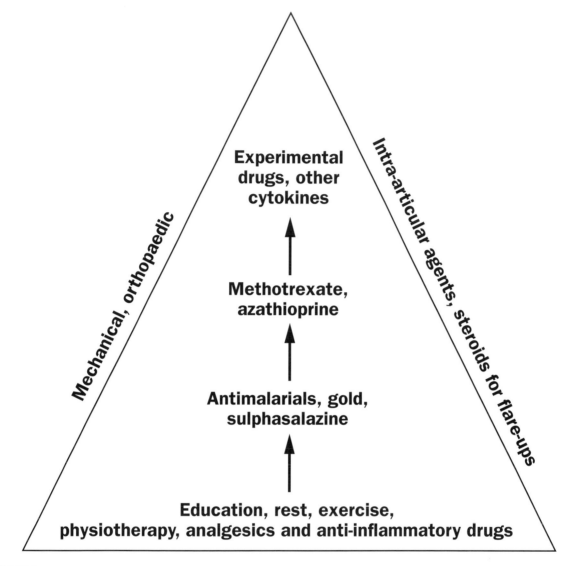

Figure 1

The pyramidal approach to treatment

Destructive arthritis of the shoulder

Recently an uncommon form of destructive arthritis of the shoulder has been re-described by several authors under various names such as Milwaukee shoulder (McCarty et al 1981), cuff tear arthropathy (Neer et al 1983) and apatite-associated destructive arthritis of the shoulder (Dieppe et al 1986).

There is no specific therapy; treatment is extremely difficult. Some patients suffer persisting severe pain unresponsive to analgesics and NSAIDs. Local steroid injections provide little, if any, benefit.

Suprascapular nerve block

Vecchio et al (1993) undertook a double-blind placebo-controlled study to investigate the effectiveness of suprascapular nerve block using steroid and local anaesthetic in patients with defined rotator cuff lesions. They found it to be an effective but temporary form of analgesia for rotator cuff lesions. It reduced pain in patients with tendonitis and in the tear group. The suprascapular nerve provides sensory fibres to about 70% of the shoulder joint, mostly to the superior and posterior–superior positions of the joint. It would seem that a suitable block to treat a majority of rotator cuff lesions (the supraspinatus and infraspinatus muscles) are supplied by the suprascapular nerve.

There is little available literature on suprascapular nerve blocks in the painful shoulder. One study reported the use of this procedure in glenohumeral arthritis with moderate success (Brown et al 1988). This study utilized image intensifiers to assist localization of the suprascapular notch and nerve, an encumbrance to simple outpatient use. Emery et al (1989) demonstrated better success than for intraarticular steroid with a similar method to ones in patients with RA.

Complications are rare; the most significant is a pneumothorax resulting from the needle passing over the superior scapular border or through the notch and penetrating the posterior lung. The technique of the ipsilateral hand being placed on the contralateral shoulder (Parris 1990) is said to reduce this low risk further. There are small risks of intramuscular injection and nerve trauma.

It is uncertain whether it is necessary to inject the solution of bupivacaine into the suprascapular notch: the main nerve trunk is situated here and then divides distal to this, and it has been thought that blocking the main nerve trunk results in the best chance of success. There is anecdotal evidence of good analgesia using 10 ml of bupivacaine injected deep into the suprascapular fossa in scapular fracture when the needle point has not closely related to the suprascapular notch, as confirmed with dye studies through the needle (Gado and Emery 1991). When the volume is large (i.e. 10 ml), the injected solution fills the suprascapular fossa, so bathing the majority of the nerve and its branches. Consequently less accurate localization may produce good results. Our volume (2 ml) was small and may require better positions for effectiveness; conversely, poor results may indicate unsatisfactory localization of the solution.

It has recently been shown (Gado and Emery 1991) that the steroid is not essential to the success of suprascapular nerve block in patients with chronic shoulder pain due to RA. The authors demonstrated good improvement in pain scores and movement ranges using bupivacaine (10 ml) alone.

Although the gains are small and relatively short-lived, these patients are a refractory group who have had minimal or no benefit from standard therapy of rotator cuff lesions. It would be useful in treating pain while awaiting surgery and can be performed appropriately in an out-patient setting.

Shoulder disorders of the elderly

Hospital-based studies have suggested that non-traumatic symptomatic shoulder disorders, although common in middle-aged adults, are relatively rare in the elderly (Hazleman 1972, Wright and Haq 1976, Kessell and Watson 1977). One community survey found a less marked difference in prevalence, but the maximum age of the study subjects was only 74 years (Allander 1974). These findings contrast with those of pathologic studies, which have suggested that there is progressive degeneration of the rotator cuff with age (Skinner 1937, Lindblom 1937, Wilson and Duff 1943), with tendon rupture being found in 20% or more of shoulders from patients of all ages, examined postmortem (Fowler 1933, Keynes 1935, Codman and Akerson 1939). One study suggested that there was no true relationship between clinical symptoms and pathologic changes (Olsson 1953).

It was considered that physically fit middle-aged people were more likely than the elderly to stress their tendons and, hence, produce symptoms. However, a recent hospital study of elderly patients (over age 70) who were admitted to an acute-care geriatric unit found that 21 of the 100 surveyed had a symptomatic shoulder disorder, mostly related to the rotator cuff (Chard and Hazleman 1987). Not only was the frequency greater than might have been expected, but only three of these subjects had sought medical treatment for those symptoms.

A community survey of identifiable symptomatic shoulder disorders in a sample of 644 elderly people over age 70 (318 male and 326 female) revealed a prevalence of 21%. Shoulder disorders were more common in women (25% versus 17% in men). Approximately 70% of the cases of shoulder pain involved the rotator cuff. Fewer than 40% of the subjects sought medical attention for these symptoms. Increased medical awareness is needed, since the elderly often do not volunteer information about such symptoms.

A follow-up study of this group of patients 3 years later showed no significant improvement with therapy (Vecchio et al 1995).

References

Allander E (1974) Prevalence, incidence and remission rates of some common rheumatic diseases or syndromes, *Scand J Rheumatol* **3:**145–53.

Brown DE, James DC, Ray S (1988) Pain relief by suprascapular nerve block in glenohumeral arthritis, *Scand J Rheumatol* **17:**411–15.

Chard MD, Hazleman BL (1987) Shoulder disorder in the elderly (a hospital study), *Annals Rheum Dis* **46:**684–7.

Codman EA, Akerson IB (1939) The pathology associated with rupture of the supraspinatus tendon, *Ann Surg* **93:**348–59.

Dieppe PA, Alexander GM, Jones HE (1982) Pyrophosphate arthropathy: a clinical and radiological study of 105 cases, *Annals Rheum Dis* **41:**371–6.

Dieppe PA, Campion G, et al (1986) Destructive arthritis of the shoulder joint, *Br J Rheum* **25:**99.

Doherty M, Dieppe PA (1981) Effect of intra-articular yttrium 90 on chronic pyrophosphate arthropathy of the knee, *Lancet* **11:**1243–6.

Emery P, Bowman S, Wedderbury L, et al (1989) Suprascapular nerve block for chronic shoulder pain in rheumatoid arthritis, *Br Med J* **299:**1077–80.

Fowler E (1933) Stiff painful shoulders exclusive of tuberculosis and other infections, *JAMA* **101:**2106–8.

Gado K, Emory P (1991) Suprascapular nerve block with Marcain alone effectively controls chronic shoulder pain in patients with rheumatoid arthritis, *Br J Rheumatol* **30**(suppl 2):77.

Hazleman BL (1972) The painful stiff shoulder, *Rheumatol Phys Med* **11:**413–21.

Kerr R, Resnick D, et al (1985) Osteoarthritis of the glenohumeral joint: a radiologic–pathologic study, *J Roentgenol* **144:**967–72.

Kessell L, Watson M (1977) The painful arc syndrome: clinical classification as a guide to management, *J Bone Joint Surg* **59B:**166–72.

Keynes EL (1935) Anatomical observations on senile changes in the shoulder, *J Bone Joint Surg* **17A:**953–60.

Lindblom K (1937) On the pathogenesis of rupture of the tendon aponeurosis of the shoulder joint, *Acta Radiol* **20:**563–77.

McCarty DJ, Halverson PB, Carrera GF, et al (1981) Milwaukee shoulder – association of microspheroids containing hydroxyapatite crystals, active collagenases, and neutral protease with rotator cuff defects, *Arth Rheum* **24:**464–91.

Menkes CJ, Simon F, Debrieu F (1976) Destructive arthropathy in chondrocalcinosis articularis, *Arth Rheum* **19**(suppl): 329–48.

Neer CS, Craig VE, Fukada H (1983) Cuff-tear arthropathy, *J Bone Joint Surg* **65A:**1232–44.

Olsson O (1953) Degenerative changes in the shoulder joint and their connection with shoulder pain: a morphological and clinical investigation with special attention to the cuff and biceps tendon, *Acta Chir Scand* **181**(suppl):1–13.

Parris WCV (1990) Suprascapular nerve block: a safe technique, *Anaesthesiology* **72:**580–1.

Petersson CJ (1986) Painful shoulders in patients with rheumatoid arthritis, *Scand J Rheumatol* **15:**275–9.

Rothfield N (1985) Systemic lupus erythematosus: clinical aspects and treatment. In: McCarty DJ, ed. *Arthritis and Allied Conditions*, 10th edn. Lea & Febinger: Philadelphia: 915.

Skinner HA (1937) Anatomical considerations relative to rupture of the supraspinatus tendon, *J Bone Joint Surg* **19A:**137–51.

Vecchio PC, Adebajo AO, Hazleman BL (1993) Suprascapular nerve block for persistent rotator cuff lesions, *J Rheumatol* **20:**453–5.

Vecchio PC, Kavanagh RT, Hazleman BL, et al (1995) Community survey of shoulder disorders in the elderly to assess the natural history and effects of treatment, *Ann Rheum Dis* **54:**152–4.

Wilde A (1984) Osteoarthritis of the shoulder and elbow. In: Moskowitz RW et al, eds. *Osteoarthritis: Diagnosis and Management*. WB Saunders: Philadelphia: 377–87.

Wilson CL, Duff GL (1943) Pathological study of degeneration and rupture of the supraspinatus tendon, *Arch Surg* **47:**121–35.

Wright V, Haq AMMM (1976) Periarthritis of the shoulder: aetiological considerations with particular reference to personality factors, *Ann Rheum Dis* **35:**213–19.

Yocum D (1994) Aggressive therapy versus conservative treatment. In: Klippel J, Dieppe P. eds. *Rheumatology* Mosby: London. 313–9.

5
Assessment
Christopher Constant

Introduction

In assessing the stiff shoulder an attempt must be made to identify the cause of the problem, as well as the functional disability associated with it. Appropriate management of the condition can only be considered once the diagnosis has been made, and the results of any treatment undertaken can only be assessed if ongoing repeated functional assessments are undertaken.

The diagnostic assessment of the stiff shoulder is different to the assessment of shoulder function in this condition. Since shoulder stiffness may be a manifestation of a variety of conditions affecting the shoulder, or may be an idiopathic problem with an unidentifiable cause, it is necessary to undertake a systematic diagnostic assessment in order to confirm or exclude the presence of conditions associated with shoulder stiffness. In the assessment of shoulder function painless active range of motion (ROM) will be significantly affected in a stiff shoulder, and the effect that this will have on shoulder function will be discussed later in the chapter.

In considering the assessment of the stiff shoulder, therefore, it is necessary briefly to outline the clinical problems associated with shoulder stiffness, the clinical history associated with these problems, and the examination findings one is likely to encounter. Supplementary to the detailed history and examination are the investigations that confirm the clinical impression, and these will be outlined. A knowledge of the natural history of the stiff and painful shoulder is essential when assessing shoulder stiffness, and this will be considered. Finally, a brief comment on the management of the stiff shoulder and the functional outcome as assessed by using the Constant shoulder functional score will be presented.

Causes of shoulder stiffness

The majority of cases of shoulder stiffness, frequently referred to as adhesive capsulitis or a frozen shoulder, have no known associated cause, and are therefore described as idiopathic. There are, however, a number of conditions associated with the occurrence of adhesive capsulitis or shoulder stiffness: these include diabetes mellitus, trauma, and visceral neoplasm in which there appears to be a significant association with adhesive capsulitis. For the purposes of this discussion I will exclude local conditions of the shoulder resulting in severe stiffness of glenohumeral motion such as primary or secondary osteoarthrosis, rheumatoid arthritis, avascular necrosis and so on.

Adhesive capsulitis is frequently a symptom and a finding in degenerative acromioclavicular joint and subacromial/rotator cuff disease. Along with pain and weakness, shoulder stiffness is a common presenting symptom in such patients, and the history, examination and assessment of patients with a stiff shoulder must include either a confirmation of an exclusion of these diagnoses.

Following shoulder trauma, in the form of either a fracture or a severe soft tissue injury, stiffness may be an ongoing persistent and troublesome problem, and clearly the treatment in such instances will be to deal with the problems associated with the injury.

An important cause of shoulder stiffness is shoulder surgery. Following shoulder surgery, stiffness of the shoulder or postoperative adhesive capsulitis can often be prevented by a structured rehabilitation programme. Failure on the part of the patient to comply with such a programme in many instances will result in a significant and frequently severe postoperative adhesive capsulitis which may be very difficult to treat satisfactorily.

Diagnostic assessment

The first part of the diagnostic assessment of a stiff shoulder is to record a detailed history. This should include a history of the chronology of events in the onset of pain and stiffness. History of injury should be recorded, the patient's general health should be noted and a history of diabetes or significant systemic illness questioned. In the absence of any significant history to account for shoulder stiffness, a diagnosis of an idiopathic adhesive capsulitis may be considered. The history in such cases is usually one of a spontaneous and unexpected onset of either pain or stiffness. In the initial stages the restriction of motion is first observed in internal rotation with the patient being unable to take their hand behind their back, and frequently being unable to reach above their waist from a very early stage. There is associated pain which is frequently present at night, and may be localized to the front of the shoulder or generalized around the shoulder. Radiation to the periscapular region, down the arm to the area of the deltoid insertion, and up towards the neck, is not uncommon. A history of associated shoulder weakness is often unreliable because of the presence of pain and stiffness.

The natural history of the condition is to go from a painful and increasingly stiff phase (first phase), into a very stiff but less painful phase (second phase), followed by resolution of the stiffness over a further period of time (third phase). Once the stiff but less painful phase is reached, pain is particularly a problem only with sudden movements and often in the resting position where the scapula is felt to protrude posteriorly on account of the fixed flexion deformity that is present in the shoulder during this stage. During the third phase, pain may frequently be considerable, but the increasing useful ROM that occurs is often gratifying. A careful history will often indicate the transition between the first, second and third phases, and will help to confirm the diagnosis, often without the need for further more specific investigations. This is particularly the case where the diagnosis is being made during the third phase and where the patient is often satisfied with the reassurance that resolution is about to occur.

Physical examination as part of the assessment of the stiff shoulder must include an examination of the neck for signs of stiffness or pain, and bilateral shoulder examination. Assessment of the other joints of the upper limb as well as a neurological assessment of the upper limbs should be undertaken, and general physical assessment should not be forgotten. Examination of the shoulders themselves should also include inspection for signs of associated subacromial and acromioclavicular joint disease, as well as rotator cuff pathology, and should furthermore assess the presence or absence of glenohumeral joint pathology as a cause for the stiffness. Presence of any scars, indicative of previous surgery, should be noted, as sometimes a history of previous surgery is omitted by the patient, despite the fact that this may be very relevant to the ongoing problems the patient has. An unusual but not uncommon cause of a severe and frequently protracted adhesive capsulitis is a sternotomy for open heart surgery; this association may not be apparent to the patient, who may omit to mention that his or her symptoms began shortly after such surgery was undertaken.

The degree of glenohumeral stiffness, scapulothoracic movement and therefore overall shoulder movement should be recorded both in terms of the initial assessment of the condition and in order to assess the progress being made during the various stages of the disease.

Investigations

The diagnosis of a frozen shoulder is a clinical one. Assuming that all conditions associated with adhesive capsulitis have been excluded, the diagnosis of idiopathic adhesive capsulitis can be made. In order to exclude local shoulder problems resulting in stiffness and pain, a series of investigations is advocated before the diagnosis of idiopathic adhesive capsulitis is accepted.

Plain radiography

A series of plain x-rays of the shoulder should be undertaken to exclude glenohumeral arthritis, significant AC joint osteoarthrosis, avascular necrosis, evidence of old trauma or severe subacromial or rotator cuff disease. Idiopathic adhesive capsulitis is frequently associated with a normal plain x-ray of the shoulder. The use of multipositional x-rays, with the arm in as much elevation as possible and at rest, and the use of C-arm fluoroscopy in the diagnosis of adhesive capsulitis are probably unnecessary. Calcification may be seen to be present in the cuff, but its presence is neither diagnostic nor exclusive of a diagnosis of adhesive capsulitis.

Contrast radiography

A single contrast arthrogram is a useful investigation in the confirmation of the diagnosis of adhesive capsulitis. Varying degrees of stiffness are associated with a number of radiological findings (Fig. 1). A saw-toothed appearance, small capsular volume, lack of filling of the inferior recess, and early filling of the lymphatics around the shoulder with the contrast medium are all suggestive of capsulitis. Of equal importance to these findings is the description by the radiologist at the time of injection of contrast: a careful note should be made at the time of injection, the pressure perceived within the joint, the occurrence of back flow of contrast out through the needle or cannula, the volume of contrast used, and the degree of pain experienced by the patient at the time of injection. The presence of a rotator cuff tear may be apparent on the arthrogram.

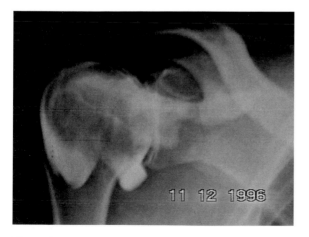

Figure 1

Arthrogram of shoulder, showing features of adhesive capsulitis

Bone scanning

A nuclear bone scan frequently shows evidence of diffuse changes consistent with capsulitis but, of itself, is not a specific means of investigation.

MRI scanning

MRI scanning is not good at showing the presence or absence of adhesive capsulitis. Whilst it is useful in demonstrating associated pathology, it is likely to be normal in cases of adhesive capsulitis.

Diagnostic arthroscopy

Diagnostic arthroscopy is not necessary to make a diagnosis of adhesive capsulitis. Where there are associated conditions of the shoulder or where the diagnosis is uncertain, despite the use of the other non-invasive tests already described, the use of a diagnostic arthroscopy may be considered. More likely, however, an arthroscopic examination of the shoulder is used as part of a therapeutic arthroscopic capsular release in the treatment of the condition. There are, in these circumstances, frequently seen to be excessive adhesions in the subacromial bursa and tightness of the capsule of the glenohumeral joint. The posterosuperior joint is particularly tight in many of these patients, and capsular release of this part of the capsule is an important part of the arthroscopic release.

Functional assessment

In discussing the assessment of shoulder function in the patient with a stiff shoulder I will use the Constant shoulder functional score (Constant and Murley 1987, Constant 1991, Constant 1997). This scoring system, now widely used in the field of shoulder surgery, consists of a 100-point score made up of 15 points for pain (i.e. the lack of pain), 20 points for activities of daily living (ADL), 40 points for functional ROM, and 25 points for strength (Table 1).

Using the Constant shoulder functional score, a painful stiff shoulder will lose functional points in

Table 1 Functional parameters in the Constant score

Parameter	Points
Pain	15
ADL	20
ROM	40
Power	25
TOTAL	100

respect of the pain, the limitations in ADL, and the limited ranges of active painless functional shoulder motions. Severe pain in association with inability to undertake recreational and occupational activities, together with disturbed sleep, will have a significant effect on shoulder functional score. Restricted ROM may be as much as 70% or more of normal in a patient with severe adhesive capsulitis and this in turn will severely affect shoulder function. Furthermore, the inability to abduct the arm to 90° will result in 0 points for strength assessment. The functional loss associated with adhesive capsulitis may therefore vary from a mild loss of function to a severe and disabling loss. The functional disability associated with a frozen shoulder increases during the first stage, remains virtually static during the second stage, and then usually worsens prior to resolution and improvement in the third stage. An example of a Constant assessment in a case of adhesive capsulitis is seen in Table 2.

Table 2 Example of a completed assessment in a patient with adhesive capsulitis of the right shoulder, using the Constant shoulder functional score system

Parameter Score	Right Description	Score	Left Description	Score
Pain	Severe	0	None	15
ADL: work	None	0	Full	4
ADL: recreation	Nil	0	Full	4
ADL: sleep	Poor	1	Unaffected	2
ADL: position	Neck	6	Above head	10
ROM: flexion	95°	6	180°	10
ROM: abduction	90°	4	180°	10
ROM: external	Limited	0	Full	10
ROM: internal	Thigh	0	DV 12	10
Power	20 lb	20	20 lb	20
TOTAL		37		95

Treatment of the condition of adhesive capsulitis should aim to shorten the overall natural course of the condition, and result in an improvement of function sooner than would otherwise be expected to occur. The use of repeated functional assessments following active treatment for adhesive capsulitis can demonstrate the improvement of function.

Conclusion

The assessment of the stiff and painful shoulder is a complex combination of a good history and examination, radiological investigations, general assessment of the patient, and a functional assessment of the shoulder to determine disability. The effective management of adhesive capsulitis can only be possible once appropriate assessment of the patient with a stiff and painful shoulder is undertaken and the correct diagnosis made.

References

Constant CR (1991) Assessment of the shoulder. In: Watson M, ed. *Surgical Disorders of the Shoulder.* Churchill Livingstone: London: 39–45.

Constant CR (1997) Assessment of shoulder function. In: Copeland S, ed. *Shoulder Surgery.* WB Saunders: Philadelphia: 56–63.

Constant CR, Murley AHG (1987) A clinical method of functional assessment of the shoulder, *Clin Orthop Rela Res* **214:**160–4.

6
Post-traumatic stiffness

Herbert Resch and Herbert Maurer

The stiff shoulder has been the subject of many investigations over the years. Duplay (1872) believed that the pathology in these shoulders was in the periarticular tissues. He coined the term 'periarthritis humeroscapularis'. Codman (1934) attributed the pathology of the stiff shoulder at least initially to adhesions in the subacromial bursa. Neviaser (1945) concluded that the essential pathology in the stiff shoulder was a thickening and contraction of the shoulder joint capsule. He coined the term 'adhesive capsulitis' and felt that this term better describes the pathology than 'frozen shoulder'. He describes a contracted thickened capsule that seems to be drawn tightly around the humeral head with a relative absence of synovial fluid. He also notes cellular changes of chronic inflammation with fibrosis and perivascular infiltration in the subsynovial layer of the capsule. From this condition the stiffness caused by trauma has to be differentiated. Lundberg (1969) therefore classified the stiff shoulders into two groups:

1 Primary frozen shoulder.
2 Secondary frozen shoulder.

In the case of primary frozen shoulder no findings in the history, on clinical examination or on X-rays exist which could explain the decrease in shoulder motion. Patients who developed restricted shoulder motion after traumatic injury were classified as having secondary frozen shoulder. According to Reeves (1966), the post-traumatic stiff shoulder group had a decreased joint volume and abnormal filling of the subscapular bursa at arthrography. In the primary frozen shoulder group arthrography showed a markedly decreased joint volume. There was no filling at arthrography of the subscapular bursa, the biceps tendon sheath or the inferior recess. In the secondary frozen shoulder group we do not find changes in the capsule as described by Neviaser (1945) for adhesive caspulitis which is typical for the primary frozen shoulder.

Secondary frozen shoulder

In this group stiffness of the shoulder joint is caused by non-surgical or surgical trauma. Various conditions can be responsible for the stiffness. The classic phases typical for primary frozen shoulder (1 painful phase, 2 stiffening phase, 3 thawing phase) are not found in this group.

According to the aetiology of stiffness it can furthermore be classified into two subgroups:

1 Extracapsular stiffness or contracture.
2 Capsular stiffness or contracture.

Extracapsular contracture

This type of stiffness is caused by changes of the gliding mechanism in the subacromial space due to a traumatic impingement syndrome, a partial or full thickness rotator cuff tear, a fracture of the greater or lesser tuberosity. Pain caused by the impeded gliding mechanism in the subacromial space causes decrease of motion of the shoulder joint and consequently shrinking of the capsule, particularly of the axillary recess. When abductional or flexional movement is attempted by the patient, the shrinked capsule of the inferior recess causes increased pressure on the coracoacromial arch and increases pain. The same mechanism is seen after long-term immobilization of the shoulder joint. Due to the inactivity of the shoulder, the capsule is subjected to a shrinking process, causing pain in the subacromial space when moving the arm in the saggittal, abductional or rotational plane.

Capsular contracture

The capsular contracture is almost always caused by surgery. This condition is often seen after an open stabilization operation of an unstable shoulder joint when the anterior capsule was tightened too much causing marked loss of external rotation as well as flexion and abduction.

Treatment of post-traumatic stiffness

Extracapsular contracture

The treatment depends on the underlying pathology and the degree of movement in the shoulder joint. It aims to restore the subacromial gliding mechanism. Arthroscopy has proven to be a very helpful tool for diagnostic as well as therapeutic purposes.

Traumatic impingement syndrome

After having performed arthrography or ultrasound examination to exclude any partial or complete tear of the rotator cuff, physiotherapy is performed with stretching exercises in forward flexion, external and internal rotation. If these measurements do not provide improvement, arthroscopy is performed aiming at the excision of adhesions in the subacromial space sometimes together with acromioplasty. In cases with very advanced contracture, additional manual manipulation or inferior capsular release is performed to detach the capsule from the inferior glenoid rim. The capsule is detached from the glenoid labrum using an electrosurgical knife. An intensive exercise programme follows.

Rotator cuff tear

Stiffness due to rotator cuff rupture usually disappears by conservative measurements within two or

three months. When passive motion has reached more than 130°, reconstructive surgery of the rotator cuff can be performed. If stiffness has not improved, arthroscopy is performed following the same guidelines as mentioned above with excision of adhesions, release of the axillary recess, manual manipulation and sometimes subacromial decompression (attention: manipulation of the arm should never be done after subacromial decompression has been performed, because this can cause fracture of the acromion).

Avulsion fracture of the greater tuberosity

Conservative treatment mainly based on physiotherapy is performed first. If motion does not improve surgery is performed within 3 months. The surgical treatment depends on the degree of displacement of the tuberosity. For displacements of less than 3 mm in any direction (superior or posterior direction) gentle manipulation and acromioplasty is performed. If the displacement is more than 3 mm, correction osteotomy of the tuberosity associated with acromioplasty is the treatment of choice. Fixation of the greater tuberosity with screws will allow early passive movement exercises.

Comminuted fracture of the humeral head

The regimen to improve motion depends on the type of fracture. In any case the gliding mechanism in the subacromial space should be restored. Whether subacromial decompression and/or correction osteotomy is performed will depend on the degree of displacement and deformity of the humeral head.

Capsular contracture

Post-traumatic capsular contracture is usually caused by surgery during stabilization operations when the anterior capsule has been tightened too much preventing external rotation. If stretching exercises fail, the anterior capsule has to be lengthened surgically. This is best performed by arthroscopy with the patient in the beach chair position allowing controlled external rotation of the arm. The anterior capsule has to be released step-by-step about 5 mm away from the glenoid labrum or rim using an electrosurgical knife. The amount of external rotation gained is steadily controlled by moving the arm. Of course, an overextended release has to be avoided to prevent initiating instability again.

References

Codman EA (1934) *The Shoulder.* Thomas Todd: Boston

Duplay ES (1872) De las périotwite scapulohumérale et des raideurs de l'épaule et la consequence. *Arch Gen Méd* **20**:513–24

Lundberg BJ (1969) The frozen shoulder. *Acta Orthop Scand* (Suppl) **119**:1–59

Neviaser JS (1945) Adhesive capsulitis of the shoulder. *J Bone Joint Surg* **27**:211–22

Reeves B (1966) Arthrographic changes in frozen and posttraumatic stiff shoulders. *Proc R Soc Med* **59**:825–30

7
Rehabilitation of the stiff and postoperative shoulder

Didier Mailhe and Veronique Aurand

Restoration of shoulder function by rehabilitation is gained by complete recuperation of passive mobility.

Sectors of shoulder mobility

Without dedicating a complete chapter to functional anatomy, one can identify two important groups:

- passive mobility of the glenohumeral joint
- mobility of the scapulothoracic sliding joint.

Glenohumeral joint mobility

Testing is only possible when the scapula is immobilized. Mobility is in three planes:

- flexion – extension
- abduction – adduction
- rotation – internal
    – external.

Internal rotation is tested with the elbow close to the body and movement is recorded by noting which vertebral level is reached.

External rotation is tested in three positions:

- the arm in neutral position with the elbow close to the body (ER1)
- arm held at 90° of abduction (ER2)
- arm in forward flexion of 90° (ER3).

Mobility of the scapulothoracic joint

The mobility of the scapulothoracic joint occurs between the scapula and the dorsolateral part of the thoracic cage. This allows a greater range of motion at the glenohumeral joint, particularly of flexion–extension and internal rotation, as well as the combined movement of circumduction.

The integrity of the pericapsular spaces, e.g. the subacromial space, is important for good function. Proper assessment of the stiff shoulder must differentiate between stiffness originating from either of these joints.

Stiffness of the shoulder

Shortly after surgery, a passive limitation of movement often occurs at the glenohumeral joint. This may also occur in adhesive capsulitis.

The degree of stiffness maybe classified accordingly:

1 Slight stiffness
   - forward flexion is limited, but exceeds 135°
   - external rotation, with the elbow close to the body, is minimally limited
   - external rotation in abduction is diminished
   - internal rotation combined with extension allows the hand to reach the level of the lumbar vertebrae.
2 Average stiffness
   - forward flexion is limited, but allows greater than 90° of motion
   - external rotation with the elbow close to the body usually allows at least one segment of rotation

- external rotation in abduction is severely limited and usually no movement occurs
- internal rotation is restricted such that the hand just reaches the buttock.

3   Severe stiffness
  - forward flexion only just reaches 90°
  - rotation is restricted to such a degree that no movement occurs, particularly that of internal rotation.

4   Pain

The presence of pain often reduces the range of motion achieved, irrespective of the degree of actual stiffness present. A complete assessment must therefore include examination after pain has been abolished, e.g. by using the Neer test.

Treatment of the stiff shoulder

Treatment of the stiff shoulder may be divided into three phases:

- postoperative prevention
- treatment of early onset stiffness
- treatment of established stiffness.

Postoperative prevention

From the time of surgery, analgesia is imperative, irrespective of the surgery performed. Oral or intramuscular analgesia or, preferably, nerve blocks may be used. Adequate analgesia will allow passive mobilization to commence, under the guidance of the physiotherapist. The rehabilitation programme is divided into three phases:

1   Immediate passive mobilization. The arm is rested in a sling for three weeks when not being mobilized by the patient and physiotherapist.
2   After three weeks, more active mobilization is commenced, the level of which is determined by the level of pain. This allows a greater range of motion to be achieved and allows the muscles around the shoulder girdle to regain their strength. The arm is allowed out of the sling outside the periods of physiotherapy.
3   After approximately six weeks, cuff strengthening exercises are commenced. Again, this is dependent on the level of pain experienced by the patient. Initially static exercises are performed, progressing to dynamic exercises as pain allows. Thereafter the upper limb may be used for activities of daily living.

Immobilization phase

Early passive mobilization is necessary to maintain motion. Exercises must be performed in all planes of motion. Physiotherapy may begin with a warm-up period of approximately 10 minutes by means of an infra-red lamp.

Massage plays an important role for two reasons:

- Passive – relaxation of contracted muscles
- Active – proprioceptive activation.

This is performed with the patient seated and the limb elevated to approximately 70° in the scapular plane. This allows the muscles of the shoulder girdle to relax effectively.

Passive role

Identification of the state of contraction of the shoulder girdle muscles is important. A lengthy slow deep massage will relax the muscles. The patient should feel the mechanical effect of the physiotherapist's massage. Voluntary relaxation aids this process.

Active role

The mechanical effect of the physiotherapist stimulates the proprioceptors and is important to differentiate movements occurring at the glenohumeral and scapulothoracic joints.

The massage continues with the elbow close to the body, the position at which the trapezius muscle is under greatest tension. When the patient is able to internally rotate and extend the shoulder, passive mobilization may commence.

Mobilization phase

Primary phase: passive mobilization

This is initially performed with the patient in the lying position followed by the seated position. Again, the patient must be completely relaxed and without pain. Mobilization commences with ER1 by controlling the scapulothoracic contribution. The arm is elevated in the neutral position. Once the arm has reached the maximum degree of elevation the position of the scapula is verified. The arm is then lowered either actively or passively if pain is experienced.

The level of ER2 regained depends on the pain experienced and may also be limited by the surgical procedure performed. This may be the most difficult motion to rehabilitate. Return of extension is delayed until the second month. This movement often induces pain due to the forward projection of the humeral head at the level of the rotator interval.

Primary phase: passive-assisted mobilization

If the patient progresses such that the humeral head remains central within the joint, then assisted active movements may be performed.

ER1 The external rotation in ER1 can be maintained by fixing the elbow, flexed to 90°, to the body by a strap. The scapula is pushed backwards. External rotation may be achieved by the aid of a stick.

Elevation Simple to and fro movements allow repeated passive elevation in the scapula plane and in neutral rotation. When the arm has reached maximum elevation the patient is requested to move the scapula down and inwards to stretch the lower scapular ligaments.

Suspension Axial suspension, by pendular movements, allows abduction and adduction, and maintains anteroposterior capsuloligament elasticity. This is useful in the initial phase of rehabilitation to actively centralize the humeral head. The physiotherapist guides the relaxing of the trapezius and scapular movements. This phase of therapy should not induce pain.

Any inflammatory reaction produced may be treated by ultrasound or by application of ice packs. Electrical stimulation improves muscular tone particularly of the deltoid.

Secondary phase: active mobilization

This secondary phase of rehabilitation is enhanced by previously learnt proprioceptive feedback during the initial stages of physiotherapy. Centralization of the humeral head occurs during all movements of the upper limb without conscious effort by the patient. Goals are set for the patient to achieve, for example placing the hand behind the head with the arm in full elevation. Active mobilization induces muscular fatigue, which may be treated by massage. Mobilization should not continue to bring about pain.

At this stage of rehabilitation only light use of the arm is allowed. The shoulder should still be protected, with repetitive and prolonged movements avoided.

Tertiary phase: restoration of strength

The functional potential of the shoulder is evaluated in this phase. More sustained effort is now required to restore power to the shoulder girdle. The muscles of the rotator cuff must be strengthened particularly to maintain balanced function. A ratio of 1 : 3 (internal rotators : external rotators) has previously been demonstrated to be necessary (Codine et al 1993). Exercises must increase in number and intensity. Initially this is by static exercises, with particular attention to internal and external rotators in 0° and 45° of external rotation. Progressive resistance is used, taking care not to induce pain or inflammation. Exercise should be stopped if these develop. A muscle evaluation chart may be used to chart progress. This can be repeated on a monthly basis until the strength of the shoulder matches that of the contralateral side.

Four muscle groups are evaluated isometrically. With the external and internal rotators in position ER1 at 0° force can be assessed by the palm up test and the Jobe test and compared with the contralateral shoulder. Should the strength be decreased then the patient should be advised to continue with protected activities.

Onset of stiffness

This tends to occur in the first three weeks after surgery. Factors that may be significant in the development of stiffness include:

1 Pain – this may limit postoperative mobilization, particularly if also present during periods of rest.
2 Articular limitation – this is usually directly due to the surgery and may be graded as previously outlined. Treatment includes administration of analgesia and maintaining movement within the limits of pain. Any stiffness that subsequently develops is usually reversible. Progression to the next phases of rehabilitation may be delayed by this. If the stiffness does not resolve then this may be termed established stiffness.
3 Established stiffness – during this phase pain has usually resolved and the patient is left with a shoulder that has a reduced range of active motion. The level of stiffness may be graded as

moderate or severe. Manipulation under anaesthetic (MUA) is indicated at this stage to restore the passive range of motion to normal values. Arthroscopy may also be performed in conjunction with the MUA to diagnose any other pathology. Rehabilitation of active motion is then commenced.

We performed arthroscopy on 32 patients who had MUA of their shoulder. This allowed us to diagnose pathology within the glenohumeral joint and the subacromial space.

Materials and methods

Between June 1988 and June 1993, 32 patients, 18 female and 14 male, had arthroscopy of the glenohumeral joint and subacromial bursoscopy after MUA had been performed.

Technique of manipulation

The following technique allows restoration of external rotation and forward flexion as well as adduction and internal rotation (Caillens 1980, Neviaser 1987). The upper limb is prepared, draped and traction applied, and then (under aseptic conditions) the arthroscope is introduced into the glenohumeral joint via a posterior portal. Following diagnostic arthroscopy, manipulation of the joint is then performed. The arthroscope is then reintroduced into the glenohumeral joint and subacromial bursoscopy performed. At the end of the procedure bupivacaine hydrochloride solution is injected into the subacromial space. Once the patient has recovered from the anaesthetic, passive and assisted active mobilization is commenced. A sling may be used as a support during the initial convalescent period.

Results

Three subgroups of patients were included in the study:

- those with post-traumatic stiffness
- post-surgical stiffness
- adhesive capsulitis.

Post-traumatic

This group of patients had stiffness after fracture or after glenohumeral dislocation. There were nine males and five females and the average age was 50 years (48 years for males and 52 years for females). The non-dominant side was affected more frequently than the dominant side (eight non-dominant, six dominant). The stiffness had been present for an average of 5 months before MUA was performed. All patients had received physiotherapy immediately after the injury was sustained. Pain was not a significant symptom in these patients.

At arthroscopy inflammation was not seen in the main joint or in the subacromial bursa. Four patients had fractures of the tuberosities not involving the articular surface. In these patients a fibrous band was seen within the subacromial space, and its presence limited forward flexion. Rotation was not limited. A good result was achieved after approximately 4 months post-manipulation.

Postoperative stiffness

Six patients were included in this group. All had operative treatment for calcific tendinitis. There were five females and one male, the average age was 45 years (range 38–54 years). There were three left and three right shoulders. Stiffness of the joint began soon after operation, usually during the first 3 weeks.

Arthroscopy did not diagnose any abnormality in the glenohumeral joint. Subacromial bursoscopy demonstrated many adhesions, mainly anteriorly, and a fibrous band running vertically. Bursectomy was often necessary. Complete restoration of movement was achieved at an average of 3.5 months after MUA.

Adhesive capsulitis

The 12 patients included within this group complied with previously defined diagnostic criteria (Neviaser 1945, Troisier 1958, Wiley 1991). Eight females and four males were studied, with an average age of 51 years (females) and 54 years (males). Eight joints were on the dominant side and four on the non-dominant side. Patients had had stiffness for an average of 11 months before MUA was performed (phase IV as defined by Neviaser 1945). A detailed history from each patient identified a particular repetitive manoeuvre which preceded the onset of pain and stiffness in nine of the 12 patients.

A number of observations were made at arthroscopy:

1 Penetration of the glenohumeral joint is difficult due to a contracted capsule.

2   There is often hyperaemia of the anterior gleno-humeral capsule, which may include the long head of biceps.
3   The capsule is thickened and the subacromial bursa has a small capacity.
4   Hyperaemia of the tissue may be seen. There is always pathology in the subacromial bursa, with the presence of adhesions – in nine of the 12 cases there were signs of attachment to the acromial insertion of the coracoacromial ligament.

When arthroscopy is performed after MUA a haemarthrosis is seen. Capsular tearing is noted anteriorly, extending along the posterior aspect of subscapularis and between the middle and inferior glenohumeral ligaments. The aponeurosis of subscapularis is not damaged. The antero-inferior aspect of the glenoid labrum was not affected in any of the cases. Bursoscopy also demonstrated tearing of tissue and blood within the bursa. Bursectomy to remove adhesions was performed in some cases. Washout was also performed. Restoration of mobility was achieved in nine patients, usually within 4 months of the manipulation. Three patients required a second manipulation. Results were not as satisfactory compared with the other two patient groups.

Discussion

The term 'stiff shoulder' should be used if a specific diagnosis can be made regarding the aetiology (Wiley 1991). The term 'capsulitis' should be avoided in these patients. Manipulation under anaesthetic is simple to perform, is effective and relatively free from complications. None of the lesions to subscapularis described by de Palma (1950) were seen in our series of patients. Full mobility is achieved between the second and fourth month after manipulation in patients with postoperative or post-traumatic stiffness.

In our series of patients with capsulitis, manipulation was useful, allowing patients to restore their range of motion within four months. Arthroscopy after manipulation is useful. It did not demonstrate subscapularis rupture, as previously demonstrated by de Palma (1950), but did confirm that the long head of biceps tendon may be involved (Uitvlugt et al 1993).

Previously noted changes within the inferior recess were not noted in this series (Wiley 1991). This series did demonstrate a thickened capsule with retraction of the anterior capsule and diminution of the subscapularis bursa. Hyperaemia of the capsule within the joint and within the subacromial space confirmed previous descriptions (Wiley 1991, Uitvlugt et al 1993). Our findings confirm those by Duplay (1872), that the involvement of the subacromial bursa could explain the stiffness seen in capsulitis.

Conclusion

Rehabilitation of the postoperative stiff shoulder is essential. Restoration of passive motion is achieved in a patient who is free of pain. Progression to assisted active motion followed by active motion may then follow. Finally, increase in strength may be achieved. Normal use of the shoulder is then allowed.

Manipulation under anaesthetic, whether combined with arthroscopy or not, can be of therapeutic value. The degree of involvement of the anterior capsule and inferior recess may be defined. It also allows the contribution of adhesions within the subacromial bursa to be assessed as a cause for the stiffness.

A systematic programme of progressive, pain-free rehabilitation, adapted to each individual patient, reduces the need for surgery and enables the patient to restore mobility to the shoulder.

References

Caillens JP (1980) La manipulation de l'épaule sous anesthésie générale. In: Simon L, ed. *Actualité en rééducation Fonctionnelle et Réadaptation*, 5th edn. Masson: Paris: 172–82.

Codine P, Leroux JL, Pocholle M (1993) Apport de l'isocinétisme dans le bilan et le traitement du conflit sous-acromial. In: Simon L, Pelissier J, eds. *Pathologie de la Coiffe des Rotateurs*. Masson: Paris: 199–206.

de Palma AF (1950) *Surgery of the Shoulder*. JB Lippincott: Philadelphia: 143.

Duplay S (1872) De la péri-arthrite scapulo-humérale et des raideurs de l'épaule qui en sont la conséquence. *Arch Gen Med* 513.

Neviaser J (1945) Adhesive capsulitis of the shoulder. *J Bone Joint Surg* **27**:211–22.

Neviaser J (1987) The frozen shoulder, diagnosis and management. *Clin Orthop* **223**:59–64.

Troisier O (1958) Les capsulites de l'épaule, techniques de mensuration des mouvements et applications techniques. *Rhumatologie* **3**:113–34.

Uitvlugt G, Detrissac DA, Johnson LL (1993) Arthroscopic observation before and after manipulation of frozen shoulder. *Arthroscopy* **9**(2):181–5.

Wiley AM (1991) Arthroscopic appearance of frozen shoulder. *Arthroscopy* **7**(2):138–43.

8
The frozen shoulder

Brian Hazleman

Frozen shoulder is a descriptive term used to indicate a clinical syndrome characterized by the spontaneous onset of shoulder pain followed by a restricted range of active and passive glenohumeral movement for which no other cause can be found (Basland et al 1990). It is the second most common cause of shoulder pain and disability, while the exact prevalence and incidence is unknown, it has been estimated that 2–5% of the population and 10–20% of diabetics will present with at least one episode of frozen shoulder (Pal et al 1986).

Definition

One of the major stumbling blocks for most people is the confusing terminology. Initially, periarthritis of the shoulder was used as an all-encompassing term to describe painful shoulders for which the symptoms could not be explained on the basis of arthritis of the glenohumeral joint (Duplay 1872). In the early literature, calcifying tendinitis, adhesive subacromial bursitis, biceps tendinitis, supraspinatus tendinitis and partial tears of the rotator cuff were all included under the diagnosis of periarthritis of the shoulder. The inclusion of such heterogeneous clinical disorders makes the interpretation of the early literature difficult.

The aetiology and pathology of frozen shoulder is poorly understood, the pathological studies are few and usually are representative of late stage disease. Nevaiser (1987a), describes four stages of pathology from arthroscopic observations.

Stage I   A mild fibrinous synovial inflammation is seen especially in and around the dependent (axillary) fold of the joint

Stage II   The synovium is red, thickened and inflamed and adhesions can be visualized extending from the dependent fold to the humeral head

Stage III   The synovium is less inflamed but the dependent fold is reduced to half of its original size

Stage IV   No synovitis is present, but adhesions are pronounced and the humeral head is compressed against the glenoid and the biceps tendons.

The observations support the long held contention that primary inflammation may be responsible for the fibrosis seen in this condition, but a number of investigations have found little evidence of inflammation or even adhesions in this condition (Wiley 1991). Macroscopically the capsule is thickened and contracted and there is infiltration of the subsynovial capsule by chronic inflammatory cells, fibrosis and focal degeneration of collagen. However, these changes are non-specific and have been seen at autopsy in normal shoulders (Nevaiser 1945).

Frozen shoulder is the second most common cause of shoulder pain and disability, females are affected slightly more often than men and the condition is most common in the fifth and sixth decade. Bilateral involvement occurs in 4–40% of affected individuals (Nash and Hazleman 1989). Many predisposing conditions have been associated with the development of frozen shoulder. These include: immobility that may be the result of trauma, stroke, cardiac disorder, diabetes, thyroid disorders and intrathoracic pathology.

Natural history

Reeves (1975) prospectively studied 41 patients,

treated with a sling, analgesics and exercises alone over a 5–10 year follow-up period. He demonstrated that frozen shoulder evolves through three phases. The first painful phase lasted 10–36 weeks, the second adhesive phase 4–12 months and the resolution phase 5–26 months). The total duration of symptoms lasted 12–42 months (with a mean disease duration of 30.1 months. Binder and colleagues (1984) followed up 40 patients for 40–48 months. Objective restriction was severe in five patients and mild in a further 11 patients. Patients were often unaware that shoulder range was impaired. Dominant arm involvement, manual labour and mobilization physiotherapy was associated with a less satisfactory outcome. However, although objective restriction persisted, there was little functional impairment in the late stage of frozen shoulder.

Symptoms vary throughout the three phases. In the first painful phase patients gradually and insidiously develop diffuse and disabling shoulder pain which is worse during the night and is exacerbated by lying on the affected side. Physical examination shows pain and limitation of all movements of the shoulder. During the second phase the pain is less pronounced and stiffness and severe restrictions of shoulder movement predominates. Some disease atrophy and wasting of the deltoid muscle can be seen. The recovery phase is associated with gradual disappearance of pain and return of movement.

Diagnosis

The diagnosis is made largely from the clinical history and physical examination. While many conditions can cause shoulder pain, few are associated with severe passive restriction of movement of the shoulder. The impingement syndrome typically causes pain and limitation of active movement but the range of passive movement is usually normal. Local anaesthetic blocks can help clarify the situation in cases of apparent limitation of passive movement. Plain radiographs show either no abnormality, minor periarticular osteoporosis or minor degenerative changes in the shoulder and acromioclavicular joints, present in the same frequency as on the unaffected side. The main value of radiographs is to exclude other pathologies.

Arthrography remains the main investigation of choice. Characteristically, there is difficulty in needling the shoulder joint for arthrographic purposes because of joint contracture and restricted range of movement. Classical features include limitation of joint capacity, a small or non-existent dependent axillary fold and irregularity about capsular insertion on to the anatomical neck of humerus. The insistence of the presence of these characteristic findings by some American authors before a diagnosis of frozen shoulder is made may result in missing 'early' disease, a point when the study of aetiological agents is more likely to be fruitful. Between 10 and 30% of patients with the disorder undergoing arthrographic examination prior to any joint manipulation demonstrate rotator cuff perforation with free flow of contrast into the subacromial space (Binder et al 1984). The diagnostic role of bone scintigraphy (Binder et al 1984), thermography (Vecchio et al 1992) and ultrasound (Ryu Ku et al 1993) appears limited.

Treatment

The following list of suggested treatments emphasizes the unsatisfactory nature of treatment for this disorder:

- analgesics
- non-steroidal anti-inflammatory drugs
- heat and ultrasound
- physiotherapy and graded exercises
- corticosteroids (oral and intra-articular)
- stellate ganglion blockade
- magnetic necklace
- dimethyl sulphoxide (topical)
- arthrographic distension
- joint irradiation
- manipulation under anaesthetic (early/late).

Assessment of trial data is fraught with difficulties. Adequate patient numbers are often lacking and few studies are blinded or controlled. Patient selection is often poor, with inadequate disease definition, and treatment comparisons are made on groups of patients at differing stages of the disease process.

The objectives of treatment of frozen shoulder are to relieve pain and restore motion and function of the shoulder. Of all the treatment approaches suggested, corticosteroid injections and physiotherapy remain the treatments most commonly used.

Table 1   Controlled trials of corticosteroid injections in patients with adhesive capsulitis

Author (year)	n	Nature of the intervention. No. in parentheses indicates no. of patients	Duration of follow-up	Results
Bulgen et al (1984)	45	1 MP shoulder + bursa × 3 (11) 2 Maitland's mobilizations (11) 3 Ice packs (12) 4 Non-treatment (8)	6 months	Pain and ROM improved most in group 1 at 1 month but no difference at 6 months
Corbeil et al (1992)	45	1 TA shoulder (20) 2 TA shoulder + distension (25)	3 months	Pain improved in 80%; ROM improved 17–22 degrees. No difference between 1 and 2
Dacre et al (1989)	66	1 TA around shoulder (22) 2 'Individualized' physiotherapy (20) 3 Both (20)	6 months	Pain improved by 57–86% ROM improved by 10–34% No difference between 1, 2 and 3
Hollingworth et al (1983)	25	1 MP shoulder 2 MP 'trigger point'	2 months	Success in 1, 26%; 2, 0%
Jacobs et al (1991)	47	1 TA shoulder × 3 (15) 2 Distension (14) 3 Both (18)	3 months	Pain improved in 90% of patients No difference between 1, 2 and 3 ROM improved more in 1 and 3 than in 2
Lee et al (1973)	80	1 Infra-red + exercises (20) 2 HC shoulder + exercises (20) 3 HC bicipital tendon + exercises (20) 4 Analgesics (20)	6 weeks	ROM improved in 1, 2 and 3, but not 4 No difference between 1, 2 and 3
Lee et al (1974)	65	1 Heat + exercises (17) 2 HC shoulder + exercises (15) 3 HC bicipital tendon + exercises (18) 4 Analgesics (15)	6 weeks	ROM improved in 1, 2 and 3, but not 4 No difference between 1, 2 and 3
Murnaghan and McIntosh (1955)	51	1 HC capsular and pericapsular (24) 2 Lignocaine (27)	3 months	Pain and ROM improved in 1 and 2 No difference between treatments
Quinn (1965)	9	1 HC shoulder and periarticular × 2 + heat and exercises 3/week × 4 weeks (14) 2 Heat and exercises 3/week × 4 weeks (15)	3 months	Pain improved in 100% of 1 and 2 ROM increased in 78% of 1 and 72% of 2
Richardson (1975)	37	1 PA shoulder and bursa × 2 (17) 2 Saline shoulder and bursa × 2 (2)	6 weeks	Pain improved in 1, 38%; 2, 61% ROM improved in 1, 50%; 2, 33%
Rizk et al (1991)	48	1 MP shoulder (16) 2 MP bursa (16) 3 Lidocaine shoulder (8) 4 Lidocaine bursa (8)	6 months	Transient pain relief in 65% of 1 and 2 (mean 2.2 weeks) ROM improved minimally in 1, 2 and 3

HC = hydrocortisone acetate
MP = methylprednisolone acetate
PA = prednisolone acetate
ROM = range of movement
TA = triamcinolone acetate

Injection therapy

The use of intra-articular or periarticular corticosteroid injections for the treatment of 'periarthritis' of the shoulder was first reported by Hollander et al (1954) and Crisp and Kendall (1955). The percentage of patients reporting 'beneficial results' following the injections ranged from 70–90% depending on the stage of evolution of the condition (acute versus chronic). Eleven controlled studies have been published (Murnaghan and McIntosh 1955; Quinn 1965; Lee et al 1973 and 1974; Richardson 1975; Hollingworth et al 1983; Bulgen et al 1984; Dacre et al 1989; Jacobs et al 1991; Rizk et al 1991; Corbeil et al 1992). The characteristics of these studies and a summary of their results are shown in Table 1.

Despite the controlled nature of these studies

and that the assessments were carried out by blind observers, a number of methodological errors prevent firm conclusions about the efficacy and role of corticosteroid injections in frozen shoulder. Only four of the studies are placebo controlled, one with saline injections, two with analgesics and one with no treatment. Case definition varies among the studies and it is difficult to ascertain if patients suffered from frozen shoulder as arthrography was used on only one of the trials to select the patients. The duration of symptoms in the patients studied varied from 1 week to more than 5 years. Co-interventions were reported in only one study. Treatment of the non-responders was important in one study where non-responders were injected with steroids after 1 week. Finally, the number of patients studied on all of these studies were small and negative results could be explained by a type II error.

Physiotherapy

The value of physiotherapy in the management of established frozen shoulder also remains unproven. The only available controlled trials are those listed in Table 1. Lee et al (1973 and 1974) showed that heat and exercises alone or in combination with corticosteroid injections in the shoulder or the bicipital groove provided considerably more improvement of range of movement at six weeks than analgesics alone. However long-term follow-up was not examined. Bulgen et al (1984) found that Maitlands' mobilizations given three times weekly for 6 weeks had no long-term advantage over steroid injections, ice packs application or no treatment. Dacre et al (1989) compared physiotherapy, steroid injections or a combination of both. They found a similar improvement of pain and range of movement at 6 weeks and 6 months in all three treatment groups. However, this study did not include a placebo group, the physiotherapy programme used is not described and the number of patients in the study is small.

Ongoing encouragement of the patient by the therapist is invaluable in management. As pain is brought under control, a stretching programme of exercises is initiated in forward elevation, external rotation and internal rotation. Patients have to be motivated to participate in such an exercise programme. All patients have to withstand some physical discomfort. It is advisable to avoid stretching into abduction initially as many patients will develop impingement-like symptoms until the joints become supple enough to allow the humeral head to slide under the coraco-acromial arch.

Distension arthrography

Distension of the shoulder joint at the time of arthrography by progressive injection of fluid may have a beneficial effect (Andren and Lundberg 1965). Progressively more fluid is injected, generating intra-articular pressures of 1000–1500 mmHg. In patients with frozen shoulder and a very restricted joint volume, the capsule may rupture at these pressures. Andren and Lundberg (1965) observed that it is necessary to achieve moderate joint distension for a more favourable outcome.

Distension arthrography is thought to be most useful in patients with slight to moderate shoulder restriction. Pain relief may occur without significant change in range of motion. Distension arthrography can be repeated as there is little post-distension pain.

Manipulation

Manipulation under anaesthetic remains a controversial treatment for the frozen shoulder. The aim of treatment is to shorten the symptomatic course of the condition. Lundberg (1969) noted an increased rate of return of shoulder mobility but there was no effect on the total duration of the condition.

There are risks from the procedure which include fractures, dislocation, post-manipulation pain, haemarthrosis, tears of the joint capsule and rotator cuff and traction injury to nerves around the shoulder. Manipulation should therefore only be considered in patients with long-standing restricted range of movement who have failed to respond to a supervised exercise programme. For shoulder manipulation to be successful, the patient must be co-operative and capable of carrying out an intensive post-manipulation exercise programme. Post-manipulation care is most important as patients may be reluctant to move their shoulders into full abduction for several days following manipulation. Ongoing support of the arm in 90° of abduction at night for 3 weeks is recommended (Nevaiser 1987b).

At manipulation, the joint capsule is torn in a significant proportion of cases. The most frequent capsular tear is along the inferior capsule, but tears have been observed to involve the intra-articular long head of the biceps and the subscapularis tendon (McLaughlin 1961).

Reports of the results of manipulation are variable. No well-controlled studies have substantiated claims of superiority for this method of treatment. Kessel and colleagues (1981) felt that patients with symptoms lasting more than 6 months before treatment had a more dramatic response than those with symptoms of less than 6 months, but this observation was not supported by another study (Haines and Hargadon 1982).

Contraindications to manipulation of the shoulder include: (a) frozen shoulders that result from dislocation or fracture of the proximal humerus; (b) patients with moderate osteoporosis on X-ray; (c) patients unable to co-operate with a post-manipulation exercise programme. A relative contraindication to manipulation is patients who are in the acute and irritable phase of frozen shoulder.

Manipulation and corticosteroid injection

Several authorities have suggested injection of corticosteroid into the shoulder at the time of manipulation in an attempt to reduce post-manipulation pain and inflammation. Improvement at 3 months is reported at 33–83% (Thomas et al 1980, Haines and Hargadon 1982).

Systemic steroids have also been used in conjunction with manipulation. The steroids did not diminish the post-manipulation pain and the results are conflicting.

Oral corticosteroids

Systemic steroids have been recommended for use in frozen shoulder for their anti-inflammatory effect. Binder and colleagues (1986) noted a more rapid initial recovery when compared with controls, but by 5 months follow-up there was no distinguishable difference between the patient groups.

Stellate ganglion block

Stellate ganglion blocks have been used on the premise that frozen shoulder is a type of autonomic dysfunction. When compared with other treatment, a stellate ganglion block offers no advantage (Wiley 1982).

Radiotherapy

This is of historical interest only as it has not been shown conclusively to offer any significant benefit. Quinn (1969) found no advantage of radiotherapy over heat treatment and exercises, when assessed by outcome at 2 and 3 months, or the time required for full recovery.

Pathogenesis

As treatment remains unsatisfactory it is hoped that further understanding of this condition will lead to improved therapies. The aetiopathogenesis is not known; however, those diseases associated with secondary frozen shoulder may provide pointers. Controlled studies have shown an increased prevalence of frozen shoulder in patients with diabetes (Lequesne et al 1977). Disease in diabetics occurs at a younger age, may be less painful, is more often bilateral and is associated with prolonged duration of diabetes, the development of limited joint mobility syndrome and widespread microvascular disease.

Kay and Slater (1981) examined shoulder capsular tissue from a diabetic with frozen shoulder and found an appearance identical to that seen in the fibromatosis of Dupuytren's disease (fibroblast and myofibroblast proliferation) with vascular changes suggestive of diabetic microangiopathy. They postulate that platelet derived growth factor released from abnormal or ischaemic blood vessels may act as a stimulus to local myofibroblast proliferation. Microvascular disease, abnormalities of collagen repair and predisposition to infection may link diabetes with frozen shoulder.

Associations between hypo- and hyperthyroidism and frozen shoulder have been reported (Bowman et al 1988). Resistance to any form of treatment is described until control of the thyroid disease occurs. Again, the underlying abnormalities may be abnormal connective tissue deposition of mucopolysaccharides.

Immobilization of the affected limb appears to be a common risk factor in the development of frozen shoulder. This alone is not sufficient explanation for its development, as shoulder stiffness is generally brief after prolonged shoulder immobilization in most patients.

Several studies propose an association between pulmonary disease and frozen shoulder (Saha 1966); an average incidence of 15% per hospital year in a tuberculosis sanatorium. Reflex neuro-humeral mechanisms may be of aetiological importance.

Features against frozen shoulder being a syndrome similar to algodystrophy include absence of upper limb oedema and vasospasm, lack of prominent bone demineralizations, absence of demonstrable autonomic disturbance in the affected limb, and arguable benefit of treatment by corticosteroids and stellate ganglion blockage.

Further studies in our understanding of frozen shoulder will require tissue study at early stages of the disorder using contemporary methods, such as in situ hybridization to define cytokine and growth factor profiles, and monoclonals and tissue culture to define cell types. Abnormalities at a cellular level, with malfunction in fibroblast recruitment, cytokine or growth factor production and release, may be incriminated in the initiation of frozen shoulder. Abnormalities of platelet derived growth factor release from alveolar macrophages have been demonstrated to occur in the fibrosis developing in idiopathic pulmonary fibrosis. Platelet derived growth factor, a potent mitogenic polypeptide for mesenchymal cells, has a similar structure and function to the gene product of simian sarcoma virus, the first possible link between infection and the development of fibrosis.

Conclusions

The condition remains an enigma. There is much controversy as to the most cost-effective way to manage patients with frozen shoulder. Cortico-steroid injections and physiotherapy alone or in combination have been used extensively for more than 40 years, but despite widespread use we still do not know whether they have any impact on the natural history of this condition (Binder et al 1989).

Further studies are required to understand its pathogenesis, and further clinical studies of treatment need to be performed in carefully defined groups of patients.

References

Andren L, Lundberg BJ (1965) Treatment of rigid shoulders by joint distension during arthrography, *Acta Orthop Scand* **36:**45–53.

Basland B, Thomsen BS, Jensen EM (1990) Frozen shoulder: current concepts, *Scand J Rheumatol* **19:**321–5.

Binder AI, Bulgen DY, Hazleman BL (1984) Frozen shoulder: an arthrographic and radionuclear scan assessment, *Annals Rheum Dis* **43:**365–9.

Binder A, Hazleman B, Parr G, et al (1986) A controlled study of oral prednisolone in frozen shoulder, *Br J Rheumatol* **25:**288–92.

Binder AI, Bulgen DY, Hazleman BL, et al (1989) Frozen shoulder: a long term prospective study, *Annals Rheum Dis* **43:**361–4.

Bowman C, Jeffcoate W, Pattrick M, et al (1988) Bilateral adhesive capsulitis, oligoarthritis and proximal myopathy as presentation of hypothyroidism, *Br J Rheumatol* **27:**62–4.

Bulgen DY, Binder AI, Hazleman BL, et al (1984) Frozen shoulder: prospective clinical study with an evaluation of three treatment regimes, *Ann Rheum Dis* **43:**353–60.

Corbeil V, Dusscult RG, Ledue BK, et al (1992) Capsulite retractile de l'épaule: etude comparative de l'arthrographie avec corticotherapie intra-articulaire avec ou sans distension capsulaire, *Can Ass Radiol* **43:**127–30.

Crisp EJ, Kendall PH (1955) Treatment of periarthritis of the shoulder with hydrocortisone, *Br Med J* **1:**1500–4.

Dacre JE, Beeney N, Scott DL (1989) Injections and physio-therapy for the painful stiff shoulder, *Ann Rheum Dis* **48:**322–5.

Duplay ES (1872) De la periaarthrite scapulohumerale et des raideurs de l'epaule qui en son la consequence, *Arch Gen Med* **20:**513–42.

Haines JR, Hargadon EJ (1982) Manipulation as the primary treatment of the frozen shoulder, *J R Coll Surg Edinburgh* **27:**271–5.

Hollander JL, Brown EM, Jessar RA, et al (1954) Local anti-rheumatic effectiveness of analogues and higher esters of hydrocortisone, *Ann Rheum Dis* **13:**297–301.

Hollingworth GR, Ellis RM, Hattersley T (1983) Comparison of injection techniques for shoulder pain. Results of a double blind randomised study, *Br Med J* **287:**1339–41.

Jacobs LGH, Barton MAJ, Wallace WA, et al (1991) Intra-articular distension and steroids in the management of capsulitis of the shoulder, *Br Med J* **302:**1498–1501.

Kay N, Slater D (1981) Fibromatosis and diabetes mellitus, *Lancet* **11:**303.

Kessel L, Bayley I, Young A (1981) The frozen shoulder, *Br J Hosp Med* **25:**334–9.

Lee M, Haq AM, Wright V, et al (1973) Periarthritis of the shoulder. A controlled trial of physiotherapy, *Physiotherapy* **59:**312–15.

Lee M, Haq AM, Wright V, et al (1974) Periarthritis of the shoulder, *Ann Rheum Dis* **33:**116–19.

Lequesne M, Dang N, Benasson M et al (1977) Increased association of diabetes mellitus with capsulitis of the shoulder and shoulder–hand syndrome. *Scand J Rheumatol*: 653–6.

Lundberg BJ (1969) The frozen shoulder, *Acta Orthop Scand* **119**(suppl 1):1–59.

McLaughlin HL (1961) The frozen shoulder, *Clin Orthop* **20:**126–31.

Murnaghan GF, McIntosh D (1955) Hydrocortisone in painful shoulder. A controlled trial, *Lancet* **2:**798–800.

Nash P, Hazleman B (1989) Frozen shoulder. In: Hazleman B, Dieppe P, eds. *The Shoulder Joint*. Baillière Tindall: London: 551–6.

Nevaiser JS (1945) Adhesive capsulitis of the shoulder, *J Bone Joint Surg* **27:**211–22.

Nevaiser TJ (1987a) Adhesive capsulitis, *Orthop Clin North Am* **18:**439–43.

Nevaiser TJ (1987b) Arthroscopy of the shoulder, *Orthop Clin North Am* **18:**361–72.

Pal B, Anderson J, Dick WC, Griffiths ID (1986) Limitation of joint mobility and shoulder capsulitis in insulin and non insulin dependent diabetes mellitus, *Br J Rheumatol* **25:**147–51.

Quinn CE (1965) 'Frozen Shoulder'. Evaluation of treatment with hydrocortisone injections and exercises, *Ann Phys Med* **8:**22–5.

Quinn EH (1969) Humeroscapular periarthritis. Observations in the effects of X-ray therapy and ultrasonic therapy in cases of 'frozen shoulder', *Am Phys Med* **10:**64–9.

Reeves B (1975) The natural history of the frozen shoulder syndrome, *Scand J Rheumatol* **4:**193–6.

Richardson AT (1975) The painful shoulder, *Proc Roy Soc Med* **68:**731–6.

Rizk TE, Pinals RS, Talaiver AS (1991) Corticosteroid injections in adhesive capsulitis: investigation of their value and site, *Arch Phys Med Rehab* **72:**20–2.

Ryu Ku, Lee SW, Rhee YG, Lim JH (1993) Adhesive capsulitis of the shoulder joint: usefulness of dynamic sonography, *J Ultrasound Med* **12:**445–9.

Saha N (1966) Painful shoulder in patients with chronic bronchitis and emphysema, *Am Rev Resp Med* **94:**455–6.

Thomas, D, Williams RA, Smith DS (1980) The frozen shoulder a review of manipulative treatment, *Rheumatol Rehabilitation* **19:**173–9.

Vecchio PC, Adebajo AO, Chard MD, et al (1992) Thermography of frozen shoulder and rotator cuff tendinitis, *Clin Rheumatol* **11:**382–4.

Wiley AM (1982) Arthroscopic examination of the shoulder. In: Bayley I and Kellel L, eds. *Shoulder Surgery*. Springer: Paris: 113–18.

Wilcy AM (1991) Arthroscopic appearance of frozen shoulder, *J Arthroscopy Rel Surg* **7:** 138–43.

9
Arthroscopic management

Philippe Beaufils, Thierry Boyer and Gilles Walch

Shoulder stiffness is a label that covers many different conditions. Considerable semantic and pathogenetic confusion remains. The designations 'capsulite rétractile' (Duplay 1896), 'frozen shoulder' (Codman 1934, De Palma 1952, Zuckermann et al 1994), 'adhesive capsulitis' (Neviaser 1945), 'stiff shoulder' and 'shoulder contracture' have all been used, and the resultant ambiguity makes the literature difficult to interpret.

Moreover, the mechanism of shoulder stiffness, which depends on the aetiology, is not always known and can involve: capsular contraction, capsular adhesions, capsular scarring following trauma or surgery and extracapsular changes affecting the subacromial bursa, muscles or tendons.

In this context, it is not surprising that very few studies on the surgical treatment of shoulder stiffness have been reported. Clearly, management depends directly on the cause of shoulder stiffness. This chapter clarifies the classification of shoulder stiffness and makes a number of suggestions regarding the management of this condition.

Classification of shoulder stiffness

To avoid ambiguity, the term 'stiffness' should be used only when the exact cause is not known. Shoulder stiffness can be either functional or organic.

- 'Functional stiffness' is also called 'false stiffness'.
- Organic stiffness can be extracapsular or capsular: primary frozen shoulder, bipolar stiffness, acquired postsurgical stiffness. Organic stiffness is defined as restriction of passive motion. Capsular stiffness is considerably more common than extracapsular stiffness.

Functional stiffness or false stiffness

Functional stiffness is due only to pain. Clinically there is limitation of passive motion which disappears if the shoulder is evaluated under anaesthesia.

Subacromial impingement is the most common cause of functional stiffness, with bursal inflammation being the source of pain. Functional stiffness can be difficult to differentiate from early primary adhesive capsulitis, which is a form of true organic stiffness. It is of paramount importance to distinguish between these two conditions, since their treatment is different.

When the diagnosis is in doubt, the following algorithm proposed by Boyer et al (1995) is useful:

1 Perform Neer's test, i.e. inject an anaesthetic into the subacromial bursa. A significant increase in the range of motion indicates impingement. If the test is negative go to step 2.
2 Consider arthrography. A decrease in joint capacity suggests adhesive capsulitis.
3 If the diagnosis is still in doubt, consider testing under regional or general anaesthesia. Full passive motion indicates impingement. Arthroscopy can be performed simultaneously. Inflammation of the bursa suggests impingement, whereas vascular changes in the glenohumeral capsule suggest adhesive capsulitis, as discussed later.

Organic stiffness

Organic stiffness, or true stiffness, is defined clinically as limitation of passive motion. Organic stiffness can be due to abnormalities in either extra-articular structures or the glenohumeral joint (capsular stiffness).

Extracapsular stiffness

This can be caused by:

• post-traumatic or postsurgical obliteration of the bursa
• non-traumatic obliteration of the bursa
• obliteration of the bicipital groove.

Boyer et al (1995) have reported seven cases of non-traumatic bursal adhesions consistently accompanied with a large, full-thickness tear of the cuff. This rare condition is characterized by pain and restriction of all passive motions. Arthroscopy shows tight adhesions between the stump of the retracted cuff and the undersurface of the acromion. The treatment consists in debridement of the adhesions. Range of motion improved after treatment in all seven cases reported by Boyer et al (1995).

Thomas et al (1995) recently described three cases of flexion block of the shoulder due to adhesion of the long head of the biceps to the bicipital groove. Clinically, external rotation was normal, but forward elevation was limited to 120° with a sensation of mechanical obstruction. Internal rotation was also limited. Plain films and other imaging studies were normal. There was no decrease in joint capacity on the arthrogram. Treatment consisted of manipulation under anaesthesia.

Capsular stiffness

This is the most common form of shoulder stiffness. Three patterns can be differentiated:

• primary frozen shoulder
• bipolar stiffness
• and acquired postsurgical stiffness.

Primary frozen shoulder

Many terms have been used to designate this condition, including 'capsulite rétractile' (Duplay 1896), 'frozen shoulder' (de Palma 1952, Codman 1984), and 'adhesive capsulitis' (Neviaser 1945). Primary frozen shoulder is characterized by primary contracture of the entire joint capsule. There are two phases in the development of this condition, of which the first is characterized by pain and the second by stiffness. The most important feature is that spontaneous recovery eventually occurs.

The early phase is characterized by hyperaemia. A finding of hyperaemia upon arthroscopy is pathognomonic. Hyperaemia has also been confirmed in biopsy specimens. There are no inflammatory changes.

Fibroblastic metaplasia occurs during the second stage: the capsule is contracted, white, and thick. Bunker and Anthony (1995) has shown that this fibrous metaplasia is identical with that seen in Dupuytren's contracture.

Neviaser (1945) suggested that adhesions in the pouch may explain the arthrographic abnormalities and motion restriction. However, it is our experience, and that of many other investigators, that such adhesions are rarely found upon arthroscopy. A noteworthy fact is that the lesions first develop about the rotator interval. Arthroscopically, hyperaemic changes are observed on the undersurface of the long head of the biceps and of the surrounding capsule. Many authors have underlined the role of the coracohumeral ligament (Gagey et al 1985 and 1993, Ozaki et al 1989, Harryman et al 1992, Neer et al 1992, Pollock et al 1994, Bunker and Anthony 1995), which originates from the lateral edge of the horizontal part of the coracoid process, runs forward and downward in the rotator interval, and ends on the tuberosities on either side of the bicipital groove where its fibres intermingle with those of the capsule. The coracohumeral ligament can be seen arthroscopically when the arthroscope is inserted into the bursa via a lateral approach; the ligament is visible in the anterior part of the bursa as a band that covers the superior surface of the cuff, beneath the synovial sheath. The coracohumeral ligament tightens during external rotation, restricting the range of this movement. In patients with primary frozen shoulder, the coracohumeral ligament is contracted into a thick, fibrous cord that restricts the movements of the glenohumeral joint. This may explain the early limitation of external rotation.

Bipolar stiffness

Bipolar stiffness is characterized by rotator cuff disease with secondary contraction of the glenohumeral capsule. This is a rare condition (three of 26 cases in our series of capsular contracture). The diagnosis is based on arthroscopy, which shows:

- evidence of impingement and/or a rotator cuff tear, and
- evidence of capsular contraction (hyperaemia about the rotator interval).

It is essential to differentiate bipolar stiffness from:

- functional stiffness, discussed above, which is considerably more common and does not require capsular release
- extracapsular stiffness due to adhesions of the bursa (see above), which does not require capsular release, and perhaps most importantly
- primary frozen shoulder, which is considerably more prevalent. The risk here is overdiagnosis of impingement and unnecessary decompressive treatment (two cases in our series).

Acquired postsurgical or post-traumatic stiffness

Acquired postsurgical stiffness is due to scarring of the capsule after disruption or incision of the capsule. There is no inflammation or hyperaemia, and this condition is radically different from primary frozen shoulder. In our series, acquired postsurgical stiffness was the diagnosis in 10 of 26 shoulders.

The cause can be

- a significant injury of the shoulder responsible for capsular disruption, such as a dislocation, a humeral head fracture, a fracture-dislocation, etc.
- surgery on the glenohumeral joint (shoulder stabilization, cuff surgery, or even insertion of a prosthesis as in one case in our series).

Anterior contraction is considerably more common than posterior contraction. We have never performed posterior release of the capsule. As in primary frozen shoulders, the coracohumeral ligament is contracted.

The main diagnostic difficulty is to determine whether the capsular contraction is isolated or accompanied by contraction of periarticular structures (for instance the subscapularis tendon) or with bony impingement. In the first case, arthroscopic treatment can be used, whereas in the second open surgery is required.

Treatment of capsular stiffness arthroscopic glenohumeral release

Glenohumeral release can be achieved arthroscopically. In patients who fail to respond to conservative treatment, hydraulic distension (Lundberg 1969, Hsu and Chan 1991, Ekelund and Rydell 1992, Nobuhara et al 1994, Ogilvie-Harris et al 1995), manipulation under anaesthesia (Uitvlugt et al 1993, Ogilvie-Harris et al 1995, Vastamaki 1995), and, in a few cases, surgical release (open or arthroscopic) have been proposed. Arthroscopic release has been reported by Pollock et al (1994), Ogilvie-Harris et al (1995) and Wiley (1991).

The following questions need to be answered:

- is arthroscopic release technically feasible, safe, and effective?
- do results depend on the aetiology?
- when should the procedure be done?

Some surgeons contend that there is no indication for arthroscopic release. We interviewed 14 members of the French Arthroscopy Society who had extensive experience with shoulder arthroscopy. Only eight used arthroscopic release. We conducted a multicentric study of 26 shoulders (25 patients) with the following diagnoses:

- primary frozen shoulder, $n = 13$
- bipolar stiffness, $n = 3$
- acquired postsurgical stiffness, $n = 10$.

Technique

The procedure was performed under general anaesthesia (18 cases), interscalene block (four cases), or combined anaesthesia (four cases). Range of motion was assessed before arthroscopy. The arthroscope was then inserted via a posterior approach. Despite the tightness of the joint, the difficulties in insertion of the arthroscope reported by other authors were observed in only four cases. Instruments were inserted via anterior or anterosuperior portals. Synovial hypertrophy, generally found about the rotator interval, was debrided. The capsule was then sectioned at the anterior rim of the glenoid fossa. A purely anterior section was done in six cases, and anterior and inferior section done in 20 cases. Electrocautery was used in 15 cases and laser in four cases. Gentle manipulation was then performed. When external rotation was not improved, the coracohumeral ligament was separated from the coracoid process via the anterior portal (Pollock et al 1994). Additional procedures were required in some instances: acromioplasty (five cases), bursectomy (three cases), SLAP (superior labium from anterior to posterior) lesion debridement (one case).

Physiotherapy was started immediately, if needed, under continuous interscalene anaesthesia.

Our series

Twenty-five patients (26 shoulders) aged 21–68 years were re-evaluated after a mean follow-up of 21 months using Constant's scoring system. Mean symptom duration before arthroscopy was 13 months (range, 1–27).

Passive motion before arthroscopy was as follows:

• abduction: 74° (0/180)
• external rotation: 6° (−70/20)
• forward flexion: 84° (0/160).

Mean Constant's motion score was 12.9/40 and was lower (indicating more severe motion restriction) in patients with primary disease (9.69 vs. 15.8). Mean pain score was 5.7/15. Before arthroscopic release, anaesthesia improved the range of motion in only six cases (external rotation).

Results

No intraoperative vascular or neural complications were seen. There was one case each of Sudeck disease, wound infection, and haematoma.

Mean increases in ranges of motion under anaesthesia were as follows:

• abduction: 72° (0/150)
• external rotation: 34° (20/70)
• forward flexion: 71° (0/180).

Final outcomes were assessed after a mean of 7 months. There were no differences between aetiologic groups. There was no loss of motion as compared to the intraoperative gain (Fig. 1). Constant's motion score improved more in patients with primary disease (9.69 to 34.9 vs. 15.8 to 30.6).

Subjective results are shown in Table 1 and were better in patients with primary disease. Objective results were assessed based on the absolute Constant's score, which was 70.3 points (39/85), i.e. 83.3% of the score for the contralateral, apparently healthy shoulder. There were three excellent, five very good, seven good, and 11 fair or poor results (Table 2).

The relative Constant's score was 91% in patients with primary disease versus only 76% in those with acquired disease. The difference was not due to range of motion, which was identical in the two groups, but rather to pain and strength, which improved more in the primary group.

Discussion

Arthroscopic release of shoulder contracture is feasible. This procedure should always include anterior or antero-inferior capsular section. To improve

Table 1 Subjective results

	Global series	Primary frozen shoulder	Bipolar stiffness	Acquired post-surgical stiffness
Excellent	13	7	1	5
Satisfied	5	3	1	1
Better	5	2	1	2
Same	3	1	0	2
Worse	0	0	0	0

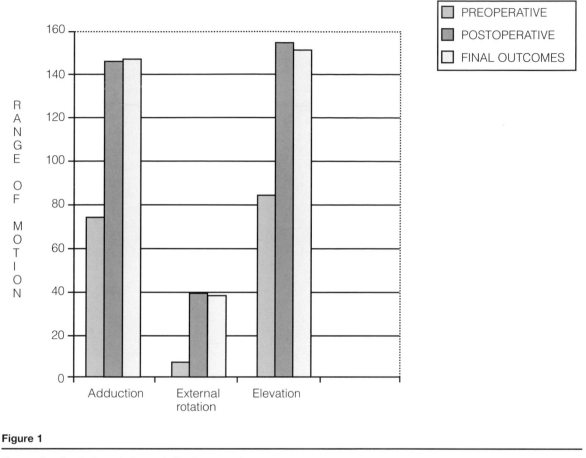

Figure 1

Range of motion before, during and after the procedure.

external rotation, Ogilvie-Harris et al (1995) suggested that the subscapularis tendon should also be severed progressively; however, we did not use this technique. Pollock et al (1994) and Ozaki et al (1989) suggested that the coracohumeral ligament and rotator interval should be cut, and did not observe secondary instability in any of their cases.

Arthroscopic release is safe. There were no intra-operative complications in our series. Arthroscopic release is effective. Improvements in motion in our series were identical with those reported by Ogilvie-Harris et al (1995) and Pollock et al (1994). However, it is important to evaluate results according to the cause of shoulder stiffness in an effort to determine the optimal indications.

Table 2 Objective results assessed based on Constant's score

	Global series	Primary frozen shoulder	Bipolar stiffness	Acquired post-surgical stiffness
Excellent	3	2	0	1
Very good	5	4	0	1
Good	7	3	2	2
Fair	7	2	0	5
Poor	4	2	1	1

Primary frozen shoulder usually resolves sponta-neously or responds to conservative management. Surgery is rarely indicated. Data reported by Ogilvie-Harris et al (1995) and our own experience suggest that arthroscopic release does not hasten recovery (in our series, symptom duration at arthroscopy was 13 months and the postsurgical recovery time was 7 months, for a total of 20 months). The goal of arthroscopic release in this condition is to improve motion until spontaneous recovery occurs. We therefore reserve this proce-dure for highly selected cases characterized by severe restriction of motion (especially external rotation). A 1-year waiting period after symptom onset is acceptable. Alternatives are hydraulic dis-tension and manipulation. Many authors have reported on the results obtained using these tech-niques (Rowe and Leffert 1988, Ekelund and Rydell 1992, Hannafin et al 1994, Pollock et al 1994, Esch 1995). Rowe and Leffert (1988) reported that manipulation has yielded conflicting results. Arthroscopic release provides similar benefits with-out tearing the capsule or damaging the cartilage.

In bipolar stiffness, arthroscopy demonstrates the exact cause of the stiffness and provides a means of treatment, particularly in patients with subacro-mial abnormalities. Bursoscopy should be per-formed and cuff lesions treated.

In postsurgical stiffness, arthroscopic release is appropriate in our view. Pollock et al (1994) have voiced the opposite opinion. Isolated manipulation is not indicated in this condition. The only effective treatment is surgical section of the scar tissue. In our experience, gain of motion is significant after arthroscopic release. Subjective and objective results are less satisfactory than in primary frozen shoulder, due to persistent pain and weakness. The alternative is open release, but morbidity is lower with arthroscopic release, which can be proposed as soon as the capsular tissue has healed (for instance after 6 months).

Conclusion

Shoulder stiffness is not synonymous with frozen shoulder. It is essential to establish the correct diagnosis. A careful history and physical evaluation are helpful. Global limitation of passive motion sug-gests a capsular origin. Limitation of abduction points to a subacromial abnormality. Limitation of

flexion and internal rotation is consistent with bicipi-tal adhesions.

The management depends on the diagnosis:

• physiotherapy in functional stiffness, followed if needed by arthroscopic decompression after restoration of a normal range of motion
• arthroscopic capsular release in refractory organic capsular contracture; however, open surgery should be done in patients who also have contraction of periarticular structures
• arthroscopic bursal release in bursal obliteration, with subacromial decompression
• manipulation under anaesthesia in bicipital adhe-sions.

References

Boyer T, Dorfmann H, Bequet R (1995) La capsulite rétractile de l'épaule et son traitement, *Act Rhum* **4**:88–98.

Bunker TD, Anthony PP (1995) The pathology of frozen shoulder, *J Bone Joint Surg* **77B**:677–83.

Codman EA (1934) *The Shoulder.* Thomas Todd Co.: Boston.

de Palma AF (1952) Loss of scapulo-humeral motion (frozen shoulder), *Ann Surg* **135**:193–204.

Duplay S (1896) La périarthrite scapulo-humérale, *Rev Trav Med* **53**:226–7.

Ekelund AL, Rydell N (1992) Combination treatment for adhesive capsulitis of the shoulder, *Clin Orthop* **282**:105–9.

Esch C (1995) Arthroscopic treatment of the frozen shoulder. In: Vastanaki, Jalovaara, eds. *Surgery of the Shoulder.* Elsevier: Amsterdam: 259.

Gagey O, Bonfait H, Gillot C, Mazas F (1985) Etude de la mécanique de l'élévation de l'épaule. Rôle du ligament coraco-huméral, *Rev Chir Orthop* **71**(suppl 2):105–7.

Gagey O, Arcache J, Welby F, Gagey N (1993) Le squelette fibreux de la coiffe des rotateurs, *Rev Chir Orthop* **79**:452–5.

Hannafin JA, Dicarlo EF, Wickiewicz TL (1994) Adhesive cap-sulitis: capsular fibroplasia of the glenohumeral joint, *J Shoulder Elbow Surg* **3**:1 part 2, S5.

Harryman DT, Sides JA, Harris SL, Matsen FA (1992) The role of the rotator interval capsule in passive motion and stability of the shoulder, *J Bone Joint Surg* **74A**:53–66.

Hsu S, Chan K (1991) Arthroscopic distension in the man-agement of frozen shoulder, *Int Orthop* **15**:79–83.

Lundberg BJ (1969) The frozen shoulder, *Acta Orthop Scand* (suppl 119)**1**:42–4.

Neer CS, Satterlee C, Dalsey RM, Flatow EL (1992) The anatomy and potential effects of contracture of the coracohumeral ligament, *Clin Orthop* **280**:182–5.

Neviaser JS (1945) Adhesive capsulitis of the shoulder, *J Bone Joint Surg* **27**:211–22.

Nobuhara K, Supapo AR, Hino T (1994) Effects of joint distension in shoulder diseases, *Clin Orthop* **304**:25–9.

Ogilvie-Harris DJ, Biggs DJ, Fitsialos DP, Mackay M (1995) The resistant frozen shoulder. Manipulation vs arthroscopic release, *Clin Orthop* **319**:238–48.

Ozaki J, Nakagama Y, Sakurai G, Tamai S (1989) Recalcitrant chronic adhesive capsulitis of the shoulder, *J Bone Joint Surg* **71A**:1511–15.

Pollock RG, Duralde XA, Flatow EL, Bigliani LU (1994) The use of arthroscopy in the treatment of resistant frozen shoulder, *Clin Orthop* **304**:30–6.

Rowe CR, Leffert RD (1988) Idiopathic chronic adhesive capsulitis ("frozen shoulder"). In: Rowe CR, ed. *The Shoulder*. Churchill Livingstone: New York: 155.

Thomas T, Gazielly D, Bruyere G, Alexandre C (1995) Réflexions sur une forme clinique particulière: l'épaule enraidie en flexion, *Rev Rhum* **62**:261–6.

Uitvlugt G, Detrisac DA, Johnson LL, Austin MD, Johnson C (1993) Arthroscopic observation before and after manipulation of frozen shoulder, *Arthroscopy* **2**:181–5.

Vastamaki M (1995) Long-term outcome of the manipulated spontaneous frozen shoulder. In: Vastamaki V, Jalovaara P, eds. *Surgery of the Shoulder*. Elsevier: Amsterdam: 265.

Wiley AM (1991) Arthroscopic appearance of frozen shoulder, *Arthroscopy* **7**:138–43.

Zuckermann JD, Cuomo F, Rokito S (1994) Definition and classification of frozen shoulder: a consensus approach, *J Shoulder Elbow Surg* **3**:S72.

10
Arthrodesis

Stephen A Copeland

As tuberculous infection of the shoulder has become less common and replacement arthroplasty has been developed, the indications for arthrodesis have become relatively rare. However, it still remains a successful and important method of management of certain specific shoulder problems. It is reliable and, once fusion has been attained, function does not deteriorate with time. All remaining movement then depends totally on the thoracoscapular articulation. Arthrodesis tends to be used when all else has failed and, therefore, each procedure must be individualized to take account of the preceding surgery, scarring, infection, loss of bone stock and specific functional requirements of the patient.

Indications

The flail shoulder

The commonest indication for arthrodesis currently is paralytic flail shoulder. Until recently this was caused by anterior poliomyelitis but is now more commonly secondary to traumatic brachial plexus lesions. Although the problems of polio have decreased, motor cycling injuries have increased with severe proximal root and upper trunk brachial plexus injuries a common indication for shoulder arthrodesis.

Patients may have good function in elbow and hand, but are unable to place the hand in space because of poor glenohumeral control. If there is good scapular control, i.e. trapezius, levator scapulae, serratus anterior and rhomboid function, then shoulder arthrodesis should allow adequate stabilization for effective hand function. Sometimes the weight of the limb causes a secondary inferior subluxation at the glenohumeral joint, purely because of

the weight of the arm. This causes an aching such that the patient may only be comfortable in a sling. The aching pain is relieved by shoulder fusion. Elbow flexor plasty in the presence of a flail shoulder can be disappointing because attempted elbow flexion can result in shoulder extension rather than flexion of the elbow. Shoulder fusion in combination with flexor plasty provides a much more useful arm.

Failed shoulder replacement

The problems presented by the failed shoulder replacement can be extremely varied and difficult to manage. Loss of bone stock may be a problem. Secondary fibrosis caused by loosening or infection may be enough to stabilize a pseudarthrosis after removal of the components. If this is inadequate, such that function remains poor and the shoulder is grossly unstable, then arthrodesis is indicated. Gaining fusion may sometimes be extremely difficult and extensive grafting may be required.

Infection

Pyogenic infection of the shoulder still occurs, but unfortunately it is frequently iatrogenic secondary to previous surgery, e.g. infection of internal fixation devices used for fracture fixation around the shoulder. A recent history of infection is an absolute contraindication to replacement arthroplasty, but may be considered when the infective episode may have happened years before without flare-ups since the original event. Sometimes further attempts at replacement arthroplasty may be unwise and fusion may be the only available option.

Trauma

As shoulder replacement has become more sophisticated, shoulder joint replacement is part of the armamentarium of the trauma surgeon in his treatment of fractures around the shoulder. Sometimes, however, the bony geometry is so grossly destroyed by malunion of a fracture that arthrodesis is the only sensible alternative because reconstruction and re-fashioning of the proximal end of the humerus may be impossible. Isolated but total loss of axillary nerve function causes variable disability. In the presence of an intact and functioning cuff, this disability may be minimal. If functional disability is a major problem, the choice will be between glenohumeral fusion and multiple muscle transfers. Muscle transfers are probably better reserved for partial axillary nerve palsy. Glenohumeral arthrodesis can provide a more reliable method of restoring function if symptoms justify.

Instability

A small percentage of patients who undergo soft tissue stabilization procedures for recurrent dislocation of shoulder, fail to gain permanent stability despite repeated procedures. Rarely, shoulder arthrodesis may be the only method to reliably regain a useful shoulder.

Contraindications

Following surgery an extensive period of immobilization of the joint is required to obtain fusion. This can be achieved either by internal fixation, by using spica casts, by using a brace or a combination of these. If the patient is unable to co-operate with immobilization, then it is unlikely that the fusion will be successful. If the patient has particularly sensitive skin, either to the materials used for the brace or the spica, or has a sensory neuropathy, then reliance must be placed totally on internal fixation devices. Arthrodesis of the shoulder relies on having a mobile thoracoscapular joint and other mobile joints in the upper limb. If the patient has a polyarthropathy, then other methods than arthrodesis should be investigated.

Position of arthrodesis

Many different positions have been described for shoulder arthrodesis and there is no one position that is universally acceptable. There must be some variation to take into account each patient's particular needs and occupation.

The 'salute' position was considered to be optimal, but now it is thought to cause an unnecessary degree of abduction and forward flexion. When the arm is lowered to the side of the body, there is a fixed winging of the scapula causing an uncomfortable strain on the thoracoscapular muscles. Rowe and Zarins (1989) advocated a modification which has been widely accepted. They recommend that the shoulder be arthrodesed with enough abduction to clear the axilla, enough internal rotation to reach the midline of the body, both anteriorly and posteriorly and enough forward flexion to reach the face and head (Fig. 1). If excessive abduction is eliminated then patients may reach their side, back pocket, gluteal area and feet with forward glide of the scapula on the chest wall. They can elevate the arm well above the head. This usually allows the patient to sleep more comfortably, even sleeping on the side of the arthrodesed shoulder.

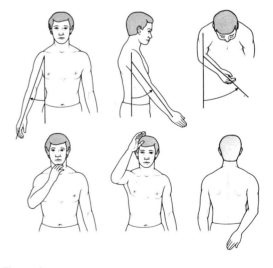

Figure 1

Rowe and Zarins (1989) modification of position for arthrodesis.

Technique

The incision extends along the spine of the scapula to the anterior acromion and down the anterolateral aspect of the shaft of the humerus. The rotator cuff is resected and the head positioned to fit snugly underneath the acromion. All bone-to-bone contact areas are decorticated and cancellous bone used to pack between bone ends and to fill any spaces.

It is important not to fracture or bend the acromion downwards to meet the humerus, but to bring the humerus up to meet the acromion. This is important for cosmetic reasons so that clothes will fit well and straps will not fall off the shoulder. The patient will look more symmetrical.

A 10-hole 4.5 mm pelvic reconstruction plate is used to secure fixing and contoured to maintain the position discussed above (Fig. 2). It is usually wise to put in one or two fixing screws and then check the position again as it can be surprisingly difficult peroperatively to get the exact position required.

a)

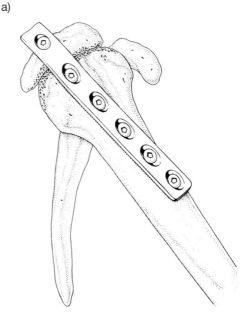

b)

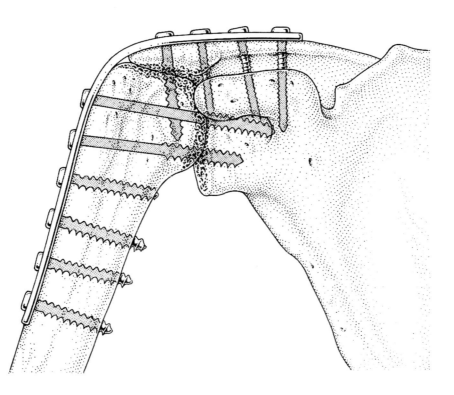

Figure 2

(a,b) Long plate used for arthrodesis of shoulder. The acromion is left intact.

Postoperative management

If a good solid fix is obtained and the patient is sensible and aware of the limitations, then any form of external fixation may not be needed. However, if fixation or the patient may not be relied upon, then it is wiser to use either a plaster spica incorporating the trunk and upper limb or a shoulder abduction brace for three months.

Complications

Non-union

It is rare to see non-union when the indication for fusion is brachial plexus palsy. Usually in this situation, the bony geometry is maintained, there has been very little bone stock loss and probably little in the way of previous bony surgery or scarring within the joint. However, in the presence of infection and bone loss, non-union rate increases. In a series of 71 arthrodeses, Cofield and Briggs (1979) had only three which resulted in non-union. These were successfully fused following a second operative procedure.

Malposition

Hyperabduction is the commonest malposition at surgery. Adult patients have great difficulty in adapting to a position of more then 45° of abduction. If too much internal rotation has been incorporated, then the patient cannot easily bring hand to mouth or reach front or back pockets, and correctional rotation osteotomy may be required.

Removal of implant

The AO Group recommends prophylactic bone grafting because of the incidence of fracture at the distal end of the internal fixation device. Cofield and Briggs (1979) also confirm this. In 10 of their 71 patients a fracture was sustained in the fused extremity.

It is recommended that the plate is removed prophylactically, but it is not known whether this reduces the incidence of fracture. Sometimes it is wise to remove the internal fixation plate because gross muscle wasting and atrophy around the shoulder may make the internal fixation device rather prominent and uncomfortable in the subcutaneous position.

In summary, arthrodesis of the shoulder can give very satisfactory functional results in specific circumstances. This whole symposium is about stiffness of the shoulder, but surprisingly this operation which gives the ultimate stiffness can lead to good results!

References

Cofield RH, Briggs BT (1979) Gleno-humeral arthrodesis, *J Bone Joint Surg* **61A**:668–77.

Rowe CR, Zarins B (1989) Improvements in arthrodesis of the shoulder. In: Post M, Morrey B, Hawkins R, eds. *Surgery of the Shoulder 353*. CV Mosby: St Louis.

11
Arthroplasty

Stephen A Copeland

Shoulder arthroplasty has developed in line with replacement of other major joints. Although not as frequently indicated as hip or knee replacement, it has been around for almost as long and the long-term results rival those of hip and knee arthroplasty. The modern approach to shoulder replacement really developed from two separate sources.

1. Some experience was gained with replacement of the proximal humerus for tumour. Initially these replacements were massive and only used as a last resort procedure. However, as these appeared to be successful, constrained-type shoulder replacements were used for arthritis. The use of constrained total joint replacements have been associated with an unacceptable mid-term failure rate due to loosening, usually of the glenoid component.

2. The other source of development arose from treatment of fractures. In the USA Charles Neer (1990) had been studying fractures at the proximal humerus and had identified a group which did very poorly. He described the four-part classification of fractures and in the four-part fracture itself, the humeral head became completely devascularized and had a high chance of undergoing avascular necrosis leading to a poor functional result.

He designed and used a stemmed hemiarthroplasty around which the humeral tuberosities could be reconstructed (Fig. 1). Having rebuilt a stable construct, rehabilitation could be started early and functional results greatly improved. Having shown that good results could be achieved with fracture, it was then only a short step to consider shoulder replacement in arthritis and a glenoid prosthesis was developed. The Neer-type stemmed prosthesis which is an unconstrained joint, is the commonest type of joint used world-wide today. There are very many modifications on this basic design which include modularity, different stem sizes, cement-less, bony ingrowth and prostheses made for left and right shoulders. However, for all these modifications, long-term results must be awaited to see if they offer advantages on the original design.

Generally it seems that the humeral component gives satisfactory long-term results if cemented. If the joint is to fail, it is usually on the glenoid side due to loss of glenoid fixation. Many different types of glenoid prostheses have been designed using bony ingrowth, metal backing, screw fixation, cement fixation or just impact fit. However, all these different designs do report a rather worrying incidence of lucent lines around the prosthesis in the mid-term. These lucent lines are not necessarily progressive and not definitely connected with clinical loosening unless they are over 2 mm in width or are non-parallel.

I have developed and used over a 10-year period, a different type of shoulder replacement (Fig. 2) (Copeland 1993 and 1995). I believe that in the majority of shoulders requiring replacement, an intramedullary stem with cement fixation around the stem is not necessary and the latter can cause problems. A cementless surface replacement design has been described which has many potential advantages. As with any joint replacement, a failure in the longer term has to be contemplated. If the joint were to fail, then some of the problems presented by revision shoulder replacement may be formidable. It therefore behoves us to consider revision surgery thus making any subsequent surgery easier. If just the surface of the joint is replaced and no bone stock is removed, relatively minimal invasive surgery is achieved.

Despite all the different types of joint replacement on the market today, the indications for shoulder replacement remain constant.

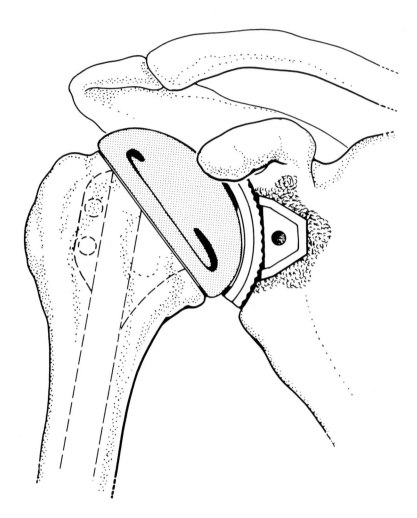

Figure 1

Neer-type total shoulder replacement.

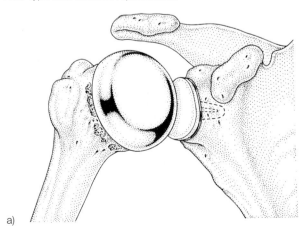

a)

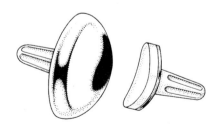

b)

Figure 2

(a, b) Copeland surface replacement arthroplasty (reproduced by kind permission from Copeland 1995).

Indications for shoulder replacement

There are two main groups:

1 rheumatoid arthritis
2 osteoarthritis primary and secondary.

Among the causes of secondary osteoarthritis are the effects of old trauma, post-dislocation arthropathy, cuff tear arthropathy, congenital dysplasia, the effects of old sepsis and osteonecrosis.

More rarely, surgery is indicated for tumour and failed surgery including revision of previous prosthesis. Whatever the cause of the destructive process on the articular surface, the net result remains the same, i.e. increasing pain and stiffness. The overwhelming indication for surgery is uncontrolled pain with loss of movement and consequent loss of function. The expectations for shoulder replacement are higher than for lower limb joint replacements. If in the hip and knee, for instance, a stable pain-free joint with two-thirds range of motion is achieved, then this is seen as an excellent result. At the shoulder however, being stable and pain free is not enough. It is the most mobile joint in the body and hence, a much greater range of mobility is expected.

The results of shoulder replacement depend almost entirely on the adequacy of soft tissues and musculature and the restoration of the anatomic geometry of the joint. This cannot be so easily achieved at the shoulder as it can at either hip or knee. When assessing a shoulder before replacement it is often thought that there is a complete loss of rotator cuff function, but this does not necessarily mean loss of continuity of the rotator cuff. Often, because of gross erosion of joint surfaces, the centre of rotation has been medialized and hence, rotator cuff function lost.

If the rotator cuff has lost its action, then the unopposed deltoid has its resolution of forces directed superiorly, and hence, upward subluxation of the humeral head results.

If this process can be reversed, that is by lateralization of the centre of rotation, by re-tensioning both cuff and deltoid, then restoration of function can be expected. Unfortunately, in the most severely affected joints, long-term adaptive changes have occurred, i.e. shortening of the rotator cuff muscles. Therefore, complete restoration of geometry by lateralization of the centre of rotation is not possible. The soft tissues cannot be elongated adequately to the anatomic position. In more severe cases, loss of rotator cuff may be true and complete. In this situation, it may be wiser to consider hemiarthroplasty alone because the incidence of glenoid loosening in the face of complete rotator cuff loss is greater (Arntz et al 1993). This can be expected on a mechanical basis alone.

If the cuff is not present, the humeral head is subluxed superiorly. If the glenoid replacement is then placed in the anatomic position, a rocking or toggle movement increases the chances of loosening (Arntz et al 1993).

Interestingly, the results of hemiarthroplasty in relation to total replacement are not too dissimilar (Bell and Gschwend 1986). It has been shown that hemiarthroplasty alone may not give the complete relief of pain experienced with total replacement.

Hence, when considering hemiarthroplasty or total replacement, it is always a question of weighing up the balance between the two. In hemiarthroplasty pain relief may not be as good, but in total replacement the risk of long-term glenoid loosening is greater.

All shoulder replacements of whatever design require good bone stock for fixation of the glenoid component. If medial erosion of the glenoid has occurred with erosion to the base of the coracoid, then it is unlikely that adequate seating of the glenoid component will be achieved. It may be better in this situation to accept hemiarthroplasty alone.

Contraindications

Contraindications are very similar to those for joint replacement anywhere.

1 Sepsis – if there is any persistent septic focus this must be dealt with before surgery. If there is any question of old deep bone infection from previous surgery, the surgeon must be certain that this has been eradicated.
2 Unstable joint – if the joint is unstable before surgery, shoulder replacement will almost certainly be unstable after surgery. For example, painful subluxation secondary to brachial plexus palsy would be better served by arthrodesis.
3 Charcot type joint – if there is loss of feeling within the joint, then the rate of long-term failure and loosening of the joint may be unacceptably high.

Postoperative management

Most advances have been made recently in postoperative management. We are now much more aggressive in trying to regain the range of motion early. At the time of surgery every attempt is made to fix everything solidly enough to allow for immediate passive mobilization. If the replacement is done for fracture, then good solid mechanical stability of the bony fragments must be achieved at the time of surgery to allow passive mobilizing to begin on the day following surgery. If the procedure is done for arthritis, then usually only subscapularis muscle has been divided and hence, rehabilitation can be started immediately avoiding external rotation until 3 weeks.

However, generally passive mobilizing only is allowed until three weeks after surgery. Passive assisted mobilization is allowed up to 6 weeks and then a full active stretching and strengthening programme from 6 weeks onwards. It is well known that improvement may be gained from shoulder arthroplasty for a year following surgery. It is therefore always worthwhile strongly encouraging patients to keep up their stretching programme vigorously and continuously for this time.

References

Arntz CT, Jackins R, Matsen F (1993) Prosthetic replacement of the shoulder for the treatment of defects in the rotator cuff and the surface of the gleno-humeral joint. *J Bone Joint Surg* **75A**:485–91.

Bell S, Gschwend N (1986) Clinical experience with total arthroplasty hemiarthroplasty using the Neer prosthesis. *Int Orthop* **10**:217–22.

Copeland SA (1993) Cementless shoulder replacement. A new design. *J Bone Joint Surg* **75**(suppl 1)42.

Copeland SA (1995) *Operative Shoulder Surgery*. Churchill Livingstone: New York: 226–48.

Neer CS (1990) *Gleno-humeral Arthroplasty in Shoulder Reconstruction*. WB Saunders: Philadelphia.

Part II
Elbow stiffness

12
Aetiology and incidence

Jens Ole Søjbjerg

Stiffness of the elbow is a common complication following fractures, dislocations, burns, surgery and other elbow traumas. The degree of stiffness is often unpredictable, although several risk factors can be identified. Prolonged immobilization, intra-articular fractures, neurotrauma and burns are well-known factors predisposing the elbow to post-traumatic contracture.

The reduction in range of motion may vary in severity ranging from loss of a few degrees of extension to a complete bony ankylosis, abolishing every movement of the joint. Elbows suffering contracture are often free of pain, but the reduced range of elbow motion causes a functional impairment of the hand because this is highly dependent on forearm rotation and elbow extension and flexion. A 50% reduction of elbow range of motion can decrease the upper extremity function by almost 80%. In practice, only a reduction of the overall range of motion to less than 100° are considered clinically important contractures, since only a range of motion less than 100° seriously interferes with the activities of daily living.

As for other joints, adequate elbow function requires a stable, pain-free joint with sufficient strength and range of motion. Morrey et al (1981) investigated the functional range of elbow motion in healthy volunteers. They studied 15 daily living activities and concluded that about 90% of these activities could be carried out in an arc of motion between 30–100° and 30° of extension and flexion. Furthermore, both supination and pronation of 50° was required. However, it must be emphasized that none of the functions studied included sports or work activities. Loss of terminal extension is less disabling than loss of the same degree of terminal flexion. In clinical practice most patients can tolerate a flexion loss of about 30° and an extension loss of 45° but if the decrease in motion reduces the

overall range of motion to less than 100°, most patients will complain of loss of function.

The specific reason that the elbow so often develops stiffness remains unclear, but one reason could be the close relationship between the capsule, especially the anterior part, and the medial and lateral collateral ligament complexes.

As the stability of the elbow joint is dependent of the soft tissues around the joint and the articular geometry, the stiffness seen in the post-traumatic elbow may be related to the constraints of the joint, and a proper knowledge of the stabilizers of the elbow is necessary to obtain good results after surgery for contracture.

The medial collateral ligament consists of two well-defined bands, one anterior and one posterior. In vitro studies have shown the anterior part of the ligament to be the prime stabilizer in valgus and internal rotation (Søjbjerg et al 1987b).

The lateral collateral ligaments are gathered in a complex and consist of the lateral collateral ligament, the annular ligament and the lateral ulnar collateral ligament (Søjbjerg et al 1987a, Olsen et al 1996). The authors also stressed the importance of this ligament complex, stabilizing the joint in varus and in external rotation. Furthermore, their study suggested that reconstruction of the ligament complex restored the stability of the elbow.

The elbow joint is a congruent joint due to its osseous geometry and, therefore, by nature rather constrained. This is due to the olecranon and coronoid process articulating tightly to the humerus, thereby stabilizing the joint in extension as well as in flexion (An et al 1986). Even minor exostosis at the tip of the olecranon or at the coronoid may increase the constraint of the joint, thereby reducing the mobility of the elbow. Also, intra-articular fractures can reduce the motion of the joint, because even minor malunions may mechanically obliterate the potentional range of motion of the joint.

The true incidence of elbow contracture after trauma is unknown, but seems to be rather common. In a previous study of former traumatic elbow dislocations, Olsen and Søjbjerg (1996) found that about 50% suffered some degree of reduction in range of motion, but only 5% had an extension lack greater than 15°. Moreover, no limitations in flexion, supination or pronation were seen. Traumatic stiffness after a severe fracture can be due to traumas of varying severity and different degrees of involvement of the joint surfaces. Mohan (1972) studied 200 cases of post-traumatic stiffness and reported that 20% were related to supracondylar, T-condylar or condyle fractures. In 20% the initial trauma was an elbow dislocation and in 38% the primary trauma was a fracture–dislocation of the joint. Finally, radial head fractures accounted for 10% of the cases.

Cooney (1993) stated that the development of post-traumatic elbow stiffness was directly related to the severity of the initial trauma. Other risk factors indicated were the degree of intra-articular involvement, the amount of periosteal stripping and the length of immobilization.

Heterotopic bone formation is a well-recognized cause of elbow contracture (Garland and O'Hollaren 1982, Kjærsgaard-Andersen et al 1992). The reasons for the development of heterotopic bone around the elbow joint after trauma remain unknown. However, recent studies have pointed out that trauma to the soft tissues initiates the stimulation of pluripotential mesenchymal cells to osteoblasts, being capable of forming heterotopic bone in the soft tissues around the elbow.

The incidence of heterotopic bone formation after trauma to the elbow is about 3%, but when the patient has also sustained a neurotrauma, the incidence seems to double (Fig. 1). Kjærsgaard-Andersen et al (1992) investigated the prevalence of heterotopic bone formation following total elbow replacement. The authors reported that clinically important ectopic bone formation was not seen in their series of 50 elbow replacements and related this to the fact that all of their patients were rheumatoids being treated with non-steroidal

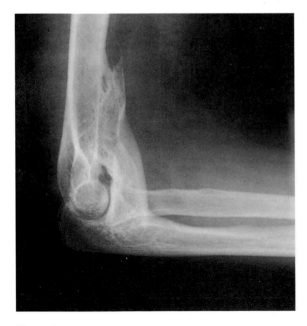

Figure 1

Extrinsic pathology causing ankylosis of the elbow. Anterior bony bridging of the elbow following severe combined thermal and head injury.

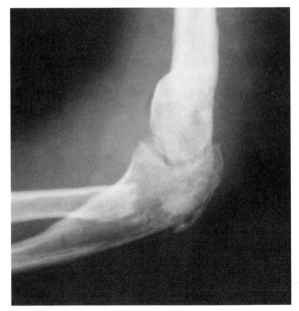

Figure 2

Intrinsic pathology of the elbow following severe intra-articular fracture causing severe reduction in elbow motion.

anti-inflammatory drugs (NSAIDs). The same authors recommended prophylactic treatment with indomethacin of the patients at risk, although such evidence concerning the prevention of heterotopic bone around the elbow, still is lacking.

Another group of elbow contractures consist of acquired cases seen in haemophiliacs, post-infectious cases or in rheumatoid arthritis. These aetiologies are seldom candidates to operative release, because pain is often the dominating symptom in these elbows.

Finally, the contractures can be congenital. Common conditions are arthrogryposis or congenital dislocation of the radial head. These patients often have a severe neuromuscular involvement causing secondary involvement of the elbow joint and therefore require a different treatment.

A proper classification of the elbow contracture is important for planning treatment and postoperative rehabilitation (Søjbjerg et al 1995, Søjbjerg 1996). A simple classification related to the position of the contracture in extension or flexion deficiency is descriptive, but insufficient for the choice of treatment. The most convenient and important classification of the post-traumatic stiff elbow is based on the pathologies responsible for the loss of motion and these can be divided into intra-articular and extra-articular causes. The intrinsic or intra-articular causes are either due to intra-articular adhesions or a deformity secondary to an intra-articular fracture, thereby mechanically limiting the elbow motion (Fig. 2). A common cause of extrinsic or extra-articular contracture is contracture of the capsule, collateral ligaments or the muscles following a severe trauma or just a simple posterior dislocation. Another category of extrinsic contracture is a bony bridging of the joint. It is well known that patients with severe head injury (Fig. 1) are at risk. Formation of heterotopic bone after a severe burn is also well documented.

In reality most cases present with a mixture of both intrinsic and extrinsic causes. Many elbow contractures due to extrinsic pathologies will present with some degree of secondary intra-articular adhesions, and many intrinsic cases demonstrate a scarring of the soft tissues, but contractures should be classified according to the major pathology.

References

An KN, Morrey BF, Chao EYS (1986) The effect of partial removal of proximal ulna on elbow constraint, *Clin Orthop* **209**:270–9.

Cooney WP (1993) Contractures of the elbow. In: Morrey BF ed. *The Elbow and Its Disorders*, Vol. 2. WB Saunders: Philadelphia: 464–75.

Garland DE, O'Hollaren RM (1982) Fractures and dislocations about the elbow in the head injured adult *Clin Orthop* **168**:38–41.

Kjærsgaard-Andersen P, Søjbjerg JO, Sneppen O (1992) Heterotopic bone formation after arthroplasty of the shoulder, elbow and knee: a review *Sem Arthrop* **3**:200–5.

Mohan K (1972) Myositis ossificans of the elbow, *Int Surg* **57**:475–80.

Morrey BF, Askew L, An KN, Chao EYS (1981) A biomechanical study of normal functional elbow motion, *J Bone Joint Surg* **63**:872–7.

Olsen BS, Søjbjerg JO (1996) Posterolateral elbow instability following a traumatic dislocation, *Acta Orthop Scand*, **67**(S272):66.

Olsen BS, Søjbjerg JO, Væsel MT, Helmig P, Sneppen O (1996) The lateral collateral ligament complex of the elbow joint: anatomy and kinematics. An experimental study, *J Shoulder Elbow Surg* **2**:103–12.

Søjbjerg JO (1996) Stiff elbow, *Acta Orthop Scand*, **67**:626–31.

Søjbjerg JO, Ovesen J, Gundorf C (1987a) The stability of the elbow following excision of the radial head and transection of the annular ligament *Arch Orthop Trauma Surg* **106**:248–50.

Søjbjerg JO, Ovesen J, Nielsen S (1987b) Experimental elbow instability after transection of the medial collateral ligament, *Clin Orthop* **218**:186–90.

Søjbjerg JO, Kjærsgaard Andersen P, Johannsen HV, Sneppen O (1995) Release of the stiff elbow followed by continuous passive motion and indomethacin treatment *J Shoulder Elbow Surg* **4**:S20.

13
Classification and assessment

Francesco Catalano, Francesco Fanfani, Giuseppe Taccardo, Antonio Pagliei and Antonio Tulli

Elbow stiffness can be distinguished in two main ways:

- non-traumatic, in which there is not a progressive local trauma directly involved with the stiffness
- post-traumatic, in which the stiffness is the result of a progressive trauma of the elbow or the surrounding anatomical region.

This stiffness presents itself in two other main ways:

- extra-articular, in which the stiffness is caused by an anatomical and/or functional lesion not strictly involved with the joint

- articular, in which the stiffness is due to defects in the bones, cartilaginous surface, synovial sheet and capsular ligaments.

On the basis of these concepts, we make the following classification (Table 1):

Extra-articular non-traumatic stiffness

Neuromuscular diseases

This group is made up of stiffness in which a reduced mobility occurs in muscle spasticity as in

Table 1. Non- and post-traumatic stiffness in the elbow

Extra-articular	Non-traumatic (with no progressive local trauma)	Extra-articular	Post-traumatic stiffness (outcome of local trauma)

	Neuromuscular diseases
	   spasticity (spastic palsy)
	   muscle imbalance
	   (outcome of obstetric palsy)
	Ossifications
	   cranial trauma/long-term coma)
	   ossifying myositis
	Skin retraction
	   epidermolysis
	   bullous
	Multifactorial causes
	   arthrogryposis
	   dermatosclerosis
			Muscular retraction (Volkmann's contracture)
			Myotendinous adherences
			   outcome of humerus fractures
			   iatrogenic
			Skin retraction
			   burns
			   retracted scars
			Ossification of extracapsular tissues
			Secondary degenerative arthritis
			Capsular retraction
			   outcome of dislocation
			   outcome of epiphyseal fracture

Articular	Primary degenerative arthritis
	Synovial chondromatosis
	Rheumatic proliferative synovitis
	Pigmented villonodular synovitis
	Haemophilic arthropathy
	Infected arthritis or its outcome
		Articular	Articular incongruity
			   articular fractures
			   incongruity of articular surfaces
			   outcome of long-term dislocation
			   osteochondral free bodies
			Capsular ossification

lesions in the upper motor neurone (Littler disease or vascular–cerebral failure). This group also includes stiffness due to a neuromuscular imbalance caused by lesions of the lower motor neurone, e.g. flexion stiffness of the elbow observed after obstetric palsy.

Heterotopic ossification

This group includes stiffness which comes after cranial trauma or long-term coma in which articular mobility is impaired by an overproduction of extra-articular ossification. Also included are ossifications observed in ossifying myositis which is now considered to be a tumor-like lesion not necessarily caused by traumas.

Skin retraction

In this group, the most serious is bullous epidermolysis in which skin retraction, in combination with synechia of flexion folds, results in very severe stiffness.

Multifactorial causes

This group includes non-traumatic stiffness of the elbow caused by many different extra-articular processes. In dermatosclerosis both the skin and the muscle are involved together with a mechanical impediment due to large deposits of calcium salts in the soft tissue (Thibierge–Weissenbach syndrome). In arthrogryposis, the mechanism is complex because the muscle imbalance can be so serious that it causes a dislocation.

Articular non-traumatic stiffness

Primary degenerative arthritis

This group includes primary degenerative arthritis where lack of mobility is the result of osteophytes, irregularity of the articular surfaces, and osteochondral free bodies.

Synovial chondromatosis

In synovial chondromatosis, cartilage metaplasia causes an enormous quantity of intra-articular cartilaginous bodies which obstruct movement. X-rays are significant only if the cartilaginous bodies are calcified or ossified, in which case many oval bodies of various dimensions and radiopacity can be observed. In the late stages of the disease, degenerative changes are evident in the articular cavity.

Rheumatic proliferative synovitis

This group includes proliferative synovitis as in rheumatoid arthritis, lupus erythematosis systemicus (LES) and psoriasis in which the reduction of mobility is a consequence of exudative and proliferative phenomena of the synovial sheet and later of destruction of the articular surface.

In two out of three cases of rheumatoid arthritis, the elbow is involved in the late stages of the disease. The elbow is stiff and swollen, extension is severely limited and painful, while flexion, although limited, does not impede lifting the hand to the mouth. There is at the same time a pronation and supination deficit. The typical signs of rheumatoid degenerative arthritis are present in the X-ray; rarely the disease results in bony ankylosis. Ankylosis, however is the rule of Still's disease; typical is the lack of growth with the increasing volume of the epiphysis which can result in shortening of the forearm.

The location in the elbow of LES is similar, for instance, to rheumatoid arthritis. In the early stages, stiffness is evident in combination with an arthralgia with no obvious signs, such as occurs in acute rheumatic arthritis.

In later stages the clinical pattern can evolve into chronic polyarthritis which is different to rheumatoid arthritis with less important radiological evidence of bony erosions and no reduction of the articular space. Sometimes the clinical pattern can be complicated by an undifferentiated connectivitis when LES and rheumatoid arthritis are combined together so that the clinical and radiological patterns are like rheumatoid arthritis.

The psoriatic location in the elbow is not typical of psoriasis (16% of cases). It is evident at the early stages, as a proliferative synovitis and then as a capsular and ligament retraction with erosions of cartilaginous and bony surfaces. Stiffness occurs very early on.

Diffuse pigmented villonodular synovitis

Restriction of elbow movement is very rare and the disease usually presents itself in a widespread way. It is typically found in adults where X-rays are not significant except in the later stages when it is possible to see oval osteolytic areas at the level of the synovial recesses.

Haemophilic arthropathy

The elbow, together with the knee and the ankle, are characteristically involved because these joints are more easily exposed to trauma and have many articular recesses. The haemarthros occurs more frequently between 4 and 10 years. The involvement of the joint becomes a chronically disabling arthropathy because of increasing stiffness. Hypomobility in the early stages is followed by a complete contractural immobility with articular cartilage damage. At the same time, muscles, articular capsule and ligaments retract. The consequence of the haemarthros and the reactive synovitis is damage of the chondral tissue accompanied by severe stiffness.

Outcome of infective arthritis

Contrary to the general expectation in these cases, stiffness is quite rare and only occurs due to late diagnosis not allowing an early treatment or when infection is by resistant bacteria. Stiffness is caused by the destruction of the joint and the severe fibrosis which remains after the infection.

Extra-articular post-traumatic stiffness

Muscular retraction

Stiffness in the elbow as a consequence of Volkmann's disease, although rare, is due to a retraction of the epitrochlear muscles that cause a limit to the extension of the elbow.

Myotendinous adherences

In these cases the stiffness occurs because of the adherence between muscles and bones, as in fractures of the diaphysis of the distal humerus. The posterior transtricipital access often used in retrograde osteosynthesis of the humerus, especially following prolonged immobilization, can be complicated by the formation of tenacious myotendinous adherences.

Skin retraction

A post-traumatic skin retraction can cause a stiffness of the elbow, e.g. retraction scars of the flexion surface or the results of burns, especially in early childhood.

Ossification of the extracapsular tissues

Ossification of the extracapsular soft tissues can frequently complicate the outcome of a fracture or a dislocation of the elbow. In such cases, damage of the extra-articular tissue leads to a bony metaplasia which is able to impair elbow movement.

Articular post-traumatic stiffness

Secondary degenerative arthritis

This condition might represent the final stage of many traumatic elbow complaints and so can be responsible for an increasing stiffness set up by the same pathogenetic movement of the degenerative arthritis (osteophytosis, roughness of the osteochondral surface, thickening and retraction of the capsule, adherences).

Capsular retraction

This cause represents the most frequent event as a result of retraction fibrosis of capsula tears (an outcome of dislocation) or traumatic haemarthros following a protracted immobilization (as in distal epiphyseal fractures of the humerus). We stress that capsular retraction occurs in every kind of long-term elbow stiffness and seldom becomes the cause of further stiffness.

Articular incongruity

This group includes the stiffness caused by anomalous incongruity of the articular surface, e.g. articular fractures, dislocations, and long-term frac-ture–dislocation. Also, the presence of many osteo-chondral free bodies might represent an impedi-ment to movement.

Capsular ossification

As mentioned before, the metaplasia of soft tissue especially involves the extra-articular tissues. Therefore, post-traumatic conditions occur in which ossification involves the capsula resulting in an impediment of movement.

14
The contribution of the elbow joint to upper limb function

William A Souter

Elbow stiffness, or indeed total loss of elbow movement, can result from various causes including rheumatoid arthritis, juvenile chronic arthritis, post-traumatic arthritis, myositis ossificans following trauma or burns, pyogenic or tuberculous infection, skeletal dysplasia, osteochondritis dissecans, synovial chondromatosis and congenital anomalies. The resulting functional disability for the patient can be of dire significance with regard to work potential and the ability to cope with the activities of daily living.

Functions and mobility of the normal elbow

The human elbow can be regarded as having three main functions:

1 As one of the joints positioning the hand in space.
2 As a fulcrum for the forearm lever.
3 As a weightbearing joint in disabled patients.

Stability is obviously required for the second and third of these functions, but mobility is vital for the realization of the first and second. No one specializing in elbow surgery can be left in any doubt as to the degree of dysfunction occasioned by elbow immobility when they experience the intensity of importunity of patients seeking remobilization of this joint.

The use which is made of the mobility of the normal elbow is indeed quite phenomenal. In a study undertaken jointly by the Bioengineering Department of the University of Strathclyde in Glasgow and my own Unit in Edinburgh on the pre- and postoperative utilization of elbow movement in relation to elbow arthroplasty (Macmillan 1988), the individual elbow movements performed in a 9-h observation period in a series of nine normal control subjects could vary as much as from 5000 to 13 000. Even more impressive are the figures for the cumulative geometric angle score through which such normal elbows might move in the observation period. Again there was great variation in different subjects by a factor of 5.8. In absolute figures, a cumulative total angle score varied from 110 000 degrees up to 620 000 degrees with a mean of 355 688 degrees (SD 166 170). Moreover, it was of interest that in rheumatoid patients with severe elbow pain who had restricted their elbow movement as much as possible preoperatively so that their mean 9-h cumulative score had fallen to 48 774 degrees (SD 37 551), successful arthroplasty resulted in a rapid return to a greatly enhanced cumulative total angle score of 126 341 degrees (SD 54 480).

Elbow movement required for activities of daily living

Very little data on the requirements of elbow movement are available in the literature. Morrey et al (1981), in their classic study on normal functional elbow movement, concluded that both with regard to the need for positioning the hand for particular functions and for executing the necessary arc of movement required in other activities of daily living, a flexion–extension arc of 30–130° in the elbow itself coupled with a 100° arc of pronation and supination would suffice. A further reductionist scrutiny of their data would suggest that a flexion–extension arc of 60–120° with 35° of pronation and 55° of supination would allow *most* activities to be performed with the possible exception at the one extreme of tying shoelaces and at the other of reaching the occiput.

Interestingly, these authors concluded that in most activities of personal care and hygiene, supination is the dominant requirement for forearm rotation. It has been the author's experience that in patients undergoing arthroplasty for virtual loss of elbow movement, it is pronation which has been relatively well preserved (mean 39°, SD 32°, $n = 16$), while supination was only satisfactorily preserved in two patients (40° and 60°, respectively), the remainder having less than 10° (four cases), 0° (six cases), or a pronation deformity varying from 5° (two cases), through 10° (one case) to 40° (one case). This observation may be due to patients tending to hold their hands for prolonged periods in pronation for desk-top activities, while the supination movements so vital to many of the activities of daily living and personal care are by comparison very transitory.

Morrey and his colleagues (1981) concluded that with activities directed at face and head, flexion of 120–145° was required, the last 25–45° of this range being necessary for combing hair or reaching to the occiput.

Personal hygiene on the other hand requires extension to a variable degree in different subjects (range 57–83°, mean 70°). Moreover attending to personal hygiene required greater supination than any other activity. Again the requirements were variable in different subjects, i.e. 36–76°, average 56°.

Overall they concluded that most activities of personal care could be accomplished provided the elbow had a range from 40° to 140° of flexion and from 0° to 55° of supination. The exception to this was tying shoelaces where extension to 16° with the forearm in 19° of pronation was required.

For activities requiring a continuous sweep of movement within the elbow and forearm, and taking eating and drinking or using a telephone as typical examples, an arc of movement from 40° to 130° within the elbow itself and forearm rotation totalling 60° was found to be required.

The most disastrous functional disability occurs with ankylosis in full extension. This can occasionally occur after fracture and, more commonly, after burns. Seth and Khurana (1985) reporting on bony ankylosis of the elbow after burns found that in 13 ankylosed elbows in 10 patients, 10 elbows were fixed in almost full extension with total functional disability of the limb. Three patients in whom this disaster had occurred bilaterally were unable to look after themselves and had to depend on others for feeding, cleaning and dressing.

Degree to which other joints can compensate

In a later study from the Mayo clinic (O'Neill et al 1992), 10 male subjects who were fitted with an adjustable brace that could simulate an arthrodesis of the elbow at 50°, 70°, 90° and 110°, were studied for compensatory movements that were invoked in shoulder, spine, forearm and wrist during normal everyday activities such as grasping or pouring from a pitcher, handling a steering wheel, tying shoelaces, and reaching to shelves, or to the mouth, occiput, shoulder or sacrum.

With simulated fusion at 50° or 70°, none of the subjects could reach their occiput, mouth or opposite shoulder. With the elbow positioned at 90° most could reach these targets. By contrast, the sacrum could be reached with the elbow fixed at all three of these positions and possibly also with as flexed a position as 110°.

Surprisingly the shoulder complex was not found to make a major contribution to compensatory movement. In activities requiring relative extension, e.g. reaching up to shelves or out to a steering wheel, touching the sacrum or tying shoes, some diminution towards zero was found in circumduction and elevation as the fusion angle increased. The compensatory shoulder movements that do occur with a stiff elbow are protraction, retraction, elevation and depression of the shoulder girdle as a whole at the scapula–thoracic joint and through movement of the clavicle. Elevation and internal rotation of the shoulder theoretically can compensate for limitation of pronation, but in practice, e.g. for pianists or keyboard operators, this position is so tiring that in the author's experience these pursuits are usually abandoned even by formerly enthusiastic performers.

The main compensatory movements allowing patients to cope with their elbow disability take place in spine, forearm and wrist. Compensatory spinal movements may be in the nature of lateral rotation or flexion and extension to compensate for lack of variability in reach.

The wrist and forearm aid in the compensation through abduction, adduction, flexion and extension in the wrist, and pronation and supination in the radio-ulnar joints. These movements can be regarded as truly complementary to flexion and extension of the normal elbow for positioning the hand in space, and thus can be called on to provide an increased contribution when elbow movement itself is lost. This normal complementary relation does not seem to exist between the elbow and shoulder, and hence the shoulder makes only a very limited contribution to compensatory movement when the elbow is stiff.

The overall conclusion of the Mayo study was that for activities in the environment or on a work-top or when reaching to the lower limbs, a 50–70° fusion angle was preferable. Any personal care activities involving reaching to the upper body, however, demanded fusion of the elbow in at least 90° of flexion. This would very much fit with traditional teaching (Russell 1987) that unilateral elbow fusion should be at 90°, while with bilateral arthrodesis one elbow should be fused at 65° and the other, probably the non-dominant, at 110°. The author would suggest that this latter figure may be rather too great as 110° can be a very uncomfortable position for the elbow since it precludes a natural lie of the arm on any work surface, nor can the hand reach with any ease into a trouser pocket.

Snider and De Witt (1973), using an experimental technique similar to that employed in the Mayo study, concluded from a review of 35 arms that a flexed position of 45–60° was best for work related activities, but that 15–30° extra were required for self-care. So critical may the fixation angle be for the individual that Rashkoff and Burkhalter (1986) have suggested that this should finally be determined by the patients themselves after trial immobilization in a series of casts fixing the elbow at differing angles and retained for a significant period. It is of interest that Young (1993) utilizing this approach found that a paraplegic patient who was a full-time manual wheelchair user, and who required an elbow arthrodesis following a severe fracture, opted for fusion at 30° rather than at 90°. Thereafter she was independent with regard to propelling and storing her wheelchair, and in all self-care and transfers including uneven transfers to heights of 9" higher and 18" lower than her wheelchair seat. This illustrates very clearly the importance of allowing the patient the final choice of fusion angle since what would be a very unattractive fusion angle for most patients proved to be ideal for this individual patient.

Conclusion

A stiff or arthrodesed elbow presents a very real functional disability for a patient as there is no ideal angle of fusion which will reconcile the very differing demands of both work-related activities and personal care and hygiene. A fusion angle of 70° or less will make work-related activities easier, but even with maximum compensatory movements from an uncompromised wrist, forearm and spine, personal care and hygiene will not be possible.

In view of the inescapable disability inherent in elbow arthrodesis, this operation should only be exhibited very rarely. When it is felt to be the only solution, very careful individual assessment of each patient with regard to their work and/or social demands, the state of the spine and the ipsilateral shoulder, forearm and wrist, and the functional status of the contralateral upper limb is required before the most useful fixation angle can be determined. In the final selection the patient's own preference must be given full consideration.

References

Macmillan FS (1988) Aspects of Biomechanics of the Upper Limb following Elbow Arthroplasty and following Phalangeal Fracture. PhD Thesis, University of Strathclyde, Glasgow.

Morrey BF, Askew LJ, An KN, Chao EY (1981) A biomechanical study of normal functional elbow motion, *J Bone Jt Surg* **63A**:872–7.

O'Neill OR, Morrey BF, Tanaka S, An KN (1992) Compensatory motion in the upper extremity after elbow arthrodesis, *Clin Orthop* **281**:89–96.

Rashkoff E, Burkhalter WE (1986) Arthrodesis of the salvage elbow, *Orthopaedics* **9**:733–8.

Russell TA (1987) Arthrodesis of the upper extremity. In: Crenshaw AH, ed. *Campbell's Operative Orthopaedics*, 7th edn. Mosby: St Louis: 1139.

Seth MK, Khurana JK (1985) Bony ankylosis of the elbow after burns, *J Bone Jt Surg* **67B**:747–9.

Snider WJ, De Witt HJ (1973) Functional study for optimum position for elbow arthrodesis or ankylosis, *J Bone Jt Surg* **55A**:1305.

Young JH (1993) Implications of elbow arthrodeses for individuals with paraplegia, *Phys Ther* **73**:194–201.

15
Arthroscopic arthrolysis

Franklin Chen and A Lee Osterman

Introduction

The primary function of the elbow is not only to position the hand in space, but also to provide power and stability for upper extremity tasks. Loss of elbow mobility can therefore lead to significant disability. While normal elbow flexion and extension is in the range of 0–145°, most activities of daily living fall within a smaller arc of motion. Morrey et al (1981) evaluated 33 normal volunteers in the performance of various activities and concluded that most activities of daily living can be performed with a flexion–extension arc of 30–130° and a rotational arc of 100° (50° supination and 50° pronation). This range of motion, however, may be insufficient for the lifestyle of certain individuals, for example, the young active, athletic population (Timmerman and Andrews 1994).

Elbow stiffness is not an infrequent sequelae following a traumatic event. Other factors have been identified which adversely affect elbow motion: prolonged immobilization, infection, inflammatory arthritis, degenerative arthritis, heterotopic bone formation, soft tissue contracture or muscular spasm (Morrey 1993). All variables considered, traumatic dislocation with or without an associated fracture is the most common cause of elbow stiffness.

The predisposition of the elbow to contracture and loss of motion compared to other major joints still remains unclear. The fundamental anatomy of the joint, composed of three bony articulations within a single synovial tissue-lined capsule (Kapandji 1982), portends this ill fate. In addition, soft tissue trauma following an event such as a fracture–dislocation will inevitably alter the interrelationship between the joint capsule and its associated intracapsular ligaments and extracapsular muscles, creating an environment for potential contracture.

Morrey (1993) has classified elbow stiffness according to extrinsic causes, intrinsic causes, and a combination of both. Extrinsic stiffness results from capsular and collateral ligament contracture or the formation of heterotopic bone with relative sparing of the joint surfaces. In contrast, intrinsic causes will involve intra-articular adhesions and distortion of articular congruency. Bony disruption usually results in intrinsic stiffness, though concomitant extrinsic contracture can also occur secondary to prolonged immobilization.

Management of the stiff elbow

The initial management of the stiff elbow involves physical therapy and the use of splints. External devices, such as the turnbuckle splint, have been shown to effectively reduce post-traumatic flexion contracture (Green and McCoy 1979, Zander and Healy 1992, Karachalios et al 1995). The objective of these non-operative methods is to achieve a painless functional arc of motion. If improvement has plateaued short of realizing this result, surgical release or reconstruction is the next best option in a well-motivated patient.

While the operative indications must be individualized according to the patient, functional disability is a generally accepted criterion. Preoperatively, the type and extent of elbow contracture must be assessed with plain radiographs, tomograms, and when indicated, computed axial tomography (CAT) scan or magnetic resonance imaging (MRI). Amelioration of intrinsic elbow stiffness in the setting of articular incongruity or ankylosis will often require more extensive procedures such as interposition arthroplasty, distraction arthroplasty, the Outerbridge–Kashiwagi procedure, or total elbow replacement. Arthrolysis of the stiff elbow is more readily successful in cases of extrinsic contracture, as the joint is relatively preserved. In the appropriately selected patient, release of contracture can be performed arthroscopically.

Since its introduction in 1932 (Burman 1932), the technique of elbow arthroscopy has been well established. The indications include both diagnostic as well as therapeutic treatment of elbow internal derangement. With respect to arthrofibrosis, elbow arthroscopy has been shown to successfully improve elbow range of motion (Andrews and Carson 1985, Nowicki and Shall 1992, Timmerman and Andrews 1994). Extrinsic components of contracture are perhaps more amenable to arthroscopic intervention than intrinsically related aspects given the associated degree of joint damage in the latter situation. Timmerman and Andrews (1994) found limited value in arthroscopic arthrolysis of patients in their series who showed radiographic evidence of post-traumatic arthritis or severe degenerative arthritis. The advantages of an arthroscopic approach over an open procedure are: 1, lower surgical morbidity; 2, more comprehensive joint visualization; and 3, ability to start early rehabilitation. The disadvantages of arthroscopy are: 1, its technical difficulty; and 2, spatial limitations imposed by an incongruent joint. If difficulties arise during arthroscopy, the operation can be converted into an open procedure in the operating theatre with relative ease.

The contraindications to arthroscopic arthrolysis include ongoing local infection, advanced arthritis or ankylosis, uncorrectable bleeding disorder, poor vascular status, and severe oedema (ElAttrache 1995). Certainly, in these situations surgery is best avoided, but if necessary, an open procedure is preferred. Previous anterior transposition of the ulnar nerve is a relative contraindication for creation of medial portals at the time of arthroscopy. This limitation can be made inconsequential with the establishment of a transhumeral window from a direct posterior portal to view the anterior compartment (Day 1995).

Familiarity with elbow anatomy and its associated neurovascular structures is paramount in avoiding major complications in elbow arthroscopy. The reported incidence of neurologic deficits following elbow arthroscopy is 2–14% (Andrews and Carson 1985, Guhl 1985, Lynch et al 1986). This percentage is likely to be higher for the arthrofibrotic elbow in lieu of capsular contracture. For example, Jones and Savoie (1993) reported one case of posterior

interosseous nerve transection in 12 patients who underwent arthroscopic release for elbow contracture. Gallay et al (1993) compared intracapsular volumes in 11 contracted elbows with 10 contralateral normal elbows in 11 patients. The mean volume capacity of the stiff elbows was markedly reduced to less than half of the normal elbows. Capsular distension was also further hampered by a 14% reduction in capsular compliance of the stiff elbow. These studies suggest that elbow arthroscopy of the contracted elbow may have a higher risk for neurovascular injury. Cadaveric studies on five non-contracted elbows have shown that the median nerve could be displaced 14 mm from the anteromedial portal with 35–40 ml of joint distension (4 mm without distension) (Lynch et al 1986). If adequate capsular distension cannot be obtained in the stiff elbow, arthroscopy should be abandoned in favour of an open approach to avoid risks of anterior neurovascular damage.

Surgical technique

The technique of elbow arthroscopy can have minor variations depending on the surgeon's preference. Either a general anaesthetic or regional block can be used. Three options exist for patient positioning: supine, prone, or lateral decubitus. Andrews and Carson (1985) advocated placing the patient supine with the arm suspended at 90°; Poehling et al (1989) and Hempfling (1983) preferred the patient placed in the prone position. The lateral position has been recently advocated by O'Driscoll and Morrey (1992). If the pathology is mainly in the posterior compartment, the prone position proves more advantageous. This is particularly true if posterior olecranon osteophytes are blocking extension.

Though portal choice may differ depending on the patient's pathology and positioning, we generally use the anterolateral, anteromedial, posterolateral, and posterior portals. Capsular distension is first obtained via the direct lateral portal. The anterolateral portal is then established at a point 2 cm distal and 1 cm anterior to the lateral epicondyle. Andrews and Carson (1985) originally described an entry point 3 cm distal and 1 cm anterior to the epicondyle, but more recent studies have suggested that the neurovascular structures are at less risk when utilizing a slightly more proximal site (O'Driscoll 1992, Stothers et al 1993). The superolateral portal as described by Stothers et al (1993) can also be used for lateral entry. From a point 1–2 cm proximal to the lateral epicondyle, the trochar is kept in direct contact with the distal humerus until it pierces the brachioradialis and distal brachialis to enter the lateral joint capsule. Safety of neurovascular structures and visualization are improved with this portal; however, joint distortion in the stiff elbow may preclude its use. The anteromedial portal is established approximately 2 cm distal and 2 cm anterior to the medial epicondyle.

If the prone position is used, this portal is established just by palpating 2 cm superior to the medial epicondyle and just anterior to the palpable medial intermuscular septum. Before making this portal it is useful to mark out the course of the ulnar nerve on the patient.

After arthroscopic examination of the anterior compartment, capsular release can be performed with the use of a full radius resector (Fig. 1). Visualization is maximized with the arthroscope placed in the portal opposite to the operative site. Through these combined anteromedial and lateral portals, the anterior capsule can be debrided to a level where the underside of the brachialis muscle fibres can be visualized. Attention can then be turned to anterior osseous structures. The burr can again be used to debride any bony prominences such as an overgrown coronoid. Throughout the procedure, elbow range of motion should be evaluated periodically. If further capsular remnants remain, a small arthroscopic knife can be introduced to incise scar tissue. If necessary, a direct lateral portal can also be established through the anatomic lateral soft spot.

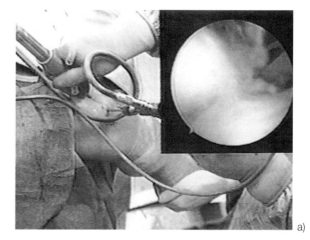

a)

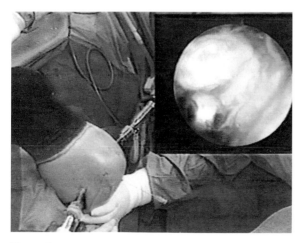

Figure 1

Patient with a 45° elbow contracture. Arthroscopic release in the prone position. Arthroscopic inset shows debridement of coronoid osteophytes and release of anterior capsular fibres. The scope is lateral and the shaver medial.

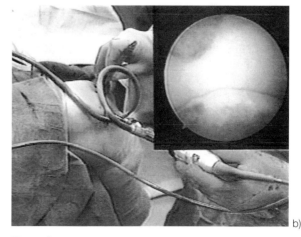

b)

Figure 2

(a) Patient with a 25° contracture and posterior osteophytes. A power burr and small osteotome are alternatively used via a direct posterior portal while viewed from the posterior lateral portal. (b) Post-debridement: the osteophytes have been debrided. Range of motion is full.

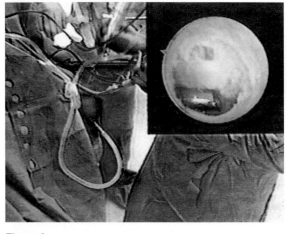

Figure 3

A transhumeral portal. If there is a great deal of bone blocking the supracondylar fossa, as can be seen in osteoarthritis, a complete debridement of the fossa can be done. When complete this allows another access to the coronoid and any spurs there. Here the scope is in the lateral portal and the burr has created a tunnel through the humeral fossa.

Posterior compartment release can be performed through either a midlateral, posterolateral, or straight posterior portal (Fig. 2a, b). The direct lateral portal can sometimes be used to visualize the posterior compartment to assist in establishing these portals; however, this may often be prohibited by extensive posterior scarring. If necessary, a transhumeral portal located directly over the olecranon fossa can be made with a 6.5-mm drill hole through the distal humerus (Stothers et al 1993). This portal not only enables visualization of the anterior compartment, but also alleviates any posterior mechanical impingement (Fig. 3).

Following completion of the surgical release and debridement, final evaluation of the elbow's range of motion is then made. It is generally accepted that a portion of the intraoperative gains will be lost postoperatively, but this is usually less than 20°.

Postoperative rehabilitation

Postoperative rehabilitation is geared towards maximizing the gains in motion attained at surgery.

Mobilization should begin within 24 hours postoperatively, which is made easier by an arthroscopic procedure. In the appropriate patient, a selected indwelling brachial or supraclavicular catheter can be used for 1–2 days postoperatively to control pain while still allowing for motor function. Another adjunct to early mobilization is the use of a continuous passive motion (CPM) device. The acceptance of this device is not universal. One study in particular has shown that there was no significance in final flexion contracture when comparing 15 patients managed with postoperative CPM to a similar group of 18 patients who were not placed in this device postoperatively (Gates et al 1992). A noteworthy benefit of the CPM device is its capability to range the elbow to the extremes of flexion and extension, hopefully matching that which was achieved at the time of surgery (Modabber and Jupiter 1995). A shortcoming of CPM, however, is its inability to provide for adequate rotational motion. Currently, we utilize the CPM device in patients who appear less motivated to begin early aggressive motion. This assessment is often made preoperatively.

A knowledgeable physical therapist is essential for the patient's rehabilitative success. Supervised physical therapy as well as a home programme is initiated in the early postoperative period. In the initial phase, pain control and range of motion are the primary goals. Subsequently, strengthening can be addressed. Turnbuckle splints or other dynamic braces, both flexion and extension, are also used in postoperative management. These can be worn for 6 weeks to 3 months after surgery if continued improvement is noted with their use (Morrey 1990). With these various techniques, a painless functional arc of motion can usually be restored.

Conclusion

Arthroscopic debridement of elbow arthrofibrosis has advantages over open arthrolysis in the well-selected patient. The most notable advantages are the diminished requisite insult of surgery and the facility towards early postoperative therapy. We do not advocate an arthroscopic approach in patients with severe joint incongruity or bony ankylosis.

Previous investigators have reported good success with arthroscopic arthrolysis. Timmerman and Andrews (1994) demonstrated good to excellent overall results in 79% of patients treated for post-traumatic arthrofibrosis via arthroscopy. In their 19 patients, elbow extension improved from a mean of 29° to 11° and flexion improved from a mean of 123° to 134°. Eleven patients were able to return to their pre-injury level of activity following surgery. More significant improvement in motion was noted in 12 patients from a study by Jones and Savoie (1993). These authors noted a postoperative reduction in flexion contracture following arthroscopic arthrolysis from a mean of 38° to 3°. Byrd (1994) reported on his arthroscopic treatment of five patients afflicted with arthrofibrosis after Type I radial head fractures. Range of motion and pain was improved in all of his patients at approximately 24 months follow-up.

Common to these studies are not only resultant improvement in range of motion, but also subjective pain relief. Though pain is usually secondary to the chief complaint of limited motion, in each afore-mentioned study, patients were noted to have decreased pain levels compared to preoperatively. This holds true in our clinical experience as well.

In summary, operative elbow arthroscopy can be techniquely demanding, especially when dealing with arthrofibrosis. Knowledge of the pertinent anatomy and attention to detail must be maintained at the time of surgery. With both an appropriate patient and a skilled physical therapist, one can achieve a successful outcome via arthroscopic arthrolysis of the stiff elbow.

References

Andrews JR, Carson WG (1985) Arthroscopy of the elbow, *Arthroscopy* **1**:97–107.

Burman MS (1932) Arthroscopy of the elbow joint: a cadaver study, *J Bone Joint Surg* **14A**:349–51.

Byrd JWT (1994) Elbow arthroscopy for arthrofibrosis after type I radial head fractures, *Arthroscopy* **10**:162–5.

Day B (1995) Arthroscopy of the elbow, *AAOS Instructional Course Lectures no. 230L, 62nd AAOS Meeting, 1995.*

ElAttrache NS (1995) Arthroscopy of the elbow, *AAOS Instructional Course Lectures no. 122, 62nd AAOS Meeting, 1995.*

Gallay SH, Richards RR, O'Driscoll SW (1993) Intraarticular capacity and compliance of stiff and normal elbows, *Arthroscopy* **9**:9–13.

Gates I IS, Sullivan ΓL, Urbaniak JR (1992) Anterior capsulotomy and CPM in the treatment of post-traumatic flexion contracture of the elbow: a prospective study, *J Bone Joint Surg* **74A**:1229–34.

Green DP, McCoy H (1979) Turnbuckle orthotic correction of elbow-flexion contractures after acute injuries, *J Bone Joint Surg* **61A**:1092–5.

Guhl J (1985) Arthroscopy and arthroscopic surgery of the elbow, *Orthopaedics* **8**:1290–6.

Hempfling H (1983) Die endoskopische Untersuchung des Ellenbogen gelenkes vom dorso radialen Zugang, *Z Orthop* **121**:331–2.

Jones GS, Savoie FH (1993) Arthroscopic capsular release of flexion contractures of the elbow, *Arthroscopy* **9**:277–83.

Kapandji IA (1982) *The Physiology of the Joints. Upper Limb. Vol. 1,* 5th edn. Churchill Livingstone: New York: 72–96.

Karachalios T, Maxwell-Armstrong C, Atkins RM (1995) Treatment of post-traumatic fixed flexion deformity of elbow using an intermittent compression garment, *Injury* **25**:313–15.

Lynch GJ, Meyers JF, Whipple TL, Caspari RB (1986) Neurovascular anatomy and elbow arthroscopy: inherent risks, *Arthroscopy* **2**:191–7.

Modabber MR, Jupiter JB (1995) Current concepts review: reconstruction for post-traumatic conditions of the elbow joint, *J Bone Joint Surg* **77A**:1431–46.

Morrey BF (1990) Post-traumatic contracture of the elbow. Operative treatment, including distraction arthroplasty, *J Bone Joint Surg* **72A**:601–18.

Morrey BF (1993) Post-traumatic elbow stiffness: distraction arthroplasty. In: Morrey BF, ed. *The Elbow and its Disorders* 2nd edn. WB Saunders: Philadelphia: 476–91.

Morrey BF, Askew LJ, An KN, Chao EY (1981) A biochemical study of normal functional elbow motion, *J Bone Joint Surg* **63A**:872–7.

Nowicki KD, Shall LM (1992) Arthroscopic release of a post-traumatic flexion contracture in the elbow: a case report and review of the literature, *Arthroscopy* **8**:544–7.

O'Driscoll SW (1992) Elbow arthroscopy for loose bodies, *Orthopedics* **15**:855–9.

O'Driscoll SW, Morrey BF (1992) Arthroscopy of the elbow. Diagnostic and therapeutic benefits and hazards, *J Bone Joint Surg* **74A**:84–94.

Poehling GG, Whipple TL, Sisco L, Goldman B (1989) Elbow arthroscopy: a new technique, *Arthroscopy* **5**:222–4.

Stothers K, Day B, Regan WR (1993) Arthroscopic anatomy of the elbow: an anatomic study and description of a new portal, *Arthroscopy* **9**:362–3.

Timmerman LA, Andrews JR, (1994) Arthroscopic treatment of post-traumatic elbow pain and stiffness, *Am J Sports Med* **22**:230–5.

Verhaar J, van Mameren H, Brandsma A (1991) Risks of neurovascular injury in elbow arthroscopy: starting anteromedially or anterolaterally? *Arthroscopy* **7**:287–90.

Zander CL, Healy NL (1992) Elbow flexion contractures treated with serial casts and conservative therapy, *J Hand Surg* **17A**:694–7.

16
Open arthrolysis with distraction

Thierry Judet, Philippe Piriou, Christian Garreau, Godfrey Charnley and
†Robert Judet

One of the most common pathological problems of post-trauma is stiffness of the elbow joint. It may be due only to soft tissue contracture (extrinsic stiffness), but within the joint there may be other features such as cartilage destruction, fibrous ankylosis, bone fusion or permanent posterior dislocation (intrinsic stiffness). While classical surgical arthrolysis is the most adequate treatment for extrinsic stiffness, in more complex cases this arthrolysis procedure may be disappointing, even with bony resection or surface arthroplasty.

Recurrent stiffness may occur with insufficient bony resection and pain, due to a lack of normal articular cartilage, and may be compounded by instability if an excessive soft tissue release or bony resection has been performed.

Since 1974, in an attempt to address such problems, Robert Judet has conceived and developed a concept of early elbow mobilization combined with temporary distraction of the joint and has used this technique not only in the elbow, but also at the knee and ankle. More recently, other articular distractors have been developed and implant surgery and prosthetic surgery has advanced.

After 20 years of distraction surgery, we need to evaluate the results of our surgery and draw lessons from our failures and successes to identify the role of distraction in the treatment of post-traumatic elbow stiffness.

The elbow distractor concept

The distractor is an external device, temporarily fixed to the bony elements across the operated elbow.

It provides:

- Stability
  Instantly because of its symmetrical design and secondly by orientating soft tissue healing
- Mobility
  Centred around the axis of rotation of the elbow allowing for immediate joint movement and rehabilitation
- Distraction
  By maintaining a permanent distance between the bony landmarks, a space is created allowing pain-free mobilization and space for fibrous tissue healing with a possibility of fibrocartilaginous metaplasia, as we demonstrated in our dog experiment.

The Judet distractor (Fig. 1) is a development of Judet's original external fixature. A rotational axis is held by two elements fixed to the humeral shaft extra-articularly by two 5-mm diameter rods. The upper rod is placed at the humeral shaft level and unilateral, while the lower one transfixes the diaphysometaphyseal junction of the humerus. The ulna is transfixed by two pins and two telescopic bars on either side kink the ulna to the distractor axis. The construction is adjusted to position with the distractor axis in line with the elbow's anatomical axis. The modulation within the device permits correction in any direction. The aim is to obtain a constant articular space between the trochlea and the ulnar notch, without any bony contact whatever the position of flexion or extension. Pronation and supination is not inhibited by the device as this motion occurs distal to the device.

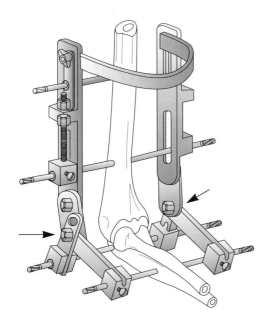

Figure 1

Judet articular distractor. All the fixator pins are at a distance from rotational axis (arrows).

Materials and method

Between 1974 and 1995 we applied an articular distractor to 38 elbows (14 women and 24 men: range 13–72 years, mean 41 years). There were three main indications for our surgery: complications following old posterior dislocation, post-traumatic joint stiffness and bony ankylosis.

Seven cases were operated upon following old posterior dislocation injuries
All the elbows were stiff with a mean lack of extension of 45° and a mean arch of motion of 48°. Four of the cases had had associated coronoid fractures and three had a radial head fracture. The time between the original injury and referral to our unit ranged between 4 weeks and 5 months.

Fourteen cases were post-traumatic joint stiffness
There was a mean extension lack of 15° and a mean range of motion of 35°. Seven cases had established post-traumatic arthritis with degenera-

tive changes and three had an inflammatory type of arthritis. The final four cases had had earlier surgery for stiffness and had postoperative instability after extensive arthrolysis and soft tissue releases elsewhere, but they had no major intra-articular lesion.

Eighteen elbows had an intra-articular bone fusion with complete destruction of the articular cartilage
Ten of these cases had previously had infection but were considered to have no persistent infection at the time of distraction surgery. One case had a congenital ankylosis. All the other cases had had previous surgical procedures ranging from one to five surgical interventions before distraction surgery. The bone stock on radiological evaluation was felt to be normal in 12 cases but deficient in the six other cases with problems including deficiency of the medial or lateral humeral epicondyle. Two cases having had problems with soft tissue cover required treatment by a covering flap prior to our surgery. The ankylosis position ranged from 20° to 100° flexion.

Operative technique

The surgery was performed in two successive stages. Firstly an arthrolysis was performed if necessary along with bone 're-fashioning'. The distractor was then positioned.

Our standard arthrolysis is performed through either a single or, more commonly, a combined medial and lateral approach. In ankylosed elbow a transosseous approach was frequently used. In all cases a complete resection of the anterior and posterior capsule was performed, and in those cases where there was bone fusion, the bone was excised and a fashioning of a new trochlear notch performed with sharp bone chisels. If necessary, a radial head resection or a radial head refashioning may be required to restore supination and pronation.

The arthrolysis must restore a complete range of motion, and if necessary the medial and lateral collateral ligaments are divided along with capsular excision and also division of the fibrous part of the epicondylar or epitrochlear musculature. The healing of this soft tissue release is protected by the distractor itself. However, we never divide the triceps brachialis or biceps brachialis in our soft tissue release procedures.

Distractor implantation

A 2.5-mm diameter pin is inserted into the exact axis of rotation of the normal or remodelled elbow. The two bodies of the distractor are located on that pin by means of cannulated bolts. These bolts carry the axis of rotation on them and are secured to a crank shaft linked to the ulna fixation. The distractor is then fixed by two Judet external fixator pins in the humeral shaft and two transfixing pins in the upper ulna, one through the olecranon and on through the ulna metaphysis.

The axial pin is then removed, the distraction nuts are tightened to create a 5–10-mm joint space. By positioning the axis and adjusting the length of the telescopic crank shaft, a full range of motion without excentric loading and with a constant width of articular space is achieved. The wounds are then closed over suction drainage.

When a transosseous approach, via the humeral condyle has been performed, the bone block is fixed back with a lag screw and washer.

Immediate postoperative rehabilitation is undertaken along with anti-inflammatory medication and constant ice packing. The distractor is removed at between 5 and 10 weeks, and over this period and for 2 months following removal of the distractor, the patient undergoes daily physiotherapy.

Complications

We had three temporary ulnar nerve palsies.

Six cases had superficial pin tract infection problems which healed uneventfully. One septic arthritis was treated by antibiotics and drainage with an excellent long-term result.

There were six cases of ulna fracture which occurred when the distal ulna pin was located too posteriorly in the ulna crest. Three of these cases required no further treatment, but three cases needed an external fixator on the ulnar diaphysis to permit rehabilitation.

Results

The patients were evaluated postoperatively at between 6 and 12 months. The evaluation took into account mobility, stability, pain and strength. The postoperative results were related to the preoperative condition of the elbows, many of which had been operated upon several times previously.

In those cases operated upon for restricted elbow mobility with intrinsic stiffness or instability we had 13 cases of which one has been lost to follow-up. The cases remaining have a range of follow-up between 1 and 18 years. There have been six cases with good results, four fair results and two poor results where there was excessive instability requiring an elbow arthrodesis.

The series of patients operated upon with old dislocations have provided four good results with a complete range of motion and no pain, two fair results and one poor result. In this last case there was an untreated coronoid process fracture along with a resected radial head and this led to continuing dislocation following surgery.

Finally in the 18 cases of bony ankylosis a review exists between 1 and 16 years with a mean follow-up of 4 years. Eleven have achieved good results with an average range of motion of 100°. There were four fair results and three failures. Two of the failures had persistent instability and one had a recurrent ankylosis.

Discussion

With over 20 years of experience we continue to use the Judet articular distractor on the elbow. It is a demanding technique requiring great expertise particularly in elbow surgery. The surgery was initially performed before other options were available, such as elbow arthroplasty for inflammatory and traumatic arthritis, and bipolar radial head replacement for postradial head fracture (Charnley et al 1996) and instability caused by radial head excision. We also realize now that in some circumstances a simple arthrolysis may be all that is required for post-traumatic elbow stiffness.

As well as our own distractor device, several other authors have reported different distraction devices or distraction surgery and all but one are based on the same principle. Volkov et al (1975) described a progressive and non-surgical correction whilst Deland designed the Brigham and Women's Hospital device (Deland and Walker 1987). Morrey (1990) applied distraction combined with facial arthroplasty when more than half the articular surface was not covered with hyaline cartilage or when the collateral ligaments had been divided. He emphasized in particular in his reports the complication rate and technical difficulties of this procedure. Han and Yun (1995) used our distractor in 10 patients, presenting with combined extrinsic and intrinsic stiffness as outlined by Morrey (Morrey 1990, Morrey et al 1991).

In retrospect, what is our current view on the use of an elbow distractor? The Judet distractor has not been well known outside France, but we believe it has certain advantages:

• It can easily be adapted if the landmarks of axis location (as described by us in 1978), are not precisely respected and such adjustment is simple
• All the external fixator pins are distant from the joint space lowering the risk of infection
• None of the pins transfix the flexor or extensor musculature

We would no longer use the distractor for the following indications:

• Rheumatoid arthritis where we believe a total elbow prosthesis is a simple and safe solution
• Post head injury bony ankylosis which we believe can be treated by excision of the heterotopic ossification and a simple arthrolysis, except in rare cases where the osteoma is located intra-articularly
• If there is combined bone and soft tissue instability, we prefer to treat the bony problem first, such as grafting or fixing the injured coronoid process and replacing the injured radial head by a bipolar prosthesis

We recommend the distractor in the management of persistent posterior dislocation where a simple soft tissue release would create a major instability and the distractor is used as a temporary stabilizer while rehabilitation is undertaken. In post-traumatic bony ankylosis, distraction arthroplasty is an excellent indication providing there is good bone stock and good skin coverage.

Finally, we must not forget the role of the patient who must be well informed and highly motivated to undergo such surgery. If these criteria are met we believe that Robert Judet's original concept of articular surgery with a hinge distractor device still applies in elbow surgery. We believe this concept will remain valid in the management of complex post-traumatic elbow problems until a reliable prosthesis for young patients is devised.

Acknowledgements

The authors wish to thank Dr Godfrey Charnley for his assistance.

References

Charnley G, Judet T, Garreau de Loubresse C, Piriou P (1996) Articulated radial head replacement and elbow release for post head injury heterotropic ossification, *J Orthop Trauma* **10**:68–71.

Deland JT, Walker PS (1987) Biomechanical basis for elbow hinge-distractor design, *Clin Orthop* **215**:303.

Han D, Yun H (1995) Operative treatment for post-traumatic elbow stiffness, *Orthopedic International Edition*, May–June volume 3, number 3.

Judet R, Judet T (1978) Arthrolyse et arthroplasties sous distracteur articulaire, *Rev Chir Orthop* **64**:363–5.

Judet T, Garreau de Loubresse C, Piriou P, Charnley G (1996) Floating prosthesis for radial head fracture, *J Bone Joint Surg* **78B**:244–9.

Morrey BF (1990) Post-traumatic contracture of the elbow, *J Bone Joint Surg* **72A**:601.

Morrey BF, Adams R, Bryan RS (1991) Total replacement for post-traumatic arthritis of the elbow, *J Bone Joint Surg* **73B**:607.

Volkov MV, Oganesian OV (1975) Restoration of function in the knee and elbow with a hinge distractor apparatus, *J Bone Joint Surg* **57A**:591.

17
Open arthrolysis and rehabilitation

Joachim Hassenpflug

Contractures of the elbow joint may cause severe functional impairment. The high incidence of contractures of the elbow joint results from its specific anatomical conditions, its high potential for injuries and, last but not least, inadequate treatment, especially manual mobilization of post-traumatic or post-operative contractures (Cooney 1985, Blauth et al 1990, Morrey 1990). For instance 30% of our patients with elbow arthrolyses had been passively mobilized over-aggressively before. Many of these patients reported severe pain during these passive manipulations and subsequent deterioration of their contractures. Most of our data is based on the experiences of Blauth and co-workers in the Orthopaedic Department of Kiel University (Blauth 1982 and 1991, Blauth and Jaeger 1992).

Indications

The indications for an operative treatment depend on the kind of contracture, the resulting functional disability and its duration. Loss of motion should be more than 30° in the direction of extension or flexion. Conservative treatment should have failed and adequate functional compensation of the deformity should not be possible.

Any irritation of the joint itself and the surrounding tissues should have faded away, the region of the joint should not be warm, show any tenderness or inflammatory skin reactions. Altogether, the contracture should be fixed and mature. There should not be any active osteoblastic or fibroblastic process. Surgery should be performed not before 6–9 months in adults and not before 9–12 months in children, because spontaneous improvements are possible until then. Exceptions are bony fragments which are dislocated or interposed into the joint space which should be excised earlier.

The excision of ectopic bone formation should be postponed until maturity of the ossification is achieved after about 1–1.5 years. A guideline may be a decrease of radionuclide uptake. Otherwise recurrence of the heterotopic ossifications is to be expected. On the other hand, waiting too long may also be disadvantageous. The prognosis seems to be poorer if the joint has been stiff for a very long time, e.g. more than 1–2 years.

The radiological state of the articulating surfaces is not as important in the elbow as in the weight-bearing legs where intact joint surfaces are essential, e.g. in knee joint arthrolyses, but there should be a detectable joint space between the articulating surfaces.

Decision making may be facilitated by the characteristics of the end point of the arc of motion. If there is a well-defined stiff impaction the contractures are mature for operation. If there is a soft elastic resistance at the end point, spontaneous improvements can occur if the joints are 'left alone'. Patient and surgeon should be aware of these conditions if they agree to operate despite them.

As well as local conditions, some other prerequisites are also essential for successful procedures. The personality of the patient, the qualification of the surgeon and the facilities for postoperative care have to be considered carefully. The patient should be well prepared, understand the procedures and request the intervention. Care is needed with the indications for operation in children. The upper age limit is given by the demands and vitality of the patient. Both surgeon and physiotherapist should be very experienced and collaborate very closely. Patience and sympathetic understanding are very important for the correct administration of therapeutic procedures and are important prerequisites for success.

Operative technique

Operative exposure has to be orientated according to the position of the main obstacles to mobility which may be ascertained by history and by clinical and radiological examination.

The radial approach is the most common. It is always recommended if the pathology is not exclusively at the ulnar side or if a transposition of the ulnar nerve is not necessary. The radial approach has been used in nearly half of our 95 patients. After a radial skin incision, the muscle is carefully split over the posterior margin of the radial head in the direction of its fibres. The anterior border of the incision is deflected, carefully respecting the radial nerve. The joint space is gradually freed of adhesions and fibrous scar tissue, the procedure including an anterior capsulectomy.

About one-fifth of our patients had an isolated ulnar approach, in the majority of cases together with a transposition of the ulnar nerve. When detaching the ventromedial muscles, the median nerve has to be respected, especially in severe scoring. For exposure of the posterolateral aspects the joint capsule may be incised just behind the collateral ligament. This requires transposition of the ulnar nerve. In one-third of the cases incisions at both the ulnar and the radial side were necessary. A dorsal approach is advocated in extreme stiffness only, especially in extension contractures, which are less common.

It is not always sufficient to perform only a soft tissue procedure. Three-quarters of our patients required additional procedures; a so-called 'extended arthrolysis'. Bony obstacles like prominences, ectopic bony fragments or deformed radial heads are removed. Sometimes the coronoid fossa, the olecranon fossa or the trochlear notch have to be rebuilt. Removal of osteophytes from the coronoid process, for example, may restore a better flexion in addition to deepening the coronoid fossa.

Generally the range of motion is tested during the operation. Careful manual mobilization may help to overcome additional restraints which are not directly exposed. Free mobility of the joint should never be achieved by force. The aim of an arthrolysis is to obtain sufficient flexion and extension during the procedure. An additional gain of mobility above the intraoperative range is very uncommon.

Some joint contractures may not be overcome without lengthening or extensive sectioning of scarred collateral ligaments. Instability can be avoided if the patient wears suitable braces for some weeks after the operation. Tendon lengthening or a temporary osteotomy of an epicondyle is usually not necessary.

Postoperative management

Some details of the postoperative management are important. While the patient is still under anaesthesia, three removable plaster splints are applied, one with the elbow arm in approximately less than 5° of the obtained flexion, the second in approximately less than 5° of the maximal extension, and the third in an intermediate position. Alternating positioning is also possible on movable splints.

Analgesics have to be given as needed. The wound area should be kept cool and the dressing must not be too tight. The patient should not let the arm hang down when standing or walking around. The arm is placed on a shoulder adduction splint for floating and comfortable support of the arm, and light active exercises are allowed.

Continuous passive motion (CPM) treatment may be started on the first or second day after the operation once the suction drainage has been removed. The range of motion should be adjusted in small increments initially. It may be progressively increased subsequently provided there is no unacceptable pain. Pronation and supination of the forearm may also be done on CPM devices.

Occupational therapy and hydrotherapy may begin about the third postoperative week. Initially the elbow joint should still be supported. The joint should always be free of irritation. There should be no qualms about reducing the intensity of the treatment for 1 or 2 days if there are irritations of the joint region.

Patience and realistic expectations of the level of success in the early stages is needed. A slight reduction of the range of motion reached in the second or third week postoperatively is quite common and should not be used as an indication to intensify the treatment. The final result is not reached before 1 year after the operation and improvements are possible even after the end of the clinical therapy. Overall, close guidance of the patient, understanding and dosage of applied forces are absolutely necessary for both surgeon and physiotherapist.

Results

Of 102 consecutive patients operated upon, 95 could be followed up within a mean of 5.5 years after surgery.

The preoperative amount of stiffness was within 70% of the normal range in 11 patients. Moderate stiffness with a range of 40–50% of the normal movability was found in 34 patients. A severe stiffness with less than 40% was found in 25 patients, and a very severe stiffness with less than 20% of the normal range in another 25 patients. Altogether more than half of our patients had severe or very severe contractures of their elbow joints.

Assessment of the outcome was done by measurement of the absolute and evaluation of the relative improvement, i.e. the relation between the achieved gain of motion related to the maximum possible gain (Cauchoix and Deburge 1975, Blauth and Jaeger 1992). The mean absolute gain in flexion/extension was 43° and in pronation/supination it was 30°. The relative gain compared to the maximum possible range of motion was 62% in flexion/extension and 41% in pronation/supination (Fig. 1).

Nearly 80% of the patients had a rating of good or very good according to a relative gain of more than 70% or 40%, respectively. Even those patients with a poor result still had a relative gain of 17% concerning flexion/extension or 48% considering pronation/supination. Major pain was not a severe problem after elbow arthrolysis.

Complications were observed in less than 5% of the patients. There was one wound healing disturbance. On three occasions there was a temporary radial, ulnar or median nerve lesion. Eight elbow joints were operated upon a second time because the results of the first operation were not satisfactory. A satisfactory outcome was finally achieved.

Altogether operative arthrolysis of the elbow joint has a high rate of success and is recommended for improving elbow function in suitable patients. Indispensable prerequisites include careful preoperative assessment, localization of the obstacles to motion and preoperative planning, adequate selection of patients, experience with the operative techniques, highly sensitive postoperative care and sufficient rehabilitation time.

Conclusion

Mobility of the elbow joint may be compromised mainly by loose bodies, deformation of the joint surfaces, soft tissue contractures or ectopic bone formation. If conservative treatment has failed, operative arthrolysis may improve the range of motion (ROM), but some essential prerequisites have to be respected. A radial approach which enables easy access both to the anterior capsule and to the fossa olecrani is preferred. In severe deformations resection of the radial head is advocated. Postoperative management includes local

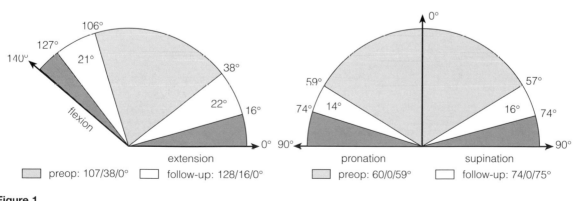

Figure 1

Mobility of the elbow joint before arthrolysis and at follow-up.

cold, anti-inflammatory drugs, alternating positioning of the joint in individual splints, early CPM in a pain-free ROM and, especially, patience.

In 95 consecutive patients the mean preoperative ROM was flexion/extension 106/38/0° and pronation/supination 59/0/57°. The ROM at follow-up was flexion/extension 127/16/0° and pronation/supination 74/0/74°.

Elbow arthrolysis is a technically demanding procedure, but nevertheless if the indication is correct, and both surgeon and physiotherapist are familiar with the procedures, good final results may be achieved in a high percentage of cases.

References

Blauth W (1982) Allgemeine Grundsätze und Techniken von Arthrolysen, *Unfallchirurgie* **8**:279–93.

Blauth W (1991) Die Arthrolyse des Ellenbogengelenkes, *Operat Orthop Traumatol* **3**:169–85.

Blauth W, Jaeger T (1992) Arthrolysis of the elbow, *Orthop Traumatol* **1**:105–21.

Blauth M, Haas NP, Südkamp NP, Happe T (1990) Die Ellbogenarthrolyse bei posttraumatischer Gelenksteife, *Orthopäde* **19**:332–42.

Cauchoix J, Deburge A (1975) L'arthrolyse du coude dans les raideurs post-traumatiques, *Acta Orthop Belg* **41**:385.

Cooney WP (1985) Contractures and burns. In: Morrey BF, ed. *The Elbow and its Disorders*. WB Saunders: Philadelphia: 433–51.

Morrey BF (1990) Post-traumatic contracture of the elbow, *J Bone Joint Surg* **72A**:601–18.

18
Arthrolysis: our experience

Francesco Catalano, Francesco Fanfani, Antonio Tulli, Antonio Pagliei and Giuseppe Taccardo

The clinical and anatomopathological patterns associated with post-traumatic and post-surgical stiffness in the elbow (Wilson 1944, Esteve et al 1971, Exner et al 1982, Morrey 1990, Catalano et al 1995, Celli et al 1995) suggest a division of the topic into two parts.

First the surgical methods routinely used either individually or in combination in the treatment of elbow stiffness are listed and analysed (Bhattacharya 1974, Judet and Judet 1975, Tucker 1978, Breifub et al 1991). Then the anatomoclinical and radiological patterns (intra- or extra-articular stiffness) are discussed individually to standardize the surgical procedures to be applied – either in combination or in sequence – and to codify methods of treatment.

The elementary surgical procedures are:

• removal of anterior extra-articular obstacles (extra-articular ossifications, e.g. the ossification of the brachialis anterior muscle or the anterior capsule) or intra-articular impediments (osteochondral loose bodies) (Roberts and Pankratz 1979)
• anterior capsulotomy with tenomyotomy of the anterior brachial muscle (Wilson 1944, Willner 1948, Urbariak et ak 1985, Breen et al 1988)
• resection of the radial head and removal of the proximal radioulnar synostosis
• posterior capsulotomy with any necessary removal of posterior extra- or intra-articular ossifications and debridement of the olecranon fossa (Glynn and Niebauer 1976, Ecke 1986)
• release of the triceps muscle from the distal metadyaphisis of the humerus
• removal of the osteosynthesis devices.

Since it is often necessary to perform not only single but also associated elementary surgical procedures, we decided not to use the usual Kocher's lateral approach, (Husband and Hastings 1990) preferring instead an anterior approach and a posterior approach which, according to circumstances could be either associated or not.

We will now analyse the various anatomoclinical and radiological patterns and determine the association or sequence in which the elementary surgical procedures must be used.

Isolated – predominant restriction of flexion or extension, with no significant radiological evidence of obstacles

This condition represents the most likely outcome of a fracture or a fracture with dislocation when stiffness is limited to either flexion or extension, but not both. In these cases, an arthrolysis is performed only on the articular side opposite to the movement requiring improvement. In this case, the impediment is due to the retraction of the soft tissues of the joint. In particular, wherever an extension deficiency exists an anterior elbow approach is performed followed by a complete capsulotomy, often in association with a brachialis anterior tenomyotomy. Alternatively, when there is only a flexion restriction, a posterior approach is used followed by a paraolecranic capsulotomy with a complete section of the subtricipital capsular expansion. This gives a complete recovery of movement, confirming our belief that the first cause of this restriction is the retraction of the opposite capsular side.

Associated flexion and extension restriction with no significant radiological evidence of obstacles

In this clinical and radiographical pattern, which is often the outcome of a dislocation of the elbow or other traumatic events, a combination of anterior and posterior arthrolysis are used. In particular, either the more restricted function or the one the patient is feeling more uncomfortable with is recovered first by performing a posterior capsulotomy to recover flexion and an anterior capsulotomy to recover extension. Then, immediate postsurgical passive kinesitherapy (Kinetec) followed by active kinesitherapy until full recovery is suggested (Dickson 1976). A second capsulotomy is performed only one or two months after initial surgical treatment to improve any movement not previously treated. In our experience, this two-step arthrolysis is essential to avoid the unbearable postsurgical trauma and pain that occur when simultaneous double approach arthrolysis is performed.

Stiffness with significant radiological evidence of obstacles

These are conditions in which a marked restriction in flexion is associated with a significant anterior ossification, or, alternatively, a restricted extension with a posterior ossification. In such cases the procedure used is the same: e.g. in flexion restriction, first we perform a posterior capsulotomy, and then, to ensure movement gain, we use an anterior approach to remove anterior ossifications by whatever method avoids an aggressive surgical approach.

Stiffness due to extra-articular causes

The most common condition occurs when restricted flexion follows a distal metadiaphyseal fracture of the humerus, mainly when it is treated by prolonged immobilization. In such cases, debridement of the sliding surface between triceps and humerus is performed according to Judet's tech-nique for the treatment of post-traumatic stiffness of the knee. A posterior capsulotomy follows only if flexion is not satisfactory after the intraoperatory detachment of the triceps.

Restriction of rotation

When the restriction of pronation and supination is due to stiffness of radiohumeral and proximal radioulnar joints, procedures are performed according to the requirements:

• resection of the radial head through a posterolateral approach for isolated impediments
• resection of the radial head through a posterolateral approach together with an anterior approach when restriction of rotation is combined with an extension impediment; resection of the radial head by an anterior approach, although possible, is believed too risky due to the presence of nearby vessels and nerves (anterior and posterior interosseous nerves)
• resection of the radial head through a posterior approach when restriction of rotation is combined with a flexion impediment.

Conclusions

From our decade of experience (Table 1) regarding the treatment of elbow stiffness, we conclude:

Table 1 Surgical treatment of stiff elbow, 1986–1995: 61 arthrolysis in 59 patients

Condition	No. of cases
Global stiffness	42
Predominant flexion stiffness	14
Predominant extension stiffness	5

• the anterior and posterior approaches, although more demanding, are more versatile
• two-step arthrolysis for global stiffness is a better treatment compared with simultaneous double-approach arthrolysis
• quality of the results depends on:
  – latency between stiffness stabilization and arthrolysis: best results occur when surgery is performed after inflammation and periarticular

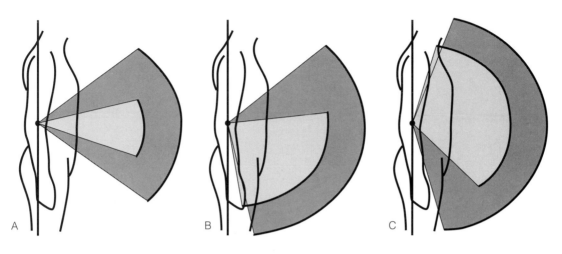

Figure 1

Results of elbow arthrolysis: mean increment of range of motion. (Light) mean value before surgical treatment; (Dark) mean value after surgical treatment. (A) Global stiffness: 45°. (B) Predominant flexion stiffness: 34°. (C) Predominant extension stiffness: 30°. Arthrolysis in predominant flexion or extension stiffness leads to a partial limitation of the opposite movement.

calcifications are completely extinguished, but before 1 year from stiffness stabilization
– quality of preservation of the articular surfaces.

Finally, we stress that for arthrolysis in predominantly flexion or extension stiffness, the gain leads to a partial limitation of the opposite movement (Fig. 1).

References

Bhattacharya S (1974) Arthrolysis: a new approach to surgery of post-traumatic stiff elbow, *J Bone Joint Surg* **56B**:567.

Breen TF, Gelberman RH, Ackerman GN (1988) Elbow flexion contractures treatment by anterior release and continuous passive motion, *J Hand Surg* **13B**:286–7.

Breifub H, Muhr G, Neumann K, Rehn J (1991) Die Arthrolyse posttraumatischer Ellenbogensteifen, *Unfall Chir* **94**:33–9.

Catalano F, Fanfani F, Pagliei A, Taccardo G (1995) Le rigidità post-traumatiche e post-chirurgiche di gomito: trattamento a cielo aperto, *G Ital Ortop Traumat* **XXI-3**:181–4.

Celli L, Mingione A, De Luise G, Rovesta C (1995) Il gomito rigido secondario: inquadramento clinico, valutazione diagnostica ed indicazioni terapeutiche, *G Ital Ortop Traumat* **XXI-3**:157–63.

Dickson RA (1976) Reversed dynamic slings. A new concept in the treatment of post traumatic elbow flexion contractures, *Injury* **8**:35–8.

Ecke H (1986) Arthrolysis of the elbow joint, *Unfall Chir* **12**:253–7.

Esteve P, Valentin P, Deburge A, Kerboull M (1971) Raideurs et ankyloses post-traumatiques du coude, *Rev Chir Orthop (Suppl)* **57**:26.

Exner G, Wisotzky W, John B, Zimmer W (1982) Therapy especially arthrolisis and its results in stiffened elbow joints after fractures, *Aktuelle Traumat* **12**:255–62.

Glynn JJ, Niebauer JJ (1976) Flexion and extension contracture of the elbow. Surgical management, *Clin Orthop* **117**:289–91.

Husband JB, Hastings H (1990) The lateral approach for operative release of post-traumatic contracture of the elbow, *J Bone Joint Surg* **72A-9**.1353–9.

Judet J, Judet H (1975) Arthrolyse du coude *Acta Orthop Belg* **41–4**:412–24.

Morrey BF (1990) Post traumatic contracture of the elbow. Operative treatment including distraction arthroplasty, *J Bone Joint Surg* **72A**:601–18.

Roberts JB, Pankratz DG (1979) The surgical treatment of heterotopic ossification at the elbow following long-term coma, *J Bone Joint Surg* **61A**:760–3.

Tucker K (1978) Some aspects of post-traumatic elbow stiffness, *Injury* **9**:216–20.

Urbaniak J, Hansen PE, Beissinger SF, Aitken MS (1985) Correction of post traumatic flexion contracture of the elbow by anterior capsulotomy, *J Bone Joint Surg* **67A**:1160–4.

Willner P (1948) Anterior capsulectomy for contractures of the elbow, *J Int Coll Surg* **11**:359–61.

Wilson PD (1944) Capsulectomy for relief of flexion contractures of the elbow following fracture, *J Bone Joint Surg* **26A**:71–86.

19

Elbow replacement arthroplasty: long-term results

Allan E Inglis

Posturing the hand in relation to the body is the essential function of the elbow joint (Morrey et al 1985). Inability to move the elbow joint gives a fixed linear position of the hand relative to the body resulting in the inability to rotate or move the hand toward or away from the body. Overall hand function is even further reduced if poor motion is accompanied by elbow pain. The cliché applied to other articulations of 'a little motion is better than no motion at all' in not applicable to the elbow joint. A 'jog' of motion does little to posture the hand in space. A stiff elbow in the presence of a functional hand and shoulder is a strong stimulus or indication for therapeutic measures directed toward improved elbow function.

Ollier in the later part of the 19th century reported excellent results with resection arthroplasty in the restoration of elbow function in a large number of patients with ankylosis of the elbow joint (Ollier 1878 and 1882). Synovectomy has also been reported to yield good results in patients with stiff elbows due to rheumatoid arthritis (Inglis et al 1971, Porter et al 1974, Bratstrom and Khudairy 1975, Bryan and Morrey 1983). Arthrodesis in patients with painful stiff elbows has also been reported (Rashkoff and Burkhalter 1986, Beckenbaugh 1993, Inglis and Figgie 1993). However, this procedure still leaves the patient with limited hand function. Early reports with distraction arthroplasty, both with and without interpositional membranes, have also been reported (Volkov and Organesian 1975). The use of total elbow replacement arthroplasty used by a single surgeon in patients with stiff or ankylosed elbow joints over the last 20 years will be reviewed.

Our experience with elbow replacement arthroplasty was sufficiently successful in movable but severely damaged elbow joints, that we judged the procedure could be extended to ankylosed or painful stiff elbows in 1975. Our indications at that time were bilaterality in the case of ankylosed elbows and pain in those patients with limited motion and poor function. The implants used in the study consisted initially of the Tri-Axial elbow that was used until 1981. This implant produced satisfactory results (Inglis and Pellicci 1980). However, because of the snap-fit design, the implant would dissociate (in 5% of cases), so we then used the Hospital for Special Surgery designed implant for the remainder of the study (Fig. 1). These two implants have the same geometrical design and the same degree of laxity at the articulation as well as the normal 15° valgus carrying angle. This later implant has an axle lined with a polyethylene sleeve. This axle is not loaded except at the extreme of tension forces across the elbow joint. Normally, all loads across the elbow joint are compressional and the small axle protects the articulation from dissociating in unusual tension load situations.

The surgical technology changed once during the study. We initially used the Campbell triceps splitting technique (Campbell 1932). Because of modest, but troublesome, wound complications and intermittent triceps weakness we changed in 1981 to the Bryan–Morrey posterior medial approach (Bryan and Morrey 1982).

We first reported our experience with total elbow replacement for completely ankylosed elbows in 1989 (Figgie et al 1989). The current report is an update on these patients and also adds the cases through to 1994. The study was expanded to include not only ankylosed elbows but also those patients with stiff (i.e. less than 10° arc of motion) elbows in 1979.

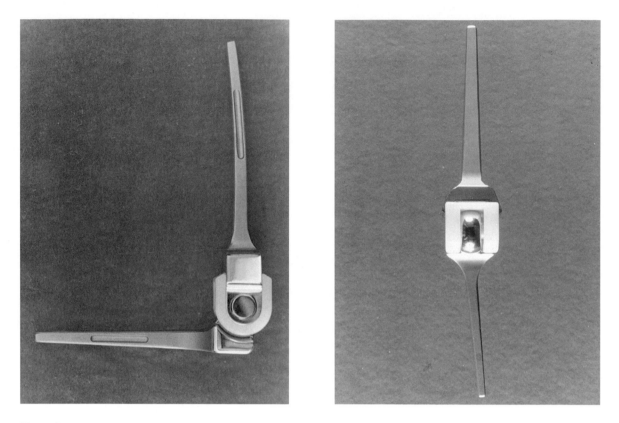

Figure 1

Illustration of the Hospital for Special Surgery design elbow. It has two sizes and can be customized by the manufacturer (Osteonics Corp., Allendale, New Jersey, USA) for special anatomic problems or circumstances.

Material and methods

Twenty patients with stiff or ankylosed elbows are reported. Fifteen with ankylosed elbows were studied (Fig. 2). Five patients studied with stiff elbows (Fig. 3) all had less than 10° arc of motion. Three patients with bilateral ankylosis required bilateral replacement arthroplasties. The current study includes all those patients operated upon between 1975 and 1994. There were 10 females and 10 males. The average age was 40 years with a range of 16–89 years. There were eight patients with traumatic arthritis and 12 patients with inflammatory arthritis. The patients were clinically evaluated initially and at regular follow-up visits with the Hospital for Special Surgery evaluation system which is heavily weighted for pain relief and restoration of motion. This system allows 40 points for pain relief, 20 points for function, 12 points for strength, and 28 points for motion (one point for each 7° of elbow motion). Additionally, the patients were evaluated radiographically for loosening, osteolysis or epicondylar fracture.

The indications for surgery for the patients with ankylosis was bilaterality or special vocational or physical needs, e.g. a poorly functioning contralateral extremity. The indications for patients with some residual painful motion was a failure of conservative therapies and a limitation of hand function due to pain.

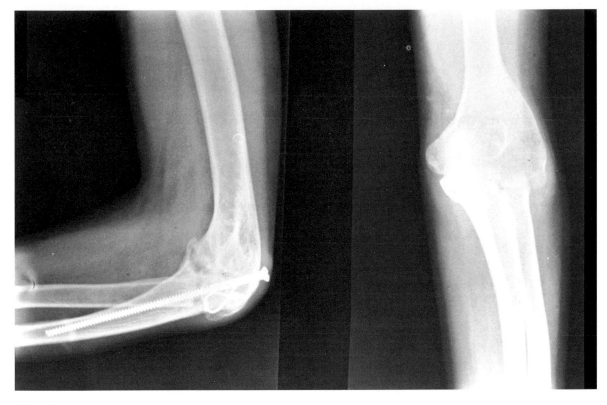

Figure 2

Illustration of one of the elbows in a patient with bilateral ankylosis who had undergone a prior synovectomy for rheumatoid arthritis. The synovectomy had been performed through a transolecranon approach. This patient was 16 years old at the time of the bilateral replacement arthroplasties.

Surgical technology

The patients were all operated in the supine position with the arm over the chest. Regional anaesthesia was preferred. Sterile tourniquets were used whenever possible for improved tourniquet control and potentially wider surgical exposure. The Bryan–Morrey approach was preferred (Bryan and Morrey 1982). This consists of a posterior medial incision directly down to the epimysium of the flexor carpi ulnaris and the triceps muscles. The ulna nerve is then identified and carefully elevated away from the triceps muscle and the ulnar nerve groove in the humerus, and away from the proximal ulna and the sublime tubercle of the ulna (Last 1966).

The ulna nerve is then held in this safe position with a small circumferential Penrose drain. The epimysium of the flexor carpi ulnaris is then dissected away from the deeper muscle and then laterally to include the periosteum of the ulna and then proximally beneath the triceps muscle containing the central tendon of the triceps insertion into the olecranon process. A single incision from the skin to the epimysium and the periosteum of the ulna is used thereby avoiding soft tissue layers and flaps. The triceps and the epimysium of the flexor carpi ulnaris as well as the periosteum of the ulna are then all carefully mobilized laterally. This allows exposure of the radial head. A sufficient amount of the radial head and neck is excised, thereby pre-

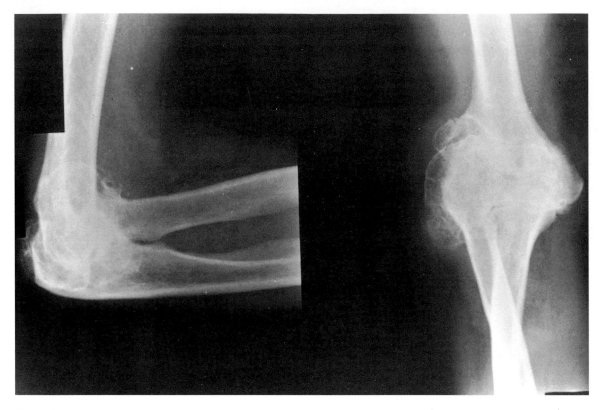

Figure 3

Illustration of a patient with traumatic arthritis of the elbow. This patient has 3° of motion and no pronation or supination. The old circumferential scarring and callus complicated the surgical procedure.

venting subsequent impingement or interference with the adjacent ulna and distal humerus. The fibrous or ankylosed joint margins between the humerus and the trochlea notch in the ulna are carefully identified and exposed medially, laterally and posteriorly. A burr or small osteotomes are then used to open the cortical margins between the trochlear groove of the ulna and the trochlea of the humerus. When these cortical margins have been incised, a minimum of gentle pressure on the arm and forearm will crack open the old articulation. A bone hook is then placed in the trochlear groove of the ulna and the proximal one-fourth inch of the brachialis muscle insertion incised. This allows complete exposure of the ulna and the distal humerus. Disarticulating the ulna and humerus in patients with a fibrous ankylosis is uniformly more difficult as the surrounding scar tissue is dense and somewhat difficult to incise and release, particularly between the damaged surfaces of the ulna and humerus. After the scar tissue between the ulna and the humerus has been incised, the anterior capsule and approximately one-fourth inch of the brachialis muscle insertion is released. This again provides good exposure of the distal humerus and the proximal ulna. After determining the centre of rotation of the trochlear notch of the ulna, the notch itself is excised with an oscillating saw. Using small burrs and reamers, the intermedullary shaft of the ulna is prepared for the ulnar implant. The ulnar implant must be positioned far enough within the ulna so that the centre of rotation of the implant corresponds to the centre of rotation of the trochlear notch of the ulna. The distal humerus is then skeletalized with the exception of the origins of both the wrist and the digital muscle. The trochlea of the humerus is excised with an oscillating saw following measurement with the templates and the jigs provided with the instruments. Again, the centre of rotation of the humeral implant must correspond to the centre of rotation of the trochlea. The reaming and broaching of the humerus is then performed. The reaming and broaching are deemed complete when the trochlear portion of the humeral component and the intermedullary portion of the distal humerus have become satisfactorily elliptified to obtain a better cement fill for humeral component rotational support. The two trial implants are then put into position and the implants articulated with the trial bearings and the elbow put through a full range of motion. Full extension and full flexion should be achieved with ease or more bone must be removed from the ulna or from the humerus. The methyl methacrylate cement is then prepared with a small amount of tobramycin antibiotic for microbial prophylaxis and a drop of methylene blue to aid in cement removal. After the cement has hardened and any excess cement has been removed, a small hole is made in the lateral epicondyle for insertion of the axle with its small high molecular weight polyethylene sleeve. The axle system is 'clicked' into place and the arc of motion is again checked to ensure that there is no bony impingement between the margins of the ulna and the humerus. The tourniquet is released to identify and to control any remaining bleeding points and then reinflated. The triceps tension is adjusted sufficiently so that full flexion and full extension is easily maintained. The central tendon of the triceps muscle is then sutured to the tip of the olecranon process with nonabsorbable sutures. A negative suction drain is then put into position and sutured to the skin to prevent an inadvertent removal in the immediate postoperative period. The ulna nerve is replaced in the humeral groove and is *never transposed*. The epimysium of the flexor carpi ulnaris muscle is closed and the remainder of the wound is then closed in a routine manner with fine absorbable sutures. The patient's arm is then put in 30° of extension and supported with a well padded anterior plaster splint, thereby preventing motion and any undue pressure by the splint on the wound. The drain is removed in 24 h. The dressings are removed on the fourth postoperative day and an active rehabilitation programme initiated.

Results

Nineteen of the original 20 patients have remained in the study group. Preoperatively, the average total Hospital for Special Surgery clinical score was 47. Postoperatively the average total score was 91. The average arc of motion of the ankylosed elbow was 0° and the average arc of motion of the stiff elbow was 5°. The postoperative arc of motion was 82°. The average flexion achieved was 117° with a range of 90–135°. The extension achieved was 31° with a range of 0–50°. There was no difference in the arc of motion achieved in the patients with ankylosed elbows and the patients with stiff elbows. No patient became re-ankylosed. Myositis ossificans was not observed.

Complications

There were four elbow infections, three of which were superficial and minor. One deep infection occurred 3 years post-operatively. A wound slough occurred in an unrecognized insensate area between two parallel incisions. The result was a healed resection arthroplasty and was deemed a failure. There were three patients with delayed healing in the early group in which the Campbell surgical approach was used. These three patients required a bipedicle skin flap with adjacent full thickness skin grafting. They went on to satisfactory function and this complication did not compromise their final result. There were two dissociations requiring an additional operation in which a new bearing was installed and a surrounding yoke to prevent bearing deformation and dissociation. There was one patient with persistent ulnar nerve dysesthesias. There are no patients with loosening or osteolysis to date.

Discussion

Limited elbow motion is functionally disabling in otherwise normal individuals. This disability is espe-

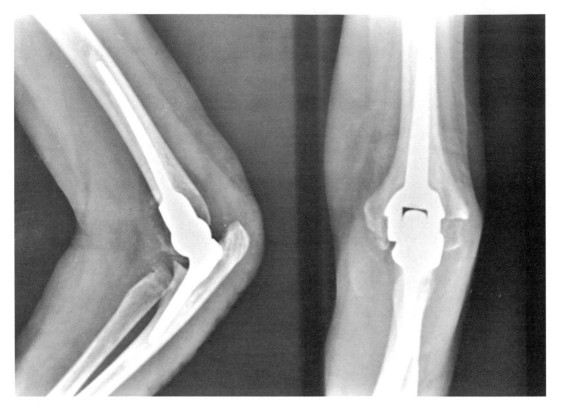

Figure 4

Illustration of the patient in Fig. 2 at the 6-years postoperative evaluation. He has flexion to 126° and extension to 10°. The opposite elbow is also fully functional. At the 19-year follow-up he was again noted to be fully active and now a 'procedural' radiologist.

cially apparent when the dominant extremity is involved as eating, grooming, toilet needs and dressing, e.g. fastening buttons, putting on stockings and tying shoe laces, all become slow and difficult. Although the individual may drive an automobile without difficulty, paying roadside tolls can be problematic if the left elbow is involved. Studies have shown that if an individual has 35° of extension and 120° of flexion, 95% of the activities of daily living can be accomplished (Morrey et al 1981). Lesser arcs of motion will involve significant compromises in the activities of daily living.

Alternative solutions to the stiff elbow should be considered, as complications can be serious with limited surgical choices for revision arthroplasty. Arthrodesis could be considered as successful operations result in a painless elbow joint (Beckenbaugh 1993). It is recognized that arthrode-sis of the elbow joint is difficult to achieve and ultimately the individual still is unable to move the hand away from the body. Resection arthroplasty has achieved excellent results with functional ranges of motion and relief of pain (Dickson et al 1976, Tillmann 1990, Ruther and Tillmann 1995). The complication rate is low, but there are two issues detracting from its success. First, there is always some degree of mediolateral instability resulting in upper extremity weakness. Second, the operation requires knowledge, skill and especially experience to obtain the best results (Ruther and Tillmann 1995). Distraction arthroplasty is a relatively new procedure used particularly in traumatic arthritis resulting in stiff joints with retained collateral ligaments (Volkov and Oganesian 1975, Deland et al 1983, Morrey 1990). It is conceded that the operation is moderately difficult and must be done accurately. The positioning of the distraction pins precisely at the centre of rotation is essential and also precise positioning of the interposition grafts is important. This new procedure should probably be restricted to those centres with experienced surgeons who will be modifying and improving the technology and evaluating and reporting the results carefully.

Joint replacement arthroplasty for stiff ankylosed joints has a history of success of over 20 years. Non-constrained implants cannot be used because the required ligament support has resorbed. A semi-constrained implant is essential. Favourable results from this procedure are reported by other centres in which elbow arthroplasty is commonly performed (Seth and Khurana 1985, Morrey 1988). Our studies show that 89% of good to excellent results can be expected in this group of patients (Fig. 4). Restoration of elbow function and pain relief are goals that can be achieved with careful planning, patient co-operation and a skilled therapeutic team.

References

Beckenbaugh RD (1993) Arthrodesis. In: Morrey BF, ed. *The Elbow and its Disorders*, 2nd edn. WB Saunders: Philadelphia: 696–703.

Bratstrom O, Khudairy HA (1975). Synovectomy of the elbow in rheumatoid arthritis, *Acta Orthop Scand* **46**:77a.

Bryan RS, Morrey BF (1982) Extensive posterior exposure of the elbow, *Clin Orthop* **166**:188–95.

Bryan RS, Morrey BF (1983) Rheumatoid arthritis of the elbow. In: Evarts CM, ed. *Surgery of the Musculoskeletal System*. Churchill Livingstone: London.

Campbell WC (1932) Incision for exposure of the elbow joint, *Am J Surg* **15**:65–7.

Deland JT, Walker PS, Slodge CB, Farberov A (1983) Treatment of posttraumatic elbows with a new hinge-distractor, *Orthopedics* **6**:732–7.

Dickson RA, Stein H, Bentley G (1976) Excision arthroplasty of the elbow in rheumatoid arthritis, *J Bone Joint Surg* **58B**(2):227–9.

Figgie MP, Inglis AE, Mow CS, Figgie HPI (1989) Total elbow arthroplasty for ankylosis of the elbow, *J Bone Joint Surg* **71A**:513–20.

Inglis AE, Figgie MP (1993) Aseptic and non traumatic conditions of the elbow. In: Morrey BF, ed. *The Elbow and its Disorders*, 2nd edn. WB Saunders: Philadelphia: 751–66.

Inglis AE, Pellicci PM (1980) Total elbow replacement, *J Bone Joint Surg* **62A**:1252.

Inglis AE, Ranawat CS, Straub LR (1971) Synovectomy and debridement of the elbow in rheumatoid arthritis, *J Bone Joint Surg* **53**:652.

Last RJ (1966) The upper limb. In: *Anatomy Regional and Applied*, 4th edn. Little, Brown and Co: Boston: 74–183.

Morrey BF (1988) Surgical takedown of the ankylosed elbow, *Orthop Trans* **12**:734.

Morrey BF (1990) Post traumatic contracture of the elbow. Operative treatment including distraction arthroplasty, *J Bone Joint Surg* **72B**:601–18.

Morrey BF, An KN, Chao EY (1985) Functional evaluation of the elbow. In: Morrey BF, ed. *The Elbow and its Disorders*. WB Saunders: Philadelphia: 73–91.

Morrey BF, Askew LJ, Chao EY (1981) A biomechanical study of normal functional elbow motion, *J Bone Joint Surg* **63A**:872–7.

Ollier LX (1878) De la resection du coude dans les cas d'ankylose, *Rev Med Chir* **6**(12).

Ollier LX (1882) Demonstration anatomique de la reconstitution du coude apres la resection souspériostée, Examen d'une série de 106 cas de cette opération, *Lentralbl Chir* **9**:548–9.

Porter BB, Richardson C, Vainio K (1974) Rheumatoid arthritis of the elbow, results of synovectomy, *J Bone Joint Surg* **56B**(3):527–37.

Rashkoff E, Burkhalter WE (1986) Arthrodesis of the salvaged elbow. *Orthopedics* **9**(5):733.

Ruther W, Tillman K (1995) Resection interposition arthroplasty of the elbow in rheumatoid arthritis. In: Ruther W, ed. *The Elbow Endoprosthetic Replacement and Non-Endoprosthetic Procedures*. Springer: Berlin: 57–67.

Seth MK, Khurana JK (1985) Bony ankylosis of the elbow after burns, *J Bone Joint Surg* **67B**:747–9.

Tillmann K (1990) Recent advances in the treatment of rheumatoid arthritis, *Clin Orthop* **258**:62–72.

Volkov MV, Oganesian OV (1975) Restoration of function in the knee and elbow with a hinge distactor, *J Bone Joint Surg* **57A**:591–60.

20
Total replacement arthroplasty in the management of the ankylosed elbow

William A Souter

Severe restriction of elbow movement can have major repercussions on the function of the arm as a whole and on a patient's ability to cope with the activities of daily living. Where the joint surfaces are reasonably well preserved and where the stiffness is due to extra-articular causes, soft tissue arthrolysis is, of course, the treatment of choice. Where the joint surfaces have been severely damaged or where there is frank fibrous or bony ankylosis, arthroplasty in one form or another will be required for the restoration of movement.

Although excision arthroplasty offers a possible solution, the results tend to be somewhat indeterminate even in post-traumatic patients (Knight and Van Zandt 1952), while rheumatoid patients may simply lack the muscle power to stabilize the pseudarthrosis. They also appear to be subject to further bone resorption, so that an originally stable pseudarthrosis may later become virtually flail (Hurri et al 1964, Dickson et al 1976). The more recently developed distraction arthroplasty (Volkov and Organesian 1975, Deland et al 1983, Morrey 1990 and 1993) may go some way to solving these problems, and consequently may well become the treatment of choice in manual workers in whom the durability of fixation of any total replacement of the elbow must be highly suspect. In patients who do *not* have to undertake significant manual work it seems worthwhile exploring the potential of total joint replacement for restoring pain-free movement coupled with stability.

To date, severe rheumatoid erosion has been by far the most common indication for total elbow replacement. Although such disease is not infrequently accompanied by *moderate* restriction of movement, very severe loss of movement or complete ankylosis of the elbow is relatively uncommon. In consequence, complete loss of elbow movement has until recently been an uncommon indication for elbow replacement. Now that interest is growing in the application of total elbow replacement to other pathologies however, gross restriction of movement or frank ankylosis is being more commonly encountered. Over the past 20 years, the author's own Unit in Edinburgh has dealt with 17 patients (four in the first decade, and 13 in the second) in whom an elbow has become totally ankylosed (13 cases), or the range of movement has been less than 10° (four cases). A breakdown of the underlying pathology of these elbows is provided in Table 1.

It must be appreciated that in many of these cases the underlying pathology may affect other joints in the upper limb and hence any attempt at remobilization of the elbow may have to be undertaken as part of a programme of reconstructive surgery for the upper limb as a whole.

Operative technique

Where the collateral ligaments remain functionally sound, the operative technique, even in the presence of complete bony ankylosis, does not differ materially from that of the standard procedure. Exposure of the elbow may be carried out by the Wadsworth (1979) or Gschwend (1991) approach,

Table 1 Underlying pathology in the 17 ankylosed elbows in present series

Rheumatoid arthritis	5
Juvenile chronic arthritis	4
Post-traumatic arthritis	4
Post-traumatic myositis ossificans	2
Infection	1
Synovial chondromatosis	1

following which the ulna and adherent trochlea, the floor of the olecranon fossa and the inner margins of the supracondylar ridges are resected *en bloc* from the humerus. Thereafter the trochlea is carved from the ulna so as to recreate a trochlear notch (Fig. 1). Next the operation proceeds as normal with excavation of the supracondylar ridges to accommodate the stirrup of the humeral component, and of the olecranon and proximal ulna for the ulnar component. If rotation is still grossly limited, resection of the ulnar head may be necessary. Obviously any radioulnar synostosis will also require resection. Where there has been very long-standing loss of

rotational movement in the forearm, tightness of the interosseus membrane may cause permanent reduction in rotational movement.

In post-traumatic cases one may encounter distortion of the supracondylar ridges to a greater or lesser degree. Where reasonably accurate reduction has been achieved at the time of the original injury, it may still be possible to burr out a channel for the insertion of the implant. In grossly comminuted cases, however, the surgeon should not attempt to be too clever in this regard. The excessive scarring surrounding such severely comminuted injuries may preclude a satisfactory return of movement. In these

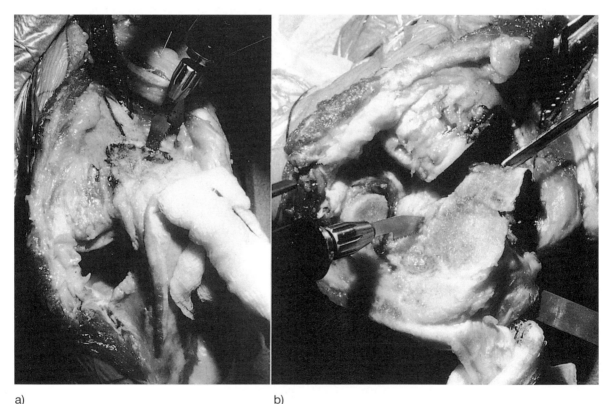

a)   b)

Figure 1

(a) Posterior view of elbow showing first stage of mobilization of bony ankylosis. The trochlea and floor of the olecranon fossa are being cut from the surrounding supracondylar ridges with a reciprocating microsaw. (b) View of ulna and ankylosed trochlea in profile. The radial head has already been removed and the stump of the radius is seen on the left just behind the microsaw. The latter is now being used to cut the trochlea from the ulna and recreate a trochlear notch.

circumstances it may be better to resect the whole of the distorted condylar mass and to have recourse to the extra long-stemmed snapfit variant of our prosthesis.

In cases resulting from juvenile chronic arthritis (JCA), complete bony ankylosis is very likely to have occurred. Moreover, there may be major growth disturbance with a relatively disproportionate development of the condyles in relation to extremely slender humeral or ulnar diaphyses. Careful preoperative assessment is required to ensure that the stirrup of our standard prototype can be accommodated within the distorted anatomy of the supracondylar ridges of the humerus. Particular attention must also be paid to the dimensions of the junctional area between the metaphysis and diaphysis of both humerus and ulna. Where it is clear on measured films that accommodation of the standard joint is not possible, a custom-built implant may be required. Alternatively, in some cases, the long stemmed model of our humeral component may be found to be more easily inserted than the standard stirrup model. Contrary to what has been suggested by Figgie et al (1989), it has been our experience that in cases of bony ankylosis arising from JCA, the ligaments are likely to be remarkably normal, so that reconstruction with an unlinked joint remains perfectly feasible. Where a linked implant is felt to be necessary, the snapfit model of our own prosthesis is likely to prove too massive, and in these cases the Stanmore, Gschwend or Morrey joints may provide very useful alternatives.

In the case of myositis ossificans, the ligaments are usually involved in the ossification process. Hence instability is likely to result if an unlinked implant is inserted. In these cases a linked joint should always be available, and in both cases in the present series where myositis ossificans was the underlying pathology, the snapfit model of our prosthesis was indeed used.

Series data

Of the 17 cases in the present series, one rheumatoid patient has been totally lost to follow-up. Full prospective data are available on the other 16 patients. This group comprises 10 female and six male patients. The age range was from 17 to 53 years (mean 37 years, standard deviation 10).

Type of prosthesis used

The standard unlinked versions of our prosthesis were used in 12 of the 16 cases. In only four cases was the linked snapfit version required, i.e. in both cases arising from myositis ossificans and in one each of the juvenile arthritic and trauma groups.

Results

Two of the 16 patients need to be dealt with separately from the rest of the series because of the peculiar nature of their pathology.

The first is an Iranian patient suffering from a very severe war injury of his forearm. Gross bone loss from both radius and ulna had been associated with major infection which had spread to involve the elbow joint resulting in total bony ankylosis. Reconstruction of the forearm had necessitated the conversion of the forearm to a single bone structure using a vascularized fibular graft. Hence any return of forearm rotation was impossible, the forearm being permanently fixed in 5° of pronation. Nevertheless, total elbow replacement undertaken 2 years after his injury and using a standard implant resulted in very satisfactory restoration of elbow movement which, at his last follow-up 3 years after surgery, was being maintained through an arc from 37° to 120°.

The second case is a young 23-year-old woman presenting with synovial chondromatosis complicated by severe arthritis of the elbow and total loss of movement. Following total joint replacement this elbow behaved quite differently from any other elbow arthroplasty in the author's experience, the joint very rapidly re-ankylosing once more and leaving the patient with little more than a jog of movement measuring certainly not more than 5°. It is of interest that histological examination of material removed at surgery suggested malignant change in the loose bodies. Fortunately the patient so far remains well 7 years after surgery.

The remaining 14 patients (four rheumatoid, four with JCA, four with post-traumatic arthritis and two with myositis ossificans following trauma) form a sufficiently homogeneous group with regard to the presenting problem and subsequent results as to warrant analysis en bloc.

Pain status before and after surgery (Table 2)

Table 2 Results in cases arising from rheumatoid arthritis, juvenile chronic arthritis, trauma and myositis ossificans

Pain Status	Preoperative	1 year	Final follow-up*
None	7	9	9
Occasional twinges	–	1	3
Mild	1	1	–
Moderate	2	1	1
Severe	4	2	1

*Follow-up was 17 months to 17 years, mean 8 years, SD5

Prior to surgery seven patients with total ankylosis of the joint had no pain. One patient was experiencing mild pain and six had moderate to severe pain. Postoperatively at the most recent follow-up (17 months to 17 years, mean 8 years, SD 5) 12 of the 14 patients had either no pain or only occasional twinges. One rheumatoid patient was still complaining of moderate pain and one of the post-traumatic group alleges that he has severe pain though no obvious cause for this can be identified.

Movement before and after surgery

The recovery of movement is set out in Table 3, and it is particularly gratifying that from a mean preoperative range of only 2°, the group as a whole achieved a mean arc of 73° at final follow-up.

Table 3 Results in cases arising from rheumatoid arthritis, juvenile chronic arthritis, trauma and myositis ossificans

	Mean movement (degrees)		
	Preoperative	1 year	Final follow-up[1]
Extension (flexion deformity)	69	56	61
Flexion	71	127	134
Range	2	71	73
Pronation	44	54	49
Supination	9	45	41

[1] As in Table 2.

Moreover, the mean flexion was restored to 134° which is likely to prove of immense value to patients in the activities of daily living. It is also noticeable that there was a very worthwhile gain in supination, which again should greatly facilitate personal care and hygiene.

Results in individual pathological groups

Rheumatoid patients

Of the four rheumatoid patients on whom data are available, the one who was completely devoid of movement in the elbow at the time of surgery had no pain preoperatively. However, the other three patients were suffering from severe pain. At the time of their most recent follow-up (average 11 years), two of the four patients were entirely painfree, one had occasional twinges of pain and one had been left with only moderate pain. This patient also had a somewhat disappointing result with regard to restoration of extension and is currently awaiting a further arthrolysis.

The preoperative range of movement in this group varied from 0° to 10° with a mean of 5.5°. Postoperatively at 1 year, the flexion deformity varied from 50° to 80°, and the range of flexion from 135° to 155°. This gave a postoperative range of movement of 50–105° (mean 76°). This situation was essentially maintained or perhaps slightly improved at the final follow-up examinations at 2, 6, and 17 × 2 years for the four patients respectively (Table 4).

Cases arising from JCA

In this group bony ankylosis was complete and all cases were painfree prior to surgery. Fortunately, after remobilization recurrence of pain was not a problem, all four patients still being painfree at the most recent follow-up (17 months, 2, 15 × 2 years – mean 8.4 years respectively).

The fused position of the elbow preoperatively varied from 20° through 60° and 68° to 80° (mean 57°). Postoperatively a very valuable arc of movement was re-established in all cases, i.e. 93°, 65°, 108° and 76°, respectively (mean 86° at final follow-up) (Table 4) (Fig. 2).

One of the cases is of particular interest in that

Table 4 Mean ranges of movement (degrees) before and after surgery in the different subgroups of the series

	Rheumatoid arthritis (4 cases)		Juvenile chronic arthritis (4 cases)		Trauma (4 cases)		Myositis ossificans (2 cases)		Infection after previous trauma (1 case)		Synovial chondromatosis (malignant) (1 case)	
	Preoperative	Final review (11 years)[1]	Preoperative	Final review (8 years)[1]	Preoperative	Final review (6.5 years)[1]	Preoperative	Final review (8 years)[1]	Preoperative	Final review (3 years)[1]	Preoperative	Final review (7 years)[1]
Extension (flexion deformity)	84	68	57	45	63	71	75	63	82	37	60	88
Flexion	89	147	57	130	64	126	75	133	82	120	60	93
Range	5.5	79	0	86	1	55	0	71	0	83	0	5
Pronation	58	64	64	58	31	46	2.5	10	5	5[2]	40	0
Supination	4.5	50	0.5	28	26	55	0	20	–5	–5	50	10

[1] Mean length of follow-up for each group; [2] One bone forearm.

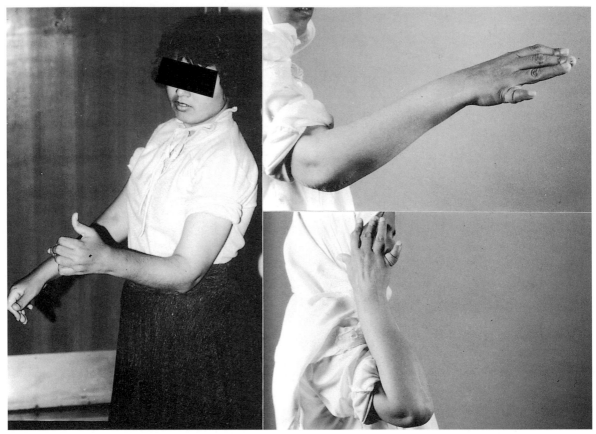

a)

b)

c)

Figure 2

(a) Preoperative problem in a 17-year-old Arab girl who, as a result of juvenile chronic arthritis, has her right elbow ankylosed at 20° and her left at 78°. (b, c) The recovery of movement in the right elbow following arthroplasty; 66–142°. Follow-up: 15 years.

initially the postoperative movement was fairly limited, i.e. 30–70°. Following excision of scar tissue and a V–Y lengthening of the triceps tendon undertaken 10 months after the original arthroplasty, the range of movement was increased to 108° (25–133° arc in absolute figures).

In both the rheumatoid and juvenile arthritic groups, pronation had been fairly well preserved preoperatively in marked constrast to supination which had been very deficient (mean figures for the two groups 4.5° and 0.5°, respectively). Postoperatively however, a marked gain in supina-

tion was achieved, the final follow-up means being 50° and 28°, respectively (Table 4).

Cases resulting from post-traumatic arthritis

In these patients, although no measurable movement persisted in any of the four cases, presumably micromovement was still present as all four were experiencing some pain, two severely.

Postoperatively at final review, one had no pain, and two had only occasional twinges. One patient, however, still complained of severe pain although no cause for this has ever been apparent.

The recovery of movement in this group, though not quite as favourable as in the patients suffering from inflammatory arthritides, was still very much worthwhile, the preoperative ranges in the individual patients changing from 5° in one patient and 0° × 3 in the other three, to 96°, 43°, 44° and 38° in these same cases individually (mean 55°) at their latest follow-up (3, 7 and 8 × 2 years respectively – mean 6.5). The recovery of flexion was not quite as good as in the other groups, but the main cause for the reduced arc of movement relative to the rheumatoid cases was a failure to achieve a gain in extension. Very satisfactory recovery of pronation and supination was obtained (Table 4).

Cases resulting from myositis ossificans following trauma

With this duo, the ossification process involved not only the elbow but also the superior radioulnar joint so that in addition to the complete ankylosis of the elbow joint itself, pronation and supination had been totally lost. It is of interest that surgery proved more successful in achieving restoration of elbow movement than of pronation and supination (Table 4), one case once more reforming a synostosis, while the other required re-operation to finally establish pronation of 20° and supination of 40°.

Complications

Three ulnar palsies occurred over the series as a whole. In the case resulting from infection, temporary paraesthesiae in the ulnar nerve distribution were experienced immediately after surgery, but this problem resolved completely after 6 months. The other two cases occurred in the post-trauma group. This is perhaps not surprising as the ulnar nerve in such patients is frequently found to be incorporated in dense scar tissue resulting from the original trauma and an extensive neurolysis may be required. In fact, one of these patients had evidence of an ulnar nerve palsy from the time of his original injury 2 years previously.

Comments and conclusions

In 1989, Figgie et al reported favourably on a series of 19 semiconstrained total elbow replacements in 16 patients suffering from complete ankylosis of the elbow. The prostheses used included four Pritchard-Walker, seven triaxial, and eight custom-built linked implants. Postoperatively the average flexion achieved was 115°, the extension 35° and the combined supination and pronation 95°. Of these, 15 were regarded as excellent or good results and all patients had relief of pain and improved function.

The results reported in the present paper substantiate the conclusions of these authors that total replacement arthroplasty has an excellent chance of providing very worthwhile and painfree remobilization of ankylosed elbows with all the attendant advantages of improved function.

All 16 patients in this series, either because of relief of pain or restoration of movement and function, aver that in the light of their experience and if the clock could be put back and they were once again in the position of making a decision for or against surgery, they would indeed opt for surgery.

Because of the good residual bone stock and the preservation of potentially functional ligaments, reconstruction with unlinked prostheses is likely to be perfectly feasible. Indeed our experience suggests that linked prostheses are likely to be necessary only in cases resulting from myositis ossificans.

It is always a matter of some concern when dealing with patients who are pain-free and who are only complaining of loss of movement, that any operative intervention might precipitate a painful joint. The results in the present series would suggest that this risk is very minimal. Although five patients did have some pain postoperatively, three of them were only experiencing occasional twinges while the fourth had much less pain than before surgery. Only one patient registered the same level of pain as that experienced preoperatively. Moreover, none of the patients who were pain-free prior to surgery have suffered pain as a result of their operation. It must be emphasized, however, that these favourable conclusions are for non-manual workers. As was stressed earlier, because of the risk of early loosening of an implant, excision or distraction arthroplasty may be the only advisable treatment in patients undertaking significant manual work.

The role of re-operation or of staged surgery in

these ankylosed joints deserves further study. There is no doubt that two of our patients in the present series gained quite appreciably from a second intervention, and a third patient with major restriction of extension is awaiting an arthrolysis. In this connection, it is of interest that Figgie et al (1989) resorted to postoperative manipulation under anaesthesia in five of their cases and achieved an increase in the range of elbow movement from a pre-manipulated mean of 35° to a post-manipulated mean of 90°.

The disappointing results for the restoration of pronation and supination in patients with myositis ossificans involving the superior radioulnar joint indicate that the restoration of forearm rotation and of elbow function should possibly be addressed at separate procedures. Certainly the results of attempting the restoration of both functions through a single operative procedure has proved very disappointing for improving forearm rotation. There might therefore be a case for attempting the restoration of forearm rotation in the first instance by an operative procedure involving excision of any synostosis and removal of the head of the radius and of the annular ligament where this has been partially or completely converted to bone. Temporary insertion of a silastic membrane and/or temporary separation of the bone surfaces through the insertion of a cortical screw as in the Brady and Jewett (1960) technique might also be worth trying. Once forearm rotation hopefully had been re-established, replacement arthroplasty of the elbow itself could be undertaken as a secondary procedure.

References

Brady LP, Jewett EL (1960) A new treatment of radioulnar synostosis, *South Med J* **53**:507.

Deland JT, Walker PS, Sledge CB, Farberov A (1983) Treatment of post-traumatic elbows with a new hinge-distractor, *Orthopaedics* **6**:732.

Dickson RA, Stein H, Bentley G (1976) Excision arthroplasty of the elbow in rheumatoid disease, *J Bone Jt Surg* **58B**:227–9.

Figgie MP, Inglis AE, Mow CS, Figgie HE (1989) Total elbow arthroplasty for complete ankylosis of the elbow, *J Bone Jt Surg* **71A**:513–20.

Gschwend N (1991) The case for a linked elbow prosthesis. In Hämäläinen M, Hagena FW, eds. *Rheumatoid Arthritis, Surgery of the Elbow, Rheumatology*, Vol. 15. Karger: Basel: 98–112.

Hurri L, Pulkki T, Vainio K (1964) Arthroplasty of the elbow in rheumatoid arthritis, *Acta Chir Scand* **127**:459–65.

Knight RA, Van Zandt IL (1952) Arthroplasty of the elbow. An end result study, *J Bone Jt Surg* **34A**:610–18.

Morrey BF (1990) Post-traumatic contracture of the elbow. Operative treatment, including distraction arthroplasty, *J Bone Jt Surg* **72A**:601–18.

Morrey BF (1993) Distraction arthroplasty. Clinical applications, *Clin Orthop* **293**:46–54.

Volkov MV, Organesian OV (1975) Restoration of function in the knee and elbow with a hinge-distractor apparatus, *J Bone Jt Surg* **57A**:591–600.

Wadsworth TG (1979) A modified postero-lateral approach to the elbow and proximal radio-ulnar joint, *Clin Orthop* **144**:151–3.

21

The GSB III elbow prosthesis

Norbert Gschwend, Hans-Kaspar Schwyzer, Beat R Simmen and Jochen F Loehr

Summary

Bony ankylosis of the elbow or severe restriction of ROM (range of motion) of this joint is mostly a sequel of extensive joint destruction with incongruency of the joint surfaces. Rheumatoid arthritis (RA) and post-traumatic conditions (intra-articular fractures or fracture dislocations) are by far the most frequent causes. Artificial joint replacement seems to be the treatment of choice for such conditions. Sloppy hinges with an inbuilt stability offer, compared to non-linked resurfacing prostheses, the advantage of allowing a more extensive soft tissue release without jeopardizing stability. Moreover, it seems easier in such cases to obtain a good ROM with a monoaxial construction.

Our experience with artificial elbow replacement is limited to the use of the GSB III elbow joint, a sloppy hinge device which we have used for 18 years in about 250 cases. In this study the results of GSB III arthroplasty in 20 ankylosed (0–40°) elbows due to inflammatory joint destruction, and 12 with post-traumatic stiffness, are presented. In all cases a marked improvement of the ROM was obtained. With few exceptions the movement was pain-free. Only one case of aseptic loosening was present, but this was due to factors not related to the procedure. Revisions were rare, and concerned the limitation of motion due to ectopic bone formation. An average follow-up of up to 8 years, the longest reaching 15 years, underlines the stability of the results obtained.

GSB III elbow arthroplasty is therefore a very reliable procedure for stiff elbow joints with a survival rate of more than 90%, 10 years postoperatively.

Indication

Independence for most daily activities requires a ROM of 100° of flexion–extension and approximately the same degree of motion for pronation and supination (Morrey and Bryan 1985). As long as the joint surface are congruent with an intact cartilage surface, it is possible to try to improve motion through an arthrolysis. Once the joint surfaces have been destroyed, an arthrolysis will only give short-lived relief, since contractures will most likely redevelop. It is in these cases that a total joint arthroplasty is indicated. Most cases will be patients with rheumatoid arthritis or post-traumatic arthrosis of the elbow. In many instances RA is a more urgent indication than the post-traumatic cases, since in RA patients a bilateral affection of the upper extremity is not uncommon, leaving the patient even more dependent on a functional joint. In our own study we could demonstrate that 85% of the RA patients will still have retained a ROM of approximately 110°, despite severe destruction of the elbow joint before seeking the attention of a rheumatoid surgeon. Assistance is sought if the degree of flexion has become reduced to less than 90–100°, or a severe instability with persistent pain forces the patient to look for help. It seems quite likely that the necessity to use the upper extremity for eating is the main cause for maintaining a residual elbow flexion, despite a quite advanced joint destruction.

The *definition of elbow stiffness* can therefore be expressed either in an anatomic way, or can be seen from a functional point of view. Mechanically, elbow stiffness describes the inability to move the elbow in flexion–extension or in pronation–supination. Functional stiffness is an elbow flexion which can not achieve 90°, thereby denying the patient any function for daily activities.

In contrast, even a severe limitation of extension will not cause a similar degree of functional loss. One can therefore conclude that to achieve a ROM of 100° which, as previously mentioned, is required for daily activities, one will need a flexion of 130–140° and can accept an extension deficit of −30 to −40°. Therefore a success in therapy can be achieved by moving the arc of ROM into the direction of improved flexion. We use these criteria to judge success in the treatment of 'stiff' elbow for our patient collective.

Joint arthroplasty

Numerous joint arthroplasties for the elbow are available today to the orthopaedic surgeon. In principle, one differentiates between two construction principles: *linked* or *non-linked* prostheses.

- linked: constrained or semiconstrained (sloppy hinges); all have stems
- non-linked: non-constrained or semiconstrained; with or without stem.

Hinged joints will either be fully constrained or they may allow a certain give between the two components, therefore being designated a so-called 'sloppy hinge' or semiconstrained device. Today the fully constrained hinges have only few indications due to the high degree of loosening found in the past. They are only used for massive tumors where the patient has a decreased life expectancy, to allow bridging of larger bony resections. A sloppy hinge will have a motion of approximately 4–8° between the two components allowing transfer of the forces in a dissipating way. The connection of the components can be constructed in various ways: either a snap-in mechanism with a metal polyethylene construct (Pritchard 1981, Risung 1995), or an ulnar component fitted loosely to a rotating axis of the humeral component (Dee 1969, Schlein 1976, Inglis 1995, O'Driscoll and Morrey 1995, etc.). A further development is a tilting extension to the distal humeral component which will then be fitted loosely into an ulnar pin, thereby allowing rotation as well as flexion–extension in a sloppy hinge mechanism (GSB III) (Gschwend et al 1988).

The other type of prostheses are so called *resurfacing prostheses* with varying degrees of anatomic resurfacing which act in a non-constrained way

(Kudo 1985, Roper et al 1986). Although the surface of the prosthetic components are kept smooth without any restriction to a gliding motion, they will still exert a certain strain on the elbow, depending on the loads applied to the surfaces by varying positions of flexion and extension. Anatomic configuration surfaces such as the Souter–Strathclyde (Souter 1987) or the Capitello-condylar-prosthesis after Ewald et al (1993) have tried to imitate the human anatomy. Here it becomes obvious that the contoured surfaces will increase the constraint even more, leading to larger shear forces in the interface between the bone and the prosthesis. It is obvious that more constrained prostheses will require additional support to act against these stresses by utilizing a medullary stem for additional anchoring, while the more smooth prostheses of a non-constrained type, except for the uncemented Kudo (1995) prosthesis, will try to do without this. The advantage of medullary anchoring systems becomes obvious when one is trying to reconstruct more damaged joints, such as might be the case in a post-traumatic arthrosis.

When comparing the different types of prostheses and the indication for their use, Goldberg et al (1988) came to the following conclusions in an article on current concepts of elbow arthroplasty:

'In RA results of sloppy hinges and resurfacing prostheses are very similar. However, resurfacing implants require the presence of intact metaphyseal bone and collateral ligaments. They are not satisfactory for patients with deficient bone stock or soft tissue or substantial flexion contracture. Sloppy hinges in elbows have for posttraumatic arthritis more predictable results than resurfacing prostheses.'

Therefore the authors draw the following conclusion from their analysis:

'Prostheses have to provide loading to the metaphyseal bone of the humerus and ulna by the use of metaphyseal configurations or by an anterior flange at the distal part of the humerus. The advantage of these prostheses would be: they allow torsional loads to be applied to the metaphyseal bone. The fatigue lifes of such prostheses are theoretically superior to those of other prostheses.'

The GSB III prosthesis (Fig. 1) is such a sloppy hinge. Ten years before the publication of the above-mentioned article, we designed this prosthesis with metaphyseal configurations on the distal and anterior part of the humeral condyles. We always try to maintain the bone stock and in a defect, attempt a reconstruction (Gschwend 1981 and 1990, Gschwend et al 1995). Our surgical technique is also different from that used with other prosthetic implants. The incision preserves the continuity of the extensor mechanism by splitting it in the middle, and by elevating it with thin bone slivers to the radial and ulnar side from the olecranon and the proximal ulna using a sharp chisel. This allows an easy transosseous reinsertion at the end of the procedure. The ulnar nerve has to be exposed and will be mobilized to its first muscular branch. In a few cases it will need to be transposed. Specially designed instruments, following the principles well established in knee arthroplasty, allow for a reproducible and exact implantation of the prosthetic components by defining the positioning for rotation as well as allowing an optimal fit between bone and prosthetic surfaces. The prosthesis has three sizes available for the humeral component which can be mated with four versions for the ulnar component.

Our patient collective

Between 1978 and the end of 1993, 197 GSB III elbow joints were implanted (Table 1):

155 were placed into the rheumatoid patient collective with
144 adult onset rheumatoid arthritis disease
  9 juvenile rheumatoid arthritis
  1 psoriatic arthritis
  1 Reiter's disease.

a)

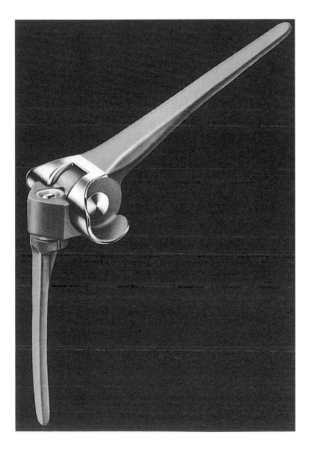

b)

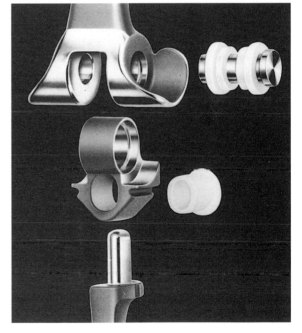

Figure 1

The GSB III elbow prosthesis, a sloppy hinge with flanges resting on the preserved or reconstructed humeral condyles with two anterior and distal flanges. HDP bushes guarantee the low friction principle.

Table 1 GSB III elbow prosthesis: 1978–93 (n = 197)

	No. of patients	Type
Rheumatoid arthritis	155	9 juvenile arthritis 1 psoriasis arthritis 1 Reiter's disease
Osteoarthritis	42	37 post-traumatic 5 non-traumatic

In 42 cases an arthrosis was the underlying indication for arthroplasty implantation with:

35 being post-traumatic lesions with intra-articular fractures
 2 with non-unions of the distal humerus
 3 for ankylosis of various history
 2 primary arthrosis with a non-traumatic history.

Of the rheumatoid patient collective, 129 patients were female (83.23%), whereas in the post-traumatic arthrosis 47.62% were female, the larger part of this group being male (52.38%). The average age in the group of rheumatoid arthritis was 56.3 years (20–81 years), whereas in the arthrotic group it was 50.9 years (23–81 years).

For the study presented here, out of this total collective only those patients which either had a complete ankylosis or a ROM of less than 40° were selected for review (Table 2). The total collective consists of 20 cases from the rheumatoid group as well as 15 patients from the post-traumatic group. In the first group 16 patients were female with four

males; in five cases a GSB III prosthesis was implanted bilaterally. In these cases only the side with less than 40° of ROM was included in the study. The age at operation varied between 30 and 83 years with a mean of 50.6 years. The average follow-up was 6.5 years (range 14 months–15 years). One patient of this collective had suffered a complete ankylosis as a sequel to joint infection after an intra-articular injection 11 years prior to arthroplasty. Three patients out of this collective (two female, one male) have since died due to unrelated causes. The follow-up time for these patients was 3, 4 and 14 years, respectively.

Of the 15 patients with post-traumatic destructed elbow joints, seven were female and eight were male. The average age was 47.8 years (range 24–66 years). In nine cases a distal intra-articular fracture resulted in the ankylosis with two patients suffering this injury as children. In three cases a fracture dislocation was the cause, one due to a distal humeral fracture and two due to forearm fractures. Two fractures were open fractures, and in two cases a polytrauma was associated with the injury. Two males of this collective have since died, and two further male patients were lost to follow-up having come from abroad for their surgery. One female patient suffering from a psychiatric disorder did not wish to be reviewed. Therefore, these last three patients were excluded from the study since no recent patient data were available. Therefore this collective consisted of 12 cases (Table 2) with six males and six females. The average age at surgery was 46.9 years with an average follow-up of 97.6 months or 8.1 years (range 40–177 months). In the cases of the two patients who died, the follow-up had been 36 and 6 months respectively.

Table 2 Ankylosed elbows (0–40°)

	No. of patients	Sex		Average age (range)	Follow-up (range)
		Female	Male		
Rheumatoid arthritis	20	16	4	50.6 years (30–83 years)	6.5 years (14 months–15 years)
Osteoarthritis	12	6	6	46.9 years (24–62 years)	97.6 months or 8.1 years (6 months–14.7 years)

The operative technique and postoperative management

This is essentially the one used for other indications besides ankylosed elbows. The patient is placed in a lateral position, the arm is bent at a right angle on a padded support, and a sterile tourniquet is applied. A slightly radially curved dorsal skin incision over the olecranon is used. Our own transtricipital approach preserves the continuity of the extensor mechanism and detaches it with thin bone slivers from the olecranon and proximal ulna using a sharp chisel thus allowing transosseous refixation at the end of the operation. Moreover, it provides us with an excellent view, which is particularly important when extensive scar formation or bony bridges have to be removed in an ankylosed elbow. The ulnar nerve is translocated only exceptionally, but it is always inspected and mobilized up to the first muscular branch. The collateral ligaments may be severed on the distal half of its origin at the humerus and detached completely with a sharp chisel and thin bone slivers only in cases with severe limitation of movement (particularly extension) after implantation of the prosthesis. The highly sophisticated special instruments allow for an exact positioning of the prosthesis between the humeral condyles; the exact centre of the prosthesis should correspond as far as possible to the rotation centre of the normal elbow. Deficient humeral condyles are reconstructed, if necessary, using autogenous pelvic bone blocks as described by Gschwend (1983). The size of the components is defined with templates before surgery, both components are fixed with cement and assembled. In the case of important flexion or extension deficit, further soft tissue release (not further proximal positioning beyond the rotation centre of the humerus) may be necessary.

The postoperative treatment

Mobilization of the elbow usually starts on the fifth postoperative day. Assisted active flexion combined with pronation and supination and purely passive extension, must be performed two to three times daily for 1 week. The use of continuous passive motion (e.g. Kinetec machine) is advisable. Initially the flexion is only 90°, but after the third week it is advanced to 110°. If the wound is healing properly, flexion is free after the fourth week. Three weeks

after surgery, the flexion should become more active, but with passive support.

Continue the therapy as an outpatient. The exercises are designed to increase the strength, and the passive stretching is supposed to increase the range of extension. Furthermore, the flexion and extension exercises require increasing strength to build up the musculature. It is our goal to achieve an active extension equalling the passive extension after 4 weeks. Otherwise the stronger flexors cause an increasing active extension deficit.

Careful exercises at the wall bar help to strengthen the muscles and to increase the ROM by passive extension.

Important: the patient has to be instructed how to do these exercises and should perform them repeatedly for 5–10 minutes every day. These exercises should further increase the strength and ROM.

Occupational therapy is an important complement to physiotherapy. It can be started on 10–14 days postoperatively with the objective of increasing strength and ROM as in physiotherapy, but also to enhance co-ordination and dexterity.

Results of the GSB III arthroplasty in ankylosis

The results concerning pain and ROM is demonstrated for both collectives in Tables 3–6. The gain in ROM can be seen in Figs 2 and 3.

Results in the rheumatoid collective (n = 20)

Pain (Table 3). Nineteen of the 20 patients did not complain about any pain or had only mild residual discomfort. One patient, who subsequently died,

Table 3 Postoperative pain

Degree of pain	Rheumatoid arthritis ankylosis n = 20	Post-traumatic ankylosis n = 12
None	19	10
Mild, occasional	–	2
Moderate	1	–
Severe	–	–

suffered a fall on to the elbow and complained of local pain after years of utilizing a cane for relief of associated pain due to arthrosis of the weight-bearing joints. She is the only patient who also demonstrated a radiographic loosening, which was not revised in view of the advanced age of the patient (>80 years), the multiple joint affections, and a poor general state of health. This patient – as mentioned – has since died.

The *range of motion* (Table 4) measured on average 20° prior to surgery and improved postoperatively to 100°. In the two cases with the least postoperative ROM (55° and 60°), flexion improved the most (140° and 110° respectively), which improved the patients' ability to participate in the activities of daily life. One case was reoperated after a flexion contracture, but could not be improved. The postoperative result did not improve significantly and pronation–supination was also limited. One patient suffered a synostosis between radius and ulna.

Table 4   Range of motion

	Rheumatoid arthritis n = 20	Post-traumatic n = 12
Preoperative	20° (0–40°)	19° (0–40°)
Postoperative	100° (55–120°)	87.3° (65–125°)
Gain	80°	68°

The average *flexion* (Table 5) for the total collective including the fixed flexion deformity of the stiff elbow was 83° preoperatively (range 20–120°), and improved to 134° postoperatively (range 110–150°). The average extension deficit improved from

−72.5° preoperatively (range −10° to −100°) to −35° postoperatively (range −10° to −85°).

Pronation–supination was not correctly documented preoperatively in all cases. The needed postoperative pronation–supination measurement is missing for two patients. One has to be aware that in most rheumatoid patients the distal radial ulnar joint is severely affected and therefore responsible for the high variation of the pronation–supination values found in this collective. This will also explain the great difference between the postoperative values for pronation–supination in the rheumatoid and post-traumatic groups (Table 6).

Table 6   Postoperative pronation–supination

	Rheumatoid arthritis n = 18	Post-traumatic n = 10
Preoperative	?	81° (0–160°)
Postoperative	113.8° (0–180°)	150.5° (100–180°)

Activity daily living (ADL) function. Sixteen of the 20 rheumatoid patients were completely independent in their daily activities while the other four had limitations due to severe deformities of the hands or shoulder joints.

X-ray evaluation. The X-ray review was done with the preoperative and postoperative X-rays as well as the last X-ray at follow-up. Incomplete lucencies were found in two patients in the area of the humeral condyles. In two further patients a radiolucency was found in the proximal humerus, one in

Table 5   Flexion–extension

	Flexion		Extension	
	Rheumatoid arthritis n = 20	Post-traumatic n = 12	Rheumatoid arthritis n = 20	Post-traumatic n = 12
Preoperative	83°	74.5°	−72.5°	−63.6°
	(20–120°)	(60–110°)	(−10° to −100°)	(−30° to −80°)
Postoperative	134°	133.6	−35°	−39.1°
	(110–150°)	(105–145°)	(−10° to −35°)	(−20° to −75°)

the distal humerus. None of the lucencies was found to be progressive and none of the cases demonstrated a radiographic or clinical loosening. This is also true for the eight patients with surgery backdating 8–15 years.

Complications and revisions. Of the 20 patients in the rheumatoid group, one patient had to be revised due to an ossification at the olecranon tip. This was the patient who had suffered a complete ankylosis after an iatrogenic infection due to a local injection into the joint. At the time of surgery the ossifications were removed resulting in a ROM of 120° flexion and 10° extension deficit, the patient having returned to work. The second revision was done for a severe extension deficit in a rheumatoid patient. Although a secondary lengthening of the flexors as well as a complete ventral capsulotomy was per-

formed, the long-term result was a similar extension deficit of −85° after an initial improvement.

It should be mentioned that in the group of the 20 rheumatoid patients, 11 patients underwent surgery of the weight bearing joints of the hip and knee as well as arthrodeses in the feet. With this they were required to walk with the aid of canes and crutches for long periods, but without any ill effect becoming evident for the implanted elbow prostheses.

If one reviews our patient collective following the *classification* proposed by Morrey (total of 100 points: total of 60 for pain, total of 30 for movement and total of 10 for stability), 16 patients in the rheumatoid group achieved 96.8 points. This is a collective excluding the deceased patients as well as the patients living overseas, where the last control dated back more than 3 years.

a)

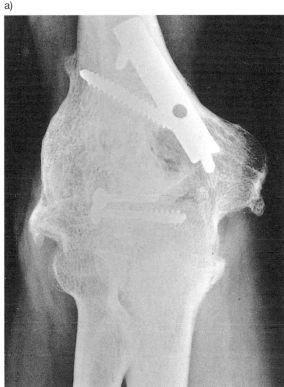

b)

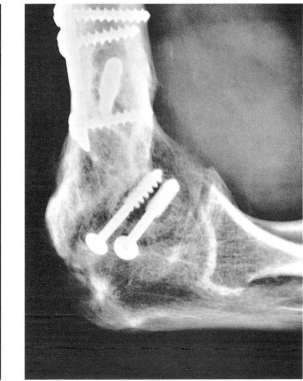

Figure 2

Example of a post-traumatic stiff elbow, having sustained a polytrauma with comminuted fracture of the distal humerus. After implantation of the GSB III prosthesis a useful range of motion has been obtained. The extension deficit is self-explanatory with all the scarring, the triceps damage and the dorsal approach for osteosynthesis and arthroplasty (see ossification at the tip of the olecranon).
(a, b) Preoperative ankylosis. Plate and screws still in place. (c, d) After GSB III arthroplasty. Excellent positioning of the prosthesis, excellent interface. Ossification at the proximal end of the olecranon limiting extension. (e) Clinical postoperative result with good flexion, (f) but with extension deficit.

c)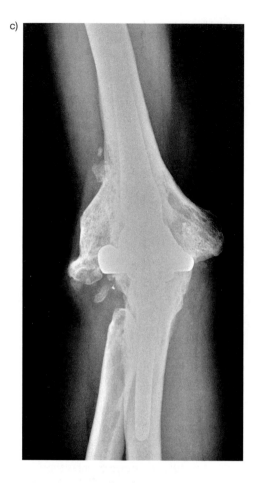

d)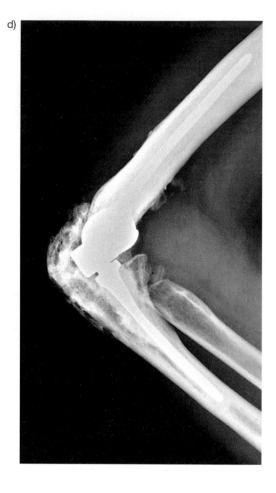

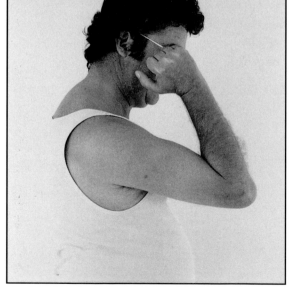 e)

f)

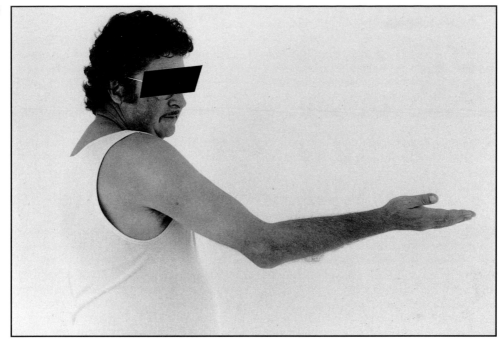

Subjective elevation. All living patients rated the results as excellent to good and would agree to the same surgery again.

Results with post-traumatic ankylosis (n = 12)

It seems important to mention that in the post-traumatic cases, eight cases had one and five cases had two previous surgeries performed prior to the implantation of the GSB III arthroplasty. In 10 cases an osteosynthesis had been performed two cases had a radial head resection, one case had a loose joint body removed, and in another a neurolysis of the ulnar nerve was performed (Fig. 2).

Pain (Table 3). Of the 12 post-traumatic cases available for follow-up, only two male manual labourers complained about pain with heavy work. All other patients considered themselves pain-free and, in comparison to the preoperative situation, much improved.

The *range of motion* (Table 4) was measured preoperatively as 19°. Postoperatively the average range of motion increased to 87.3°. The average flexion (Table 5) increased from preoperatively 74.5° (60–110°) to postoperatively 133.6° (105–145°). The average extension deficit was measured preoperatively as −63.6° (−30° to −80°) and improved to −39.1° (−20° to −75°) postoperatively.

As in the rheumatoid group, the pronation–supination was not in all cases recorded preoperatively. Therefore only the patients with values available pre- as well as postoperatively are included in this assessment. The ROM of pronation–supination increased from 81° (0–160°) preoperatively to 150.5° (100–180°) postoperatively. We feel that radial head resection which is done routinely with this procedure is mainly responsible for this improvement. It Is further fell that the much improved pronation–supination in the post-traumatic group is due to the non-involved distal radioulnar joint, which seems to be responsible for the poor motion in the rheumatoid patient collective.

ADL function. Except for one male patient, the ADL function was unimpaired for dressing, eating, combing, shaving and tying an apron, as well as for personal hygiene and touching the opposite shoulder. One patient stated partial inability to comb his own hair. None of the patients felt hampered due to elbow function during daily functions.

X-ray review. An area of lucency was found in only one female patient at the ulnar side which was incomplete and non-progressive; no other radiolucency was found. There was no radiographic loosening evident.

Complications. There were no early orthopaedic complications in this group, with one patient suffering a myocardial infarction but recovering well. Late complications were two heterotopic ossifications affecting two male manual labourers. One patient had suffered a supracondylar fracture at the age of 7 years leading to an ankylosis. The other patient had sustained a fracture dislocation of the elbow. In the first case a dorsal osseous bridge formed between the ulna and the humerus preventing flexion–extension, but not influencing pronation–supination. Prior to the implantation of the arthroplasty, flexion–extension measured 110°–45°–0°. A *revision* was performed 3.5 years after primary implantation giving the patient a range of motion of 120°–30°–0° which in the course of another two years diminished to a flexion of 110° with an extension deficit of −30°, and is now non-progressive. The second case in this group requiring *revision* was in a patient in which a bony prominence at the proximal radius had not been resected at the time of surgery, thereby impairing flexion as well as extension. The excision of this ossification was performed 5 months after the primary arthroplasty and resulted in a ROM of 130–40°, which has since been maintained.

Following the classification of Morrey (1990), all 10 post-traumatic cases which are still alive and available for follow-up could be classified as good (75–100 points). The average points awarded were 95.

Subjective evaluation. All patients reviewed expressed an excellent to good result which also included the two manual workers who complained about moderate to mild pain with heavy labour. All patients stated that they would undergo the same procedure again for the same condition.

Discussion

Our review presents two groups with severe ankylosis of the elbow and compares the results achieved to that of a general population receiving an elbow arthroplasty of the same model. One realizes that the results do not differ significantly. Pain relief could be obtained equally in the patients with RA as well as in those with post-traumatic ankylosis. In the general group, having received a GSB III arthroplasty, the ROM was 112°, the gain of the ROM postoperatively was 30° resulting in an average flexion of 139°. In those RA patients receiving an elbow arthroplasty for ankylosis, the average ROM became 100°, with a gain of 80°. The flexion achieved postoperatively reached 134°, being only 5° less than the flexion in the general group. The extension deficit postoperatively, which had improved from −72.5° to −35°, was only worse by 8° compared to the general collective. The ROM achieved in the post-traumatic group was 87.3°, which is only slightly less than that of the general group (96°). The extension deficit was slightly worse in the post-traumatic ankylosis group, being −39.1° versus −32° in the general collective, while in flexion an even better ROM was reached with 133.6° versus 128°.

The two groups presented here had a very low complication rate, with only two male patients suffering para-articular ossifications requiring revision. One of these cases already had heterotopic ossifications present preoperatively. After revision the ossification did not reoccur. While evaluating the X-ray films for loosening, one could also observe ossifications correlating to a Brooker type 1 stage (Brooker et al 1973) in the area of the dorsal approach, which might be responsible for shifting the ulnar peg slightly distally in some cases. We did not have any dislocations of the prosthetic components, with only one loosening present in a patient who had suffered a fall onto the elbow prosthesis. The loosening in this patient, who has since died from unrelated causes, was due to the fall and the stresses caused by the use of crutches because of her lower extremity involvement.

No infection was observed in this collective.

One is surprised at the high rate of success achieved with this surgery. There is no question that any fracture involving the articular surfaces of the elbow joint is best reconstructed in the most optimal anatomic way to achieve a good and long-lasting result. But it seems ill-fated to proceed with reconstructive measures after a malunited arthritic elbow has established itself, in view of the excellent results obtained by arthroplasty.

We feel that elbow arthroplasty has now established itself, in the same way as total hip or total knee arthroplasties have in the past, as an instrument allowing predictable success in over 90% of patients with proper indications. As we have seen from our past experience, it is an excellent tool for providing the patient with a pain-free and functional ROM allowing almost all the tasks of daily life to be performed.

References

Brooker AF, Bowemann JW, Robinson RH (1973) Ectopic ossification following THR, *J Bone Joint Surg* **55A**:1629–33.

Dee R (1969) Elbow arthroplasty, *Proc R Soc Med* **61**:103–5.

Ewald FC, Simmons ED, Sullivan JA, Thomas WH, Scott RD, Poss R, Thornhill TS, Sledge CB (1993) Capitello-condylar total elbow replacement in rheumatoid arthritis, *J Bone Joint Surg* **75A**:498–507.

Goldberg VM, Figgie HE III, Inglis AE, Figgie MP (1988) Current concepts review: total elbow arthroplasty, *J Bone Joint Surg* **70A**:778–83.

Gschwend N (1981) Our operative approach to the elbow joint, *Arch Orthop Traumatol Surg* **98**:143–6.

Gschwend N (1983) Salvage procedure in failed elbow prosthesis, *Arch Orthop Traumatol Surg* **101**:95–9.

Gschwend N, Loehr J, Ivosevic-Radovanovic D, Scheier H, Munzinger U (1988) Semiconstrained elbow prostheses with special reference to the GSB III prosthesis, *Clin Orthop* **232**:104–11.

Gschwend N (1990) Revision for failed elbow arthroplasty in rheumatoid arthritis. In: Hämäläinen M, Hagena FW, Schwägerl W, eds *Revisional Surgery in Rheumatoid Arthritis*, Vol. 13 *Rheumatology*. Karger: Basel: 70–82.

Gschwend N, Scheier H, Bähler A, Simmen B (1995) GSB III elbow. In: Rüther W, ed. *The Elbow*. Springer: Berlin: 83–98.

Inglis AE (1995) Elbow replacement arthroplasty for flail and ankylosed elbows. In: Rüther W, ed. *The Elbow*. Springer: Berlin: 99–110.

Kudo H (1985) Long-term follow-up study of total elbow arthroplasty with non-constrained prosthesis. In: Kashiwagi D, ed. *Elbow Joint. Proceedings of the International Seminar Kobe, Japan, Congress Series 678*. Excerpta Medica International: Amsterdam: 269–76.

Kudo H (1995) Cementless or hybrid total elbow arthroplasty – a study of interim clinical results and specific complications. In: Rüther W, ed. *The Elbow*. Springer: Berlin: 128–34.

Morrey BF, Bryan RS (1985) Total joint replacement. In: Morrey BF, ed. *The Elbow and its Disorders*. WB Saunders: Philadelphia: 546–69.

Morrey BF (1990) Posttraumatic contracture of the elbow. *J Bone Joint Surg* **72A**:601–18.

O'Driscoll SW, Morrey BF (1995) Coonrad–Morrey semiconstrained total elbow arthroplasty. In: Rüther W, ed. *The Elbow*. Springer: Berlin: 111–20.

Pritchard RW (1981) Long-term follow-up study: semiconstrained elbow. *Orthopedics* **4**:151–5.

Risung F (1995) The Norway elbow system. In: Rüther W, ed. *The Elbow*. Springer: Berlin: 121–7.

Roper BA, Tuke M, O'Riordan SM, Bulstrode CJ (1986) A new unconstrained elbow. A prospective review of 60 replacements, *J Bone Joint Surg* **68B**:566–9.

Schlein AP (1976) Semiconstrained total elbow arthroplasty, *Clin Orthop* **121**:222–9.

Souter WA (1987) Le traitement chirurgical du coude rhumatoide, *Cahiers d'enseignement de la SOFCOT. Conférences d'enseignement* **1**:159–72.

Part III
Wrist stiffness

22
Radiocarpal stiffness: introduction

Philippe Saffar

Every type of wrist pathology may lead to joint stiffness due to:

- joint malalignment
- cartilage destruction
- capsulo-ligamentous retraction
- intra-articular fibrosis.

Wrist stiffness may be of intra- or extra-articular aetiologies:

1 Intra-articular causes:
- degenerative
- post-traumatic
- postinfection
- congenital
- iatrogenic.

2 Extra-articular causes:

- tendinous adhesions after multiple and complex injuries or crush of the forearm, hand and wrist, mainly at the volar aspect of the wrist
- extensive burns mainly at the dorsal aspect of the distal upper limb
- muscular imbalance due to palsies or spasticity.

There is often a combination of extra- and intra-articular causes and a cautious preoperative examination associated with radiological investigations should differentiate these causes to allow the choice of the best treatment. The aim of all current orthopaedic practice is to regain motion and it is only when this is absolutely impossible that one has to perform an arthrodesis.

23

Radiocarpal joint: anatomy and biomechanics

Marc Garcia-Elias

In the past few years numerous investigations have been undertaken to study the functional complexities of the wrist joint. The goal of these studies was to accurately describe all the structures involved in wrist function and to identify and quantify anatomical predisposing factors that could explain the development of specific wrist pathologies. This chapter will review the findings of these investigations, in particular those emphasizing aspects of interest for the understanding of radiocarpal stiffness.

Anatomy

The radiocarpal joint consists of two elements: the antebrachial glenoid, formed by the distal articular surface of the radius in conjunction with the *discus articularis*, and the carpal condyle, formed by the convex articular facets of the proximal carpal row bones: scaphoid, lunate and triquetrum. The distal articular surface of the radius is biconcave and tilted in two planes. In the sagittal plane there is a slope of an average 10.2° palmar tilt, and in the frontal plane there is an ulnar inclination at an angle averaging 23.8° (Schuind et al 1996). The proximal joint surface of the scaphoid is more curved than that of the lunate (Kauer 1980, Boabighi et al 1988). Because of that, and to ensure articular congruency, the radius has two separated articular facets (scaphoid and lunate fossae), separated by a cartilaginous sagittal ridge, called the interfacet prominence (Berger and Landsmeer 1990, Berger et al 1991). The biconcave scaphoid fossa is triangular or oval-shaped and has a smaller radius of curvature than that of the lunate fossa. The latter is more or less rectangular in shape, also biconcave although shallower, and less inclined towards the ulnar side

than the scaphoid fossa (Boabighi et al 1988). The midcarpal joint is a combination of three different types of articulation. Laterally, the convex distal surface of the scaphoid articulates with the concavity formed by the trapezium, trapezoid and lateral aspect of the capitate. The central part of the midcarpal joint is concave proximally (scaphoid and lunate) and convex distally (head of the capitate, and sometimes the proximal pole of the hamate). The medial hamate–triquetral articulation is helicoid or screw-shaped in configuration (Weber 1984). Any alteration in the shape, orientation or surface smoothness of any one of these articular facets (radiocarpal or midcarpal) is likely to result in both incongruous motion of the overall proximal row and in abnormal stress concentration at specific points of the joint. If not corrected, these kinematic and kinetic changes will eventually induce progressive arthrosis and carpal stiffness (Knirk and Jupiter 1986). Especially important are the articular surfaces surrounding the scaphoid and lunate since they are the ones through which most of the load is transmitted (Schuind et al 1995).

The radiocarpal joint capsule is reinforced by obliquely oriented palmar and dorsal radio-ulno-carpal ligaments, the inner side of which appears resurfaced by synovial tissue (Berger and Landsmeer 1990, Siegel and Gelberman 1991). Unlike the ligaments of other articulations, the radiocarpal ligaments can be very seldom individualized. In general, they do not have clear-cut edges facilitating their differentiation from adjacent ligamentous structures. However, by analysing carefully the overall direction of the ligament bundles crossing the wrist, a number of ligament complexes with specific insertions and directions can be identified (Fig. 1). These ligamentous complexes can be classified into two categories: extrinsic and intrinsic (Cooney et al 1989) (Table 1). Extrinsic ligaments

a)

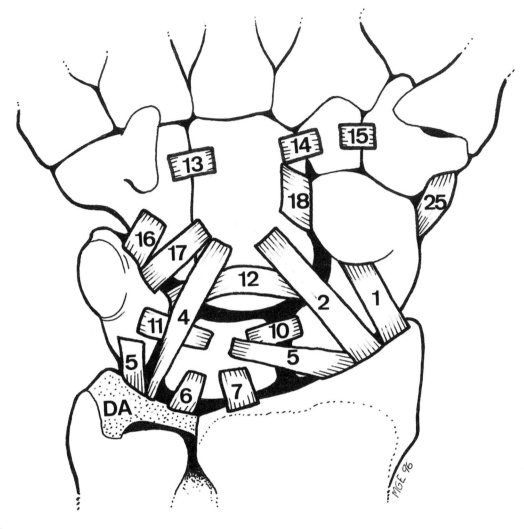

Figure 1

Schematic representation of the direction and major insertion points of the palmar (a) and dorsal (b) ligaments of the wrist, numbered as in Table 1. This figure does not represent the actual size and shape of these structures. DA, discus articularis.

are those that connect the forearm bones with the carpal bones, while intrinsic ligaments have both origin and insertion within the carpus. The intrinsic ligaments are short, stiff, and when injured, difficult to repair. By contrast, the extrinsic ligaments are longer, less stiff, and more easily repairable. Most of the stabilizing ligaments of the midcarpal joint are palmar or lateral (Cooney et al 1989). The dorsal capsule is more lax, and therefore more vulnerable to trauma, but also more exposed to any inflammatory disease affecting the adjacent extensor tendons and their corresponding synovial sheaths. Any disease or injury inducing an increased stiffness and retraction of the extrinsic ligaments usually results

b)

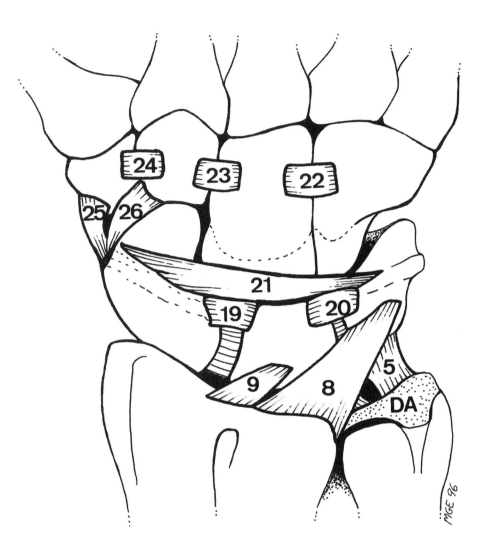

in a substantial restriction of the radiocarpal and/or midcarpal motion. By contrast, damage of the intrinsic ligaments usually does not result in stiffness but in a dissociative pattern of carpal instability.

In the radiocarpal joint, two constant synovial recesses, varying in size and shape, exist: the *recessus prestyloideus*, a synovial pouch located just palmar to the ulnar styloid process; and the *recessus prescaphoideus*, also known as interligamentous sulcus (Berger et al 1991), proximal and palmar to the scaphoid, between the long radiolunate and the radiocapitate ligaments. Between the

two deep ulnocarpal ligaments (ulnolunate and ulnotriquetral) frequently there is another synovial pouch, called *recessus pretriquetralis*. This synovial recess communicates with the pisotriquetral joint cavity in more than 30% of the population. Any disease or injury producing a chronic inflammation of these synovial structures may result in fibrosis formation with obliteration of these recesses. This may contribute to further joint stiffness.

Filling the gap between the medial non-articular aspect of the triquetrum and the joint capsule, there is a highly vascular, wedge-shaped synovial proliferation called the meniscus homologue (Taleisnik

Table 1 Ligamentous complexes of the radio-ulno-carpal joints

Category	Location	Bones connected[1]
Extrinsic	Palmar-superficial	Radius–scaphoid (1)
		Radius-capitate (2)
		Radius-lunate (long) (3)
		Ulna-capitate (4)
	Palmar-deep	Ulna-triquetrum (5)
		Ulna-lunate (6)
		Radius-lunate (short) (7)
		Radius-scaphoid-lunate[2]
	Dorsal	Radio-triquetrum (8)
		Radio-lunate (9)
Intrinsic	Palmar-intercarpal	Scaphoid-lunate (10)
		Lunate-triquetral (11)
		Triquetrum-scaphoid (12)
		Hamate-capitate (13)
		Capitate-trapezoid (14)
		Trapezoid-trapezium (15)
	Palmar-midcarpal	Triquetrum-hamate (16)
		Triquetrum-capitate (17)
		Scaphoid-capitate (18)
	Dorsal-intercarpal	Scaphoid-lunate (19)
		Lunate-triquetral (20)
		Triquetrum-scaphoid (21)
		Hamate-capitate (22)
		Capitate-trapezoid (23)
		Trapezoid-trapezium (24)
	Dorsal-midcarpal	Scaphoid-trapezium (25)
		Scaphoid-trapezoid (26)

[1] Number assigned in Fig. 1
[2] Probably not a true ligament (Berger and Landsmeer 1990)

et al 1984). This structure is continuous with the *discus articularis*, forming the roof of the prestyloid recess (Landsmeer 1976, Garcia-Elias and Domenech-Mateu 1987). The midcarpal articulation has an extensive synovial cavity including not only the interval between the two rows, but also the intervals between the bones of the two rows. Also at this level there exist synovial proliferations, which have a wedge-shaped meniscoid appearance, filling the triangular gap between the proximal and distal row bones. All these synovial structures may be the target of inflammatory systemic diseases with the consequent capsular retraction and loss of motion.

In normal subjects there should be no communication between the midcarpal and the radiocarpal joint cavities. When present, they must be regarded as either traumatic or degenerative age-related perforations. Mikic (1984) found a high incidence of scapholunate (43%) and lunotriquetral (55%) perfo-

rations among 109 wrist specimens older than 30 years. These perforations do not promote joint stiffness. By contrast, when these intercarpal joints are congenitally fused, motion may appear diminished, especially if fusion is extensive across the midcarpal joint (Delaney and Eswar 1992).

The pisotriquetral joint capsule has no supporting ligaments (Pevny et al 1995). It is a very lax structure allowing considerable motion of the pisiform during wrist motion. However, any local pathology resulting in fusion or loss of pisotriquetral motion has a secondary effect by diminishing the overall midcarpal motion.

Radiocarpal kinematics

The flexor carpi ulnaris is the only muscle inserting on the carpus. It attaches to the pisiform which, in its turn, is linked to the hamate by means of the pisihamatum ligament (Pevny et al 1995). All other wrist motor tendons are attached to the base of the metacarpals (Cooney et al 1989). The proximal carpal row bones are completely devoid of tendinous attachments. Therefore, contraction of any forearm muscle with a tendon crossing the wrist joint will generate a flexion–extension and/or a radial–ulnar deviation moment on the distal carpal row depending on the location of the tendon with respect to the centre of rotation of the carpus within the head of the capitate (An et al 1991). Unless constrained by any external force, such moments will result in motion starting always at the distal carpal row (Ruby et al 1988). The bones of the proximal row will start moving later when tightness of the ligaments crossing the midcarpal joint on the one hand, and compressive forces from the moving distal carpal bones on the other, reach a certain level (Lange et al 1990).

In normal wrists, very little intercarpal motion exists between the bones of the distal carpal row. From full flexion to extension, no more than 9° angular rotation between the bones of the distal row have been recorded by different authors (Ruby et al 1988, Sennwald et al 1993). The bones of the distal carpal row should be thought of as not a rigid structure, but as a single still functional unit. In flexion of the wrist, the bones all follow a rotation about an axis which obviously implies flexion, but also some degree of ulnar deviation. In extension the tendency of all distal carpal bones is to rotate into extension

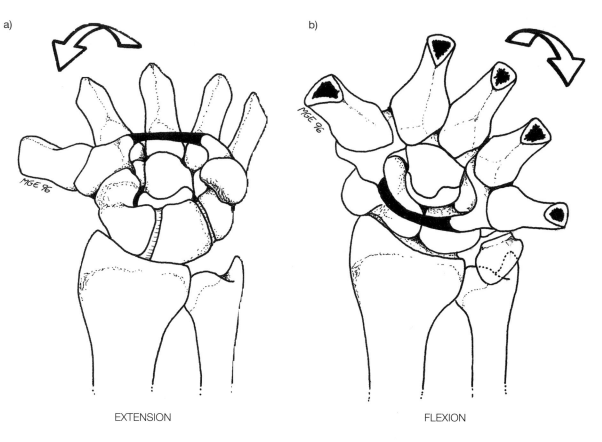

a)   b)

EXTENSION   FLEXION

Figure 2

Because of the oblique alignment of the scapho-luno-capitate joint, the unconstrained wrist extension usually implies a slight radial deviation of the distal carpal row relative to the proximal row (a) while wrist flexion usually involves some ulnar deviation (b).

with a slight radial deviation (Saffar and Semaan 1994) (Fig. 2). Because of the presence of stout interosseous ligaments between the distal carpal bones, the palmar concavity of the carpal tunnel changes little during flexion–extension of the wrist (Garcia-Elias et al 1992). The bones of the distal carpal row also move synergistically (in about the same direction) in lateral deviations of the wrist. In radial deviations of the wrist, they all radial-deviate, extend and supinate. In ulnar deviation, they flex, ulnar-deviate and pronate.

The bones of the proximal carpal row appear to be less tightly bound to one another than the bones of the distal carpal row (Ruby et al 1988, Sennwald et al 1993). Despite differences in angular rotation, however, all proximal carpal row bones move synergistically with wrist motion. Therefore, it is reasonable to consider the proximal carpal row as another functional unit, acting as an intercalated segment between the distal row and the radius (Landsmeer 1976).

According to different experiments, from full flexion to full extension of the wrist, the scaphoid has a larger amount of rotation than the lunate. This can be easily checked if one compares the relative alignment of these bones on lateral X-rays during

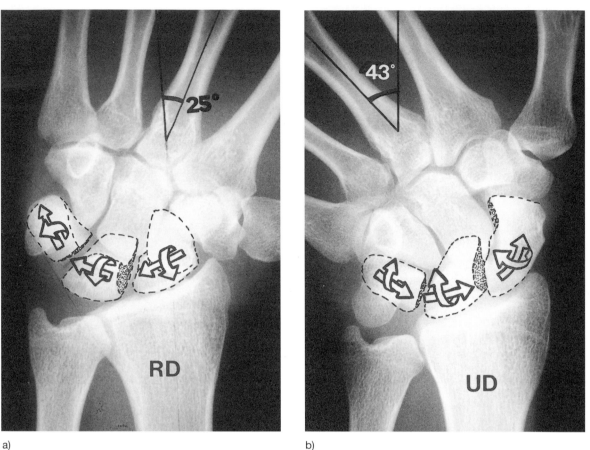

a)   b)

Figure 3

The proximal carpal row moves synergistically during wrist deviations. (a) When the wrist radial-deviates (RD) the three bones not only slide down towards the ulnar side but also rotate into flexion. (b) In contrast, wrist ulnar-deviation (UD) involves extension of the proximal row.

flexion–extension: the average scapholunate angle in full wrist flexion averages 76° while it reduces to 35° in full extension (Sarrafian et al 1977). The different radii of curvature of the proximal aspects of these bones may explain such differences in angular rotation (Kauer 1980).

The contribution of the midcarpal joint to normal wrist flexion–extension is also an interesting issue. If only the central part of the carpus (the capitate–lunate–radius linkage) is considered, the radiocarpal and midcarpal motion is equally divided in only one-third of the wrists. In the remaining two-thirds, approximately 60% of the global flexion occurs at the lunocapitate interval, while 66% of

extension is radiocarpal dependent (Sarrafian et al 1977, Garcia-Elias et al 1989). However, if motion is recorded on the lateral part (the radius–scaphoid–trapezium linkage), more than two-thirds of the global arc of movement occur at the radioscaphoid interval (Ruby et al 1988). According to that, a localized stiffness of the luno-capitate joint would result theoretically in a larger restriction of the global wrist motion than a stiff scapho-trapezial-trapezoidal joint.

During radioulnar deviation of the wrist, the three proximal carpal bones move synergistically from a flexed position in radial deviation to an extended position in ulnar deviation (Fig. 3) (Garcia-Elias et al

1989, Sennwald et al 1993). This flexion–extension adaptive mechanism, present in normal wrists, allows a constant spatial congruency between the distal carpal row and the radius no matter what wrist position is adopted. Any degeneration process secondary to injury or disease, having a direct effect on the mobility of the proximal carpal row, may prevent this adaptive mechanism and therefore block the possibility of the wrist being able to reach its maximum range of motion.

References

An KN, Horii E, Ryu J (1991) Muscle function. In: An KN, Berger RA, Cooney WP, eds. *Biomechanics of the Wrist Joint.* Springer Verlag: New York: 157–70.

Berger RA, Landsmeer JMF (1990) The palmar radiocarpal ligaments: a study of adult and fetal human wrist joints, *J Hand Surg* **15A**:847–54.

Berger RA, Kauer JMG, Landsmeer JMF (1991) Radioscapholunate ligament: a gross anatomic and histologic study of fetal and adult wrist, *J Hand Surg* **16A**:350–5.

Boabighi A, Kuhlmann JN, Guérin-Surville H (1988) Nouvelle approche radiologique de l'articulation radiocarpienne, *J Radiol* **69**:465–7.

Cooney WP, Garcia-Elias M, Dobyns JH, Linscheid RL (1989) Anatomy and mechanics of carpal instability, *Surgical Rounds Orthop* **3**:15–25.

Delaney TJ, Eswar S (1992) Carpal coalitions, *J Hand Surg* **17**:28–31.

Garcia-Elias M, Domenech-Mateu JM (1987) The articular disc of the wrist. Limits and relations, *Acta Anat* **128**:51–4.

Garcia-Elias M, Cooney WP, An KN, Linscheid RL, Chao EYS (1989) Wrist kinematics after limited intercarpal arthrodesis, *J Hand Surg* **14A**:791–9.

Garcia-Elias M, Sanchez JM, Salo JM, Lluch AL (1992) Dynamic changes of the transverse carpal arch during flexion–extension of the wrist: effects of sectioning the transverse carpal ligament, *J Hand Surg* **17A**:291–8.

Kauer JMG (1980) Functional anatomy of the wrist, *Clin Orthop* **149**:9–20.

Knirk JL, Jupiter JB (1986) Intra-articular fractures of the distal end of the radius in young adults, *J Bone Joint Surg* **68A**:647–59.

Landsmeer JMF (1976) *Atlas of Anatomy of the Hand.* Churchill Livingstone: New York.

Lange A de, Huiskes R, Kauer JMG (1990) Wrist-joint ligament length changes in flexion and deviation of the hand: an experimental study, *J Orthop Res* **8**:722–30.

Mikic ZD (1984) Arthrography of the wrist joint, *J Bone Joint Surg* **66A**:371–8.

Pevny T, Rayan GM, Egle D (1995) Ligamentous and tendinous support of the pisiform. Anatomic and biomechanic study, *J Hand Surg* **20A**:299–304.

Ruby LK, Cooney WP, An KN, Linscheid RL, Chao EYS (1988) Relative motions of selected carpal bones: a kinematic analysis of the normal wrist, *J Hand Surg* **13A**:1–10.

Saffar P, Semaan I (1994) The study of the biomechanics of wrist movements in an oblique plane – a preliminary report. In: Schuind F, An KN, Cooney WP, Garcia-Elias M, eds. *Advances in the Biomechanics of the Hand and Wrist.* Plenum Press: New York: 305–12.

Sarrafian SK, Melamed JL, Goshgarian GM (1977) Study of wrist motion in flexion and extension, *Clin Orthop* **126**:153–9.

Schuind F, Cooney WP, Linscheid RL, An KN, Chao EYS (1995) Force and pressure transmission through the normal wrist. A theoretical two-dimensional study in the posteroanterior plane, *J Biomechanics* **5**:587–601.

Schuind F, Fumière E, Sintzoff S (1996) The value of standard and functional radiographs in diagnosing wrist instability. In: Büchler U, ed. *Wrist Instability.* Martin Dunitz: London: 61–7.

Sennwald GR, Zdravkovic K, Kern HP, Jacob HAC (1993) Kinematics of the wrist and its ligaments, *J Hand Surg* **18A**:707–10.

Siegel DB, Gelberman RH (1991) Radial styloidectomy: an anatomical study with special reference to radiocarpal intracapsular ligamentous morphology, *J Hand Surg* **16A**:40–4.

Taleisnik J, Gelberman RH, Miller BW, Szabo RM (1984) The extensor retinaculum of the wrist, *J Hand Surg* **9A**:495–501.

Weber ER (1984) Concepts governing the rotational shift of the intercalated segment of the carpus, *Orthop Clin North Am* **15**:193–207.

24
Congenital radiocarpal stiffness

Ann Nachemson

Introduction

Many congenital conditions can result in wrist stiffness. One of the most important is arthrogryphosis, described in Chapter 51; others are skeletal malformations, sometimes combined with metabolic disorders, leading to a general stiffness or to a malformation with decreased motion.

Radial club hand or radial deficiency

This deformity (Fig. 1) can range from a partial absence to a total aplasia of the radius with hypoplasia of the thumb and the radial carpal bones. The hand is deviated radially, often to more

than 90° when the radius is absent. The ulna is short and also radially curved. Since the hand has no support, the carpal bones will slip over to the radial side of the distal ulna. Having poor support, the wrist feels floppy but at the same time it is stiff because of limited mobility. Active ulnar–radial motion is minimal and there is usually a limitation of extension and flexion as well.

Classification

This classification follows Bayne (1991)

- Type I: there is a short radius; the distal radial epiphysis is present but appears later than normal; there is often a thumb hypoplasia.

a)

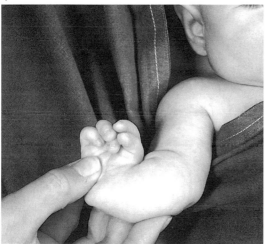

b)

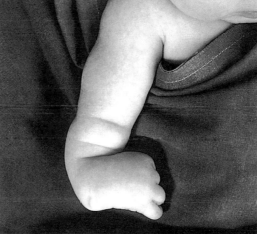

Figure 1

(a,b) Radial club hand

- Type II: there is a hypoplastic radius; both proximal and distal epiphyses are present but defective in growth.
- Type III: the radius is partially absent, most frequently in its distal one- or two-thirds; the hand is radially displaced.
- Type IV: there is total absence of the radius; the hand is unsupported and radially displaced.

Incidence and aetiology

Radial club hand has been estimated to occur in 1–3 per 100 000 births (Flatt 1994). The defect is unilateral in 50% of the patients. The aetiology is unclear. Environmental factors – such as radiation, maternal nutritional deficiencies, or compression during intrauterine life before the seventh post-ovulatory week – have been discussed, but none of these theories has been proven. Genetic factors are probably not present since the condition is seldom hereditary.

Radial deficiencies are, however, often associated with other malformations and syndromes. Cardiovascular defects are common, such as blood dyscrasias (Fanconi's anaemia), cardiac septal defects (Holt–Oram syndrome) and congenital scoliosis (Klippel–Feil syndrome).

Treatment

The aim is to stabilize the hand over the ulna and at the same time maintain some wrist motion. Treatment should start as soon as possible after birth by serial splintings in order to position the carpus over the distal ulna. Thereafter surgery is undertaken, usually when the child is around 6 months of age.

Previously ulnar implantation into carpus, as described by Riordan et al (1961) and Lamb (1977), was performed. The distal epiphyseal end of the ulna was trimmed off to a square shape and inserted into the carpus after usually the lunate as well as the capitate had been resected, followed by K-wire fixation and splinting. This resulted in a stable hand but also stiffness of the wrist.

The treatment method recommended by most authors today consists of a surgical procedure whereby the carpus is positioned over the end of the ulna – 'centralization' – as described by Bora et al (1981), Buck-Gramcko (1985), Bayne (1991) and others. There are two important steps in this procedure. One is to perform enough soft tissue release so that the carpus can be aligned over the ulna; the other is to stabilize the wrist by tendon transfers and capsular reefing. A K-wire is drilled through the ulna and the base of the third metacarpal in order to maintain the achieved reduction. Buck-Gramcko (1985) suggests an even more radical repositioning of the carpus so that the ulna is placed in line with the second metacarpal – 'radialization'. Wire fixation and a plaster cast hold the new position for approximately 6–8 weeks; thereafter a plastic splint is worn for a long period of time.

These procedures usually result in a limited but useful range of wrist motion. Recurrence of the deformity has been reported as a relatively common complication. Rarely, however, is a re-centralization indicated. Some radial deviation can result in a useful position of the wrist if the forearm is short, which is often the case.

Ulnar club hand or ulnar deficiencies

This deformity comprises a spectrum of deficiencies affecting primarily the ulnar or post-axial border of the upper extremity. The ulna is most commonly hypoplastic but can also be totally absent, sometimes together with a radiohumeral synostosis. The radius is usually short and curved with the concavity to the ulnar side. Carpal bones are often missing proximal to missing digital rays, most frequently the ulnar ones. Syndactyly occurs between the digits. Commonly, the hand is deviated ulnarwards at least 30°. However, the wrist is usually stable, in contrast to the situation in radial club hand, but is stiff, deviating in the ulnar direction and often progressively so. Commonly, the carpal bones articulate well with the radius and allow extension–flexion motion at the wrist.

Classification

This classification follows Green (1993) primarily, with a comparison of the classifications offered by Ogden et al (1976) and Riordan et al (1961).

- Type I: there is hypoplasia of the ulna (presence of distal and proximal ulna epiphyses) (Ogden type I).
- Type II: there is partial aplasia of the ulna (absence of the distal or middle one-third of the ulna) (Ogden type II, Riordan type II).
- Type III: there is total aplasia of the ulna (complete absence of the ulna) (Ogden type III, Riordan type I).
- Type IV: there is radiohumeral synostosis (fusion of the radius to the humerus) (Riordan type III).

Incidence and aetiology

The incidence is low: compared to radial club hand, ulnar deficiency occurs only once in 5–10 radial club hands (Flatt 1994). The ratio of male to female patients is approximately 3 : 2. Three out of four ulnar deficiencies are unilateral. The condition occurs sporadically and the etiology of isolated congenital ulnar deficiency is unknown. No familiar or teratogenic factors have been identified. Unlike radial club hand, ulnar deficiency is not related to anomalies of the cardiopulmonary or haematopoetic systems. Instead, it is primarily associated with musculoskeletal defects (such as scoliosis, club foot or fibular ray deficiency) and structural deformities of the other upper limb in one-third of the cases.

Treatment

Early treatment should commence as soon as possible after birth, with splinting of the wrist to correct the ulnar deviation. Surgical treatment should be decided on an individual basis. If there is a tendency to increased ulnar deviation, bowing of the radius and risk for subsequently radial head dislocation, surgical removal of the 'anlage' should be performed preferably at an early age, around 6 months. The 'anlage' is the distal portion of the ulna, made of cartilage, which has no growth potential; it arises from the dysplastic proximal part of the ulna or from the ulnar side of the humerus. As growth proceeds, this 'anlage' can exert a tethering force on the ulnar side of the forearm, resulting in increased ulnar deviation of the hand and progressive bowing of the radius. At surgery the 'anlage'

and the contracted soft tissues are resected until the hand can be moved to a neutral position over the radius. In older children, when there is a marked bowing of the radius, a wedge osteotomy on this bone is indicated together with resection of the 'anlage'. Surgery is followed by a plaster cast and later by brace treatment.

Madelung's deformity

This is an inherited (autosomal dominant) disorder, more common in females and often bilateral (Green 1993). The clinical manifestations are usually not evident until the child is 8–10 years of age. Radiographically there is early fusion of the ulnar part of the distal epiphysis of the radius resulting in ulnar and volar angulation of the shortened bone. Deformation of the wrist usually occurs with a prominent distal ulna and wrist pain.

The indication for surgery is mainly pain, while the limited motion is seldom improved by surgical intervention. The most common procedures are shortening of the ulna and epiphysiodesis of the radius. Wedge osteotomies on the latter bone, with grafting or possibly with distraction methods such as the Ilizarov device, have also been described (Lacher et al 1995).

Carpal synostosis

The most common intercarpal synostosis occurs between the lunate and the triquetrum, although many other types have been described. Sometimes an accessory bone has a coalition with one of the carpal bones (Delaney and Eswar 1992).

Most of the synostoses are isolated occurrences but some seem to be hereditary (Temtamy and McKusick 1978). Carpal fusion is often associated with other skeletal abnormalities and is also present in several syndromes (e.g. Apert–Ellis–van Creveld and Holt–Oram syndromes). The synostosis usually results in some joint stiffness, but there is rarely an indication for surgical intervention.

Multiple cartilaginous exostoses

This is a hereditary disease with autosomal dominance (Fig. 2). Exostoses can be found at the ends of the tubular bones, the vertebral bodies and the iliac crests. It is generally understood that the exostosis starts with a cartilaginous proliferation, later ossified, at the borders of the metaphyses or along the diaphysis.

The 'tumours' are often detected by the patient's parents who have noted a hard bulging process close to the joint, or sometimes because the child has a swelling and stiffness of the wrist. Exostoses can grow quickly during infancy and also cause growth disturbances of the long bones (Bock and Reed 1991). Deformity of the distal ulna can be associated with asymmetric growth of the forearm bones, resulting in stiffness and ulnar deviation of the hand (Peterson 1994). Surgical excision is indicated when the exostoses protrude so much that they cause discomfort from compression of nerves and vessels or if they inhibit joint motion. Malignant degeneration rarely occurs in childhood.

Enchondromas

Multiple enchondromas are called Ollier's disease. Enchondromas may be seen on a radiograph in early childhood. Most cases seem to be sporadic with no certain hereditary traits. The enchondromas start within either the metaphysis or the diaphysis and are usually detected because the patient complains of pain and/or because there is a swelling over the afflicted area. Enchondromas can cause severe growth disturbances and, when located in the distal ulna or radius, deformation leading to stiffness and often ulnar deviation of the wrist. Surgical excision is indicated when they cause pain or obvious deformity (Green 1993). Malignant changes are uncommon in childhood but can occur in adulthood.

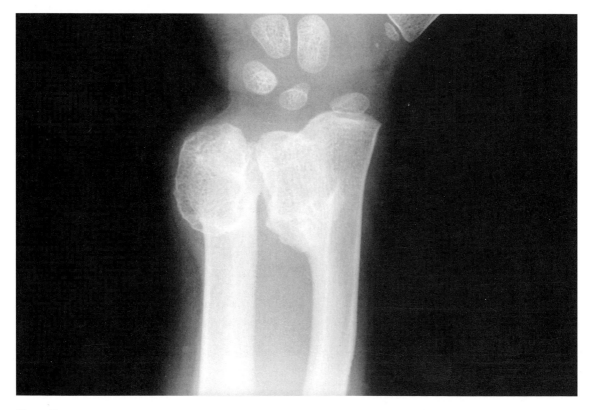

Figure 2

Multiple cartilaginous exostoses

Mucopolysaccharidosis

This is an inherited defect in the degradation and storage of mucopolysaccharides (glucosaminoglycans) in the cells of different organs, such as connective tissue and bones (dysostosis multiplex). The central nervous system may be affected, as well as tendons and joints and many other organs. The manifestations differ somewhat and are described as several different syndromes such as the following (Behrman 1992).

Hurler's syndrome

Almost every tissue in the body is affected. The children regress developmentally and the joints, including the wrists, become progressively stiff. The radius usually curves toward the ulna so that their articular surfaces are facing each other. These children die in their teens.

Scheie syndrome

This is a much milder form of mucopolysaccharidosis. The children have normal intelligence but also joint stiffness such as claw hands, often with median nerve compression at the wrist.

Hunter syndrome

This syndrome is linked to the X chromosome, affecting males only. These patients can have everything from severe mental retardation to normal brain function. Life expectancy is 20 years or in some patients even longer. The skeletal defects are usually milder than in Hurler's syndrome; classic characteristics are multiple dysostosis with short stature and joint stiffness.

There are also other mucopolysaccharidosis syndromes such as Sanfilippo syndrome and Maroteaux–Lamy syndrome which are characterized by dysostosis multiplex with mild camptodactyly and joint stiffness (in the former) and with claw hands and joint contracture (in the latter).

Diastrophic dwarfism

This is an autosomal recessively inherited syndrome, characterized by micromelia, with common involvement of both forearms and legs (Sillence et al 1978). Multiple joint deformities, especially of hands and feet (e.g. accessory carpal bones), lead to joint contractures (Stansescu et al 1984, Behrman 1992). Different types of surgical treatment may be indicated. Recurrence of the deformity after surgery is common.

Fibromatosis

In this rare condition the wrist is stiff due to either infant and juvenile aponeurotic fibroma or congenital generalized fibromatosis (Behrman 1992). This is usually a benign condition except for the congenital form, which may have a poor prognosis due to visceral involvement. Locally at the wrist there is a fibrous mass, which creates a contracture inhibiting motion. Local excision of the fibromatosis can be performed, resulting in better mobility. However, the recurrence rate can be as high as 90%.

Reference

Bayne LG (1991) Radial deficiencies. In: Carter PR, ed. *Reconstruction of the Child's Hand*. Lea & Febiger: New York: 187–97.

Behrman RE (1992) *Nelson Textbook of Pediatrics*, 14th edn. WB Saunders: Philadelphia.

Bock GW, Reed MH (1991) Forearm deformities in multiple cartilaginous exostoses, *Skelet Radiol* **20:**483–6.

Bora FW Jr, Osterman AL, Kaneda RR et al (1981) Radial clubhand deformity, *J Bone Joint Surg* **63A:**741–5.

Buck-Gramcko D (1985) Radialization as a new treatment for radial clubhand, *J Hand Surg* **10A:**964–8.

Delaney TJ, Eswar S (1992) Carpal coalitions, *J Hand Surg* **17A:**28–31.

Flatt A (1994) *The Care of Congenital Hand Anomalies*, 2nd edn. Quality Medical Publishing Inc: St Louis.

Green D (1993) *Operative Hand Surgery*, 3rd edn. Churchill Livingstone: New York.

Lacher G, Sennwald G, Frey HP (1995) Use of the Ilizarov device for correction of extensive Madelung's deformity, *Handchir Mikrochir Plast Chir* **27:**214–19.

Lamb DW (1977) Radial clubhand, *J Bone Joint Surg* **59A:**1–13.

Ogden JA, Watson HK, Bohne W (1976) Ulnar dysmelia, *J Bone Joint Surg* **58A:**467–75.

Peterson HA (1994) Deformities and problems of the forearm in children with multiple hereditary osteochondromata, *J Pediatr Orthop* **14:**92–100.

Riordan DC, Mills EH and Aldredge RH (1961) Congenital absence of the ulna, *J Bone Joint Surg* **43A:**614.

Sillence DO, Lachman R, Rimoin DL (1978) Neonatal dwarfism, *Pediatr Clin North Am* **25:**453.

Stansescu V, Stanescu R, Maroteaux P (1984) Pathogenetic mechanisms in osteochondrodysplasias, *J Bone Joint Surg* **66A:**817.

Temtamy SA, McKusick VA (1978) Carpal tarsal synostosis, *Birth Defects* **14:**502.

25

Extrinsic and intrinsic causes of radiocarpal stiffness

Philippe Saffar

Radiocarpal stiffness is a relative matter. It is rarely total and its appreciation depends on the special needs of the patient. The minimum range of motion (ROM) to perform the activities of daily living (ADL) has been defined by precise studies. The most frequently cited is Palmer's 1985 study in which an electric goniometer was used to measure the ADL. It has defined the ROM in flexion (Fl), extension (Ext), radial deviation (RD) and ulnar deviation (UD) necessary to perform ADL. Every arc of motion below the figures defined (Table 1) may be regarded as radiocarpal stiffness. Nelson (1990) has also reported a study of 24 usual activities such as personal hygiene (flexion needed), holding a telephone (extension needed), turning a tap, and so on. He has defined a minimal ROM for each activity. The study by Ryu (1991) has demonstrated the necessity of a greater ROM than the previous studies. Figures are reported in Table 1. It is evident that many occupations and sports require a significant mobility in a defined arc of motion.

Table 1 Useful wrist range of motion

	Palmer (1985)	Nelson (1990)	Ryu (1991)
Flexion	5°	28°	40°
Extension	30°	37°	40°
RD	10°	12°	10°
UD	15°	27°	30°

RD, radial deviation; UD, ulnar deviation

A hypermobile patient may complain of wrist stiffness although his ROM is still between the normal values. Wrist stiffness may be fixed in Fl, Ext, RD, UD: the most cumbersome position is a wrist in a flexed or radial-deviated position as the wrist grip strength position is in extension and ulnar deviation.

History

a   Post-traumatic stiffness is the main cause of wrist stiffness, but the initial trauma may have been forgotten by the patient because of the time elapsed since the accident.

The onset of wrist stiffness is often progressive, the evolution lasting many years, often 5–20, and patients are not always aware of this progressively evolving stiffness. Tricky movements have replaced progressively normal movements. The patients are mainly referred for wrist pain. This pain is associated with a relatively stiff wrist, but it is only comparison with the other side which allows the patient to realize that stiffness. Grip strength has progressively decreased and this is partly related to the loss of extension. Wrist extension is associated with finger flexion which is necessary to have a good grip.

A completely different presentation is a patient consulting for a recent injury and/or a prolonged immobilization. This type of patient is really affected by this recent wrist stiffness and highly demanding for treatment.

b   The pathomechanics of the initial injury has to be identified: fall, direct impact, forced rotation, crush, burn or repetitive microtraumatisms (prolonged use of pneumatic gun or drilling machines may result in a progressive destruction and stiffness of the wrist).

c   The time elapsed since injury, the medical or surgical treatments applied together with their clinical results (improvement or worsening), rehabilitation and splintage and their duration are all of great importance. Radiological records provide information on the different treatments applied.

a)

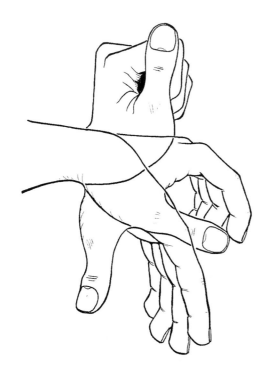

b)

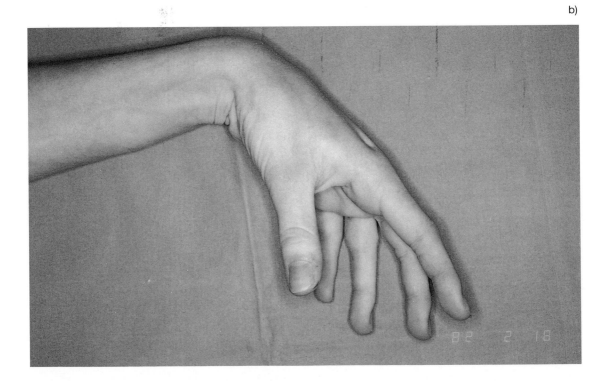

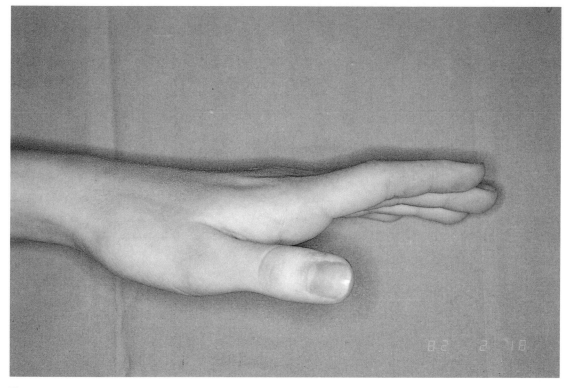

c)

Figure 1

(a) Tenodesis effect of wrist on fingers. (b), (c) Loss of tenodesis effect due to extensor tendon adherences at the dorsum of the wrist.

Diagnosis

Clinical symptoms

Skin status should be noted: scars, retractions, bands or burns sequelae. Adhesions to the underlying tendons may be evident when the skin displaces with extensor tendon movements. Adhesions of flexor or extensor tendons is displayed if finger passive motion is not provoked by wrist extension and flexion passive movements (Fig. 1).

Wrist and finger alignments may be distorted and finger stiffness and malposition may be associated. The wrist may be shortened, swollen, sometimes with an aspect of synovitis, mainly on the dorso-radial side.

Dynamic clinical examination of the wrist is performed with the elbow resting on a table, forearm vertical: motion in Fl, Ext, RD, UD and in the oblique planes and circumduction are performed actively and passively and their amplitude noted and compared with the opposite side.

Pain

This is usually the cause of the consultation. It may be intermittent or climatic, a significant or light strain or permanent. It may appear during the daytime and be related to activity or during the night as an inflammatory pain or a carpal tunnel syndrome. Evaluation should be subjectively done by the patient using the Huskinsson analogue scale from one to ten.

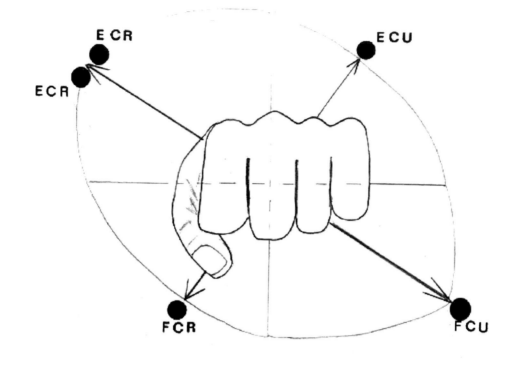

Figure 2

The oblique planes of motion of the wrist.

Palpation may elicit pain situated at the radial or ulnar part of the radiocarpal joint, on the distal radioulnar joint (DRUJ), or the midcarpal joint. Pain localization helps the diagnosis and identifies the need for complementary investigations.

Stiffness may be a reaction to pain or increased by a constant pain and should not be mistaken for a real stiffness.

Other causes of pain in this area should be eliminated, such as De Quervain's disease, carpal tunnel syndrome, tendinitis or neurosympathic dystrophy. They may be associated and take part in the pain.

Range of motion

The wrist is stiff and may be deviated in an abnormal position. Examination should elicit where the residual arc of motion is situated. Often it is in the midcarpal joint that some motion is preserved, and in this case the maximal arc of motion is situated in the oblique plane from radial deviation and extension to ulnar deviation and flexion (Fig. 2). This joint is often preserved in post-traumatic stiffness except in SLAC (scapholunate advanced collapse) type III.

A discrepancy between active and passive motion is an indication of an extra-articular problem, if passive motion is greater than active motion. It may also be due to insufficient muscular rehabilitation or tendon adhesions, or to a paresis due to nerve injury (radial nerve).

If fingers have maintained a normal motion and the normal tenodesis effect of the wrist on the fingers is present, it implies that stiffness is of intra-articular aetiology. A fixed deviated position increases the handicap.

Grip strength

This is measured with the Jamar dynamometer and compared to the opposite side. It is often decreased and this is a usual patient complaint. If there is associated finger stiffness, it is impossible to know the exact percentage of wrist stiffness in this grip loss.

Finally, extra- and intra-articular causes of stiffness are often associated and ankylosis may result from a long-standing extra-articular stiffness.

X-rays

If plain X-rays are almost normal this indicates either an *extra-articular aetiology* due to:

- tendon adhesions
- a capsular retraction due to:
  - a crush
  - a forearm ischaemia (Volkmann)
  - a neurosympathetic dystrophy (NSD)
- an ankylosis due to prolonged immobilization

or an *intra-articular fibrosis* which may be visible on the X-rays only as a decreased and less transparent joint space.

Plain X-rays can also demonstrate post-traumatic features usually situated between the two carpal arcs (Fig. 3) (where 95% of the carpal injuries are located) or at the distal radius.

Investigations

Plain X-rays

These may demonstrate features such as: post-traumatic bone defects or malalignments, decreased joint space, joint architecture anomalies which may be congenital or acquired during growth (fracture during childhood).

They allow localization of the osteoarthritic carpal joints and those which are intact. This is of the utmost importance for choosing the treatment type. An irregular joint contour may be the only abnormal feature.

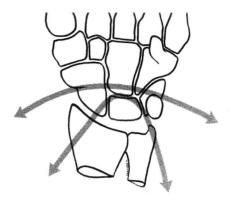

Figure 3

Johnson's carpal arcs.

The carpal height index is calculated and evaluates the carpal collapse which is associated with carpal bone malalignment. It is measured by the Youm and MacMurtry method (Fig. 4a,b) (Youm et al 1978) or Natrass method (Fig. 4c) (Natrass et al 1994). Scapholunate and radiolunate angles define the dorsal instability of the segment intercalated (DISI) and volar instability of the segment intercalated (VISI) deformities which will be useful for classifying the intracarpal or carpal bone adaptive displacements.

Dynamic X-rays

These are usually impossible to perform when wrist stiffness is total. When some motion is still present, they may provide information, mainly on the scaphoid motion.

Arthrography

The first injection should be in the midcarpal joint followed, if necessary, by radiocarpal and DRUJ injections (Fig. 5). Carpal ligament injuries suspected on plain X-rays may be confirmed and others detected. For example, an associated lunotriquetral ligament tear is demonstrated where only a scapholunate tear was suspected. It may be difficult to inject the dye and its progression is restricted by intra-articular adhesions and fibrosis

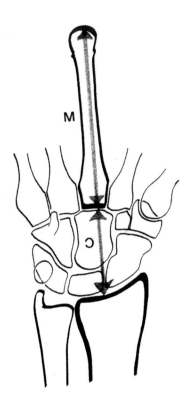

a)

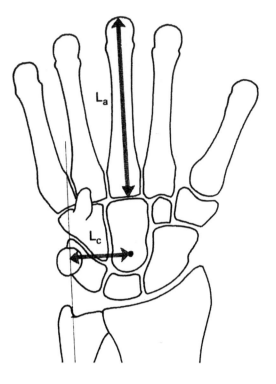

b)

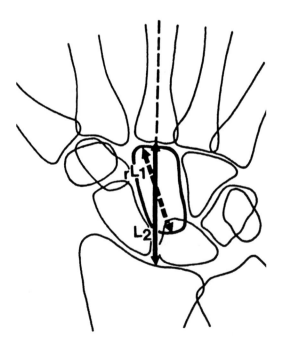

c)

Figure 4

Measurement of (a) carpal height (Youm et al 1978), (b) ulno-carpal distance (Youm et al 1978), (c) carpal height (Natrass et al 1994).

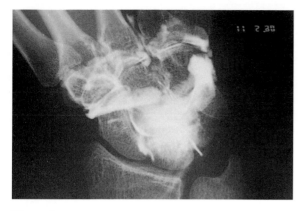

Figure 5

Arthrography: midcarpal injection.

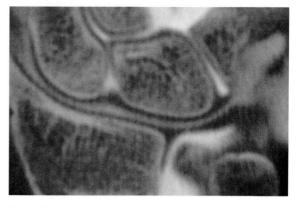

Figure 6

Arthroscan (arthrography followed by CT scan).

due to previous intra-articular haematoma, infection or surgical procedures.

Arthroscan (arthrography followed by computed tomography (CT) scan)

Millimetric cuts in different planes allow assessment of the localization and extent of ligament tears and, furthermore, for stiff joints, the extent and localization of cartilaginous defects (Fig. 6). This is essential for the choice of a reconstructive surgical procedure which is possible only in the presence of normal cartilage.

Arthroscopy

This is a semi-invasive technique (Fig. 7) and a significant distraction needs to be applied for these joints. A complete radiocarpal and midcarpal exploration is necessary in cases where stiffness is due to an intra-articular cause.

Diagnostic arthroscopy demonstrates the ligament and cartilage status and allows a dynamic examination. A probe introduced in the radiocarpal and midcarpal joint produces mobilization of adjacent carpal bones and elicits instability problems.

Therapeutic arthroscopy uses a shaver to debride

adhesions, fibrosis and articular debris. This allows a better visualization of lesions and may help the patient to regain motion.

In summary:

- where wrist bone and joints have a normal aspect (no pseudarthroses or malalignment of radio-carpal, midcarpal, carpometacarpal or metacarpal bones) this indicates *extra-articular stiffness* (extra-articular adhesions or fibrosis)
- where wrist bone and joints are partly or completely destroyed, this indicates *intra-articular stiffness*.

The two types may be associated.

Extra-articular joint stiffness

Burns

Burns of the dorsal aspect of the wrist and hand are not rare as the face and the hands are the most exposed parts of the body (Fig. 8). Depending on the burn depth, either skin or skin and tendons are injured. There is a constant and often significant involvement of the dorsal wrist skin which is retracted, resulting in a fixed extended position. Extensor tendons may also be destroyed and/or

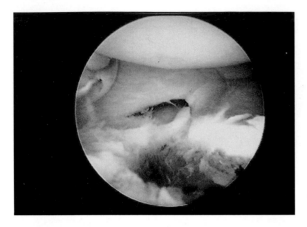

Figure 7

Arthroscopy.

adherent to the bone. Wrist stiffness may be associated with metacarpophalangeal (MCP) and proximal interphalangeal (PIP) joint stiffness. The most severe injuries combine wrist and burns as in 'power press hands'.

Complex injuries

Crush injuries

These are the consequences of, for example, the fall of a heavy object on the hand or a hand stuck in a roller machine. It is difficult to analyse the associated causes of stiffness in these hands when seen after a long delay (Fig. 9).

Care should be taken to understand the participation of each structure in the stiffness: skin, tendon, bone and joints. Radiology is not always contributive because bone injuries are usually not significant.

Complex volar wounds

At the level of the wrist or forearm these wounds combine wrist and finger flexor injuries with median and ulnar nerve sections. These injuries are caused by knife, electric saw, sheet iron and sometimes an attempted suicide. Wounds are usually transverse or slightly oblique, at the wrist or forearm and have been operated on either once or several times. Wrist and finger stiffness are associated and anaesthesia or hypoaesthesia in the median or ulnar nerve sensitive area, or both are noted. In these cases, it is difficult to know what is relevant to tendon or nerve injuries.

Long-lasting palsies

If due to distal median or ulnar nerves or proximal nerve injuries (brachial plexus), long-lasting palsies result in retractions; the consequence of palsy plus tendon imbalance. For radial nerve palsies, passive motion is preserved for a long time, except in extension. Plexus palsies result in complex wrist stiffness where palsy, retractions and fibrosis are combined.

The 'trigger' wrist

This is a rare syndrome where dorsal or palmar synovitis prevents normal gliding of extensor tendons and their synovial sheaths inside the dorsal retinaculum. Triggering and snapping at the wrist level is induced by finger or wrist motion.

Volkmann's syndrome

This acute syndrome is caused mainly by elbow fractures (supracondylar fractures) in children. It should be prevented by a careful reduction in emergency. Some patients are referred for the sequelae of an ischaemia of the forearm muscles resulting in fibrosis and retraction: the wrist is in a fixed flexed position with the fingers flexed and retracted. A certain amount of extension is possible in some cases.

Compartment syndromes are of the same origin but limited at one of the forearm compartments between two aponeuroses. It may also result in wrist stiffness.

Spasticity

Spastic wrist stiffness, usually in flexion and ulnar deviation, is treated in Chapter 45.

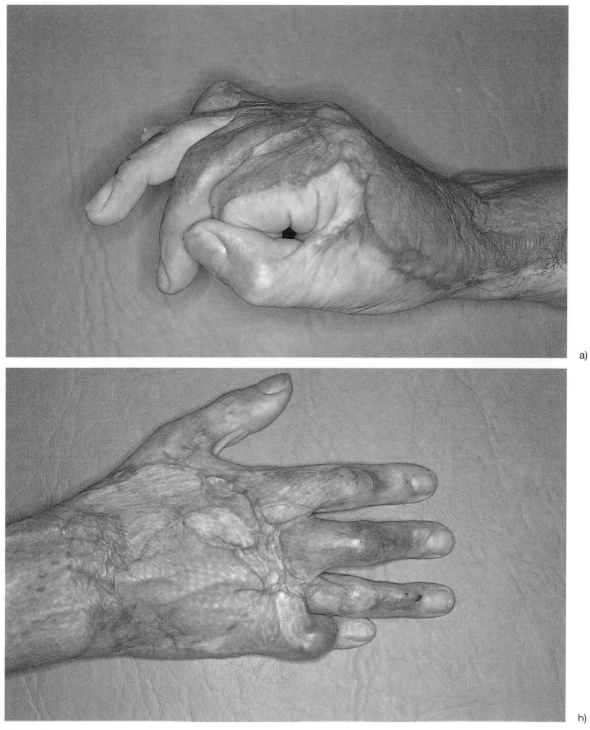

a)

h)

Figure 8

(a), (b) Sequelae of burns.

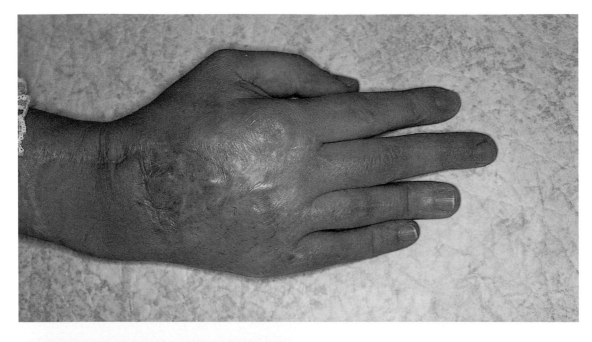

a)

b)

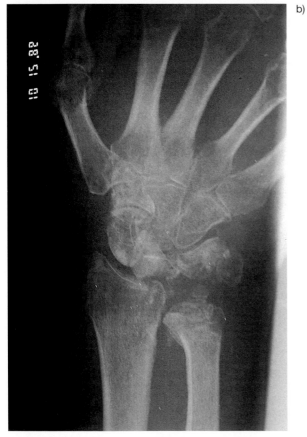

Figure 9

(a), (b) Crush injury.

Intra-articular joint stiffness

The wrist is in normal alignment or malaligned, which may be due to a complex bone fracture or crush or to a therapeutic mistake.

Early post-traumatic joint stiffness

The patient has been already treated in emergency by another surgeon and the following characteristics noted:

Bone and joint architecture is normal

It is often the consequence of a prolonged immobilization or an immobilization in a wrong position. Rehabilitation is often sufficient in most cases. An extra-articular cause should be differentiated. Intra-articular fibrosis is possible, but rehabilitation allows return of motion and arthrolysis is rarely indicated.

Bone and joint architecture is altered but may be reconstructed

Extra-articular radial malunion (Fig. 10), usually in extension and radial deviation, should be operated on to realign the distal radius in a proper position.

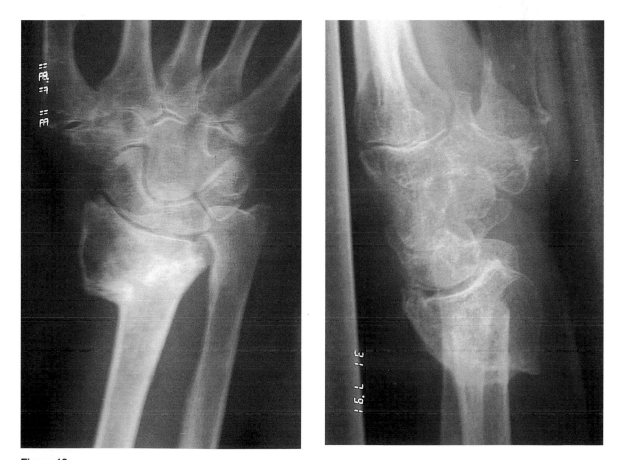

Figure 10

(a), (b) Distal radial malunion.

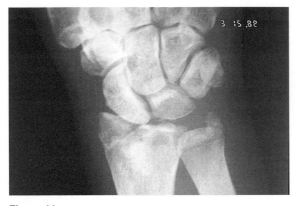

Figure 11

Intra-articular radial malunion.

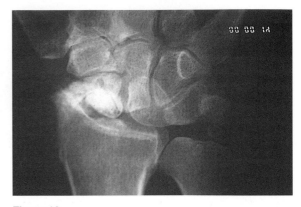
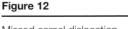

Figure 12

Missed carpal dislocation.

Radiocarpal joint stiffness is associated with a decreased pronosupination. Malunions in wrist flexion result in less stiffness. A preoperative rehabilitation is often necessary. Carpal tunnel syndrome may be present and pain should not be attributed only to malunion. Finger flexion may be altered.

Intra-articular radial malunion (Fig. 11): the wrist is in danger of early osteoarthritis if articular step-off is more than 2 mm. The wrist should be reconstructed as early as possible. Osteotomy should go through the previous fracture lines which is possible until 1 year after the fracture.

Carpal dislocations are retrolunate dislocations or anterior dislocation of the lunate bone. They combine dislocations with carpal fractures (scaphoid, capitate, triquetrum) and parcellar fractures (radial or ulnar styloid) or osteochondral fractures. They are unrecognized in 20–30% of the cases (Fig. 12). Treated by reduction and conservative treatment, they result more often in carpal instability or scaphoid non-union. When there is no or insufficient reduction, they are referred for a stiff wrist and the treatment is very difficult. They should be operated as soon as possible unless this will result in permanent stiffness with partial or total destruction of the joint spaces. Carpal ligament reconstruction or limited wrist arthrodeses are mandatory to prevent carpal instability and secondary wrist stiffness. Salvage procedures such as proximal row carpectomy or wrist arthrodeses are sometimes necessary.

Normal bone and joint relationship cannot be restored

Complex injuries or unreduced carpal dislocations, complete bone and joint crush, open complex injuries including soft tissue destruction and infection may be too complex for reconstructive surgery, and salvage procedures should be applied with skin, tendon and bone and joint reconstruction.

Chronic radiocarpal stiffness

Post-traumatic osteoarthritis (OA) secondary to carpal joint injuries is the most frequent cause of joint stiffness. Carpal injuries result in a decrease of carpal height with bone malalignment called carpal collapse. Rotatory subluxation of the scaphoid induces a horizontal position of this bone. Incongruency between the scaphoid proximal pole with the scaphoid fossa of the distal radius is then present (Fig. 13). This incongruency is the onset of radioscaphoid OA and stiffness. The lunate is in a dorsiflexed position (DISI pattern) (Fig. 14) and not incongruent with the radius lunate fossa because of its large and quadrangular area. Malalignment of the lunate on the capitate head, usually volar and ulnar subluxation, leads to a lunocapitate OA. Other joint spaces around the scaphoid may be progressively involved. Patients complain frequently at that stage of pain and stiffness. This has been called SLAC

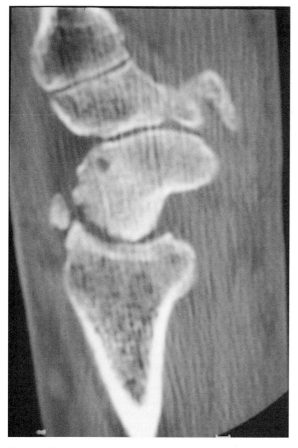

Figure 13

Radiocarpal osteoarthritis (horizontal scaphoid).

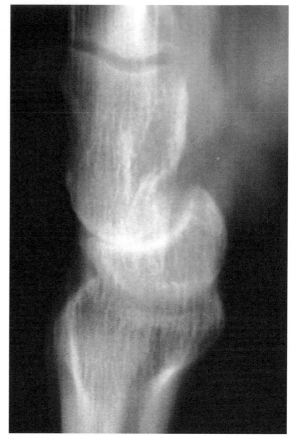

Figure 14

DISI.

(Fig. 15): scapholunate advanced collapse (Watson and Ballet 1984).

Evolution is classified in three stages:

SLAC I   Styloscaphoid OA
SLAC II Radioscaphoid OA
SLAC III Radioscaphoid plus lunocapitate OA

The two most frequent aetiologies are scapholunate dissociation and scaphoid non-union.

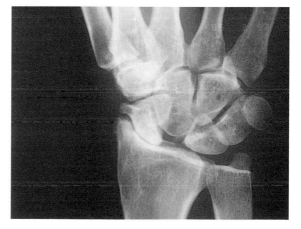

Figure 15

SLAC.

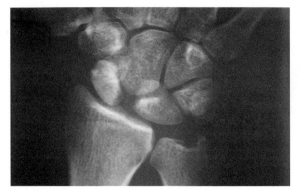

Figure 16

Capitate proximal migration.

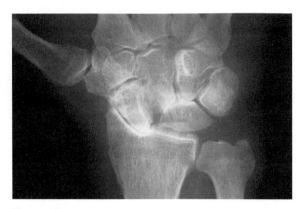

Figure 18

SLAC stage III.

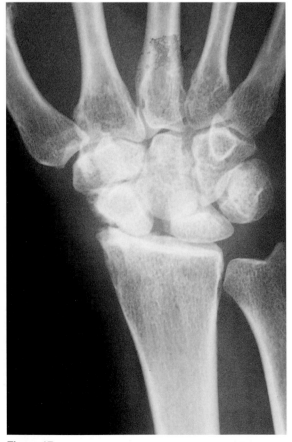

Figure 17

Scapholunate instability.

Carpal instability

This type of injury has been recognized for more than 20 years and is the cause of chronic wrist stiffness in 70% of cases.

Complete tear of the scapholunate ligament and progressive distension of the anterior ligament plane result in dissociation of the two adjacent bones, and the gap between them increases slowly. Each fist tends to produce a proximal migration of the capitate between the two bones (Fig. 16) which increases the gap and induces a carpal collapse: scaphoid in flexion, lunate in extension and carpal height decreasing (Fig. 17). This evolution toward scapholunate and lunocapitate OA defines the SLAC stage III (Fig. 18). Arthritic lesions are at times not or slightly painful during the evolution, but stiffness is present after some time.

Plain and dynamic X-rays, arthrography, CT scan after arthrography and arthroscopy have been proposed at every stage to assess the ligament tears and the cartilage defects and allow a therapeutic choice decision.

Scaphoid non-union

Evolution is slightly different and is related to the non-union location and to the use of the wrist, professional or sportive. Non-unions of the distal

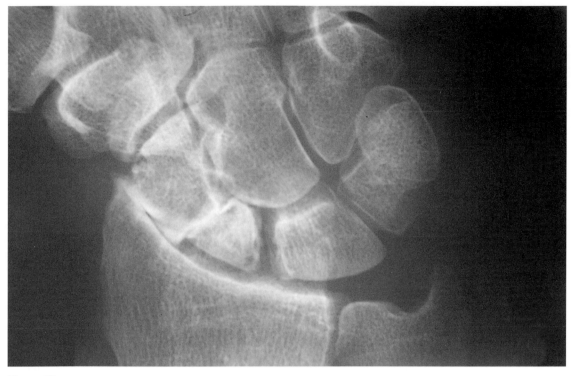

Figure 19

Scaphoid non-union with radioscaphoid osteoarthritis.

scaphoid rarely result in stiffness. Non-unions located in the proximal or middle part of the scaphoid result in OA which is always present after 5 years of evolution (Fig. 19). Stiffness may be evident only after 10–20 years and is not always significant. As scaphoid fractures occur mainly in patients aged 20 or 30 years, patients with wrist stiffness are often in their fifties and may be impaired, especially if they are manual workers.

Part of the cartilage of the scaphoid proximal pole may be preserved for a long time and this proximal pole is in extension in relationship with the lunate. It is the scaphoid distal fragment which is in flexion and is incongruent with the radial part of the scaphoid fossa. Thus, there is an extension of the OA to the scaphoid fossa and to the lunocapitate joint due to the DISI position of the lunate on the scaphoid capitate head. It is less subluxated ulnarly than in scapholunate dissociation (Fig. 20). The radiolunate joint is still intact. Osteonecrosis and fragmentation of the scaphoid proximal pole

increases carpal collapse and OA. This is mainly the case in proximal pole scaphoid non-unions (Fig. 21). This has been named scaphoid non-union advanced collapse (SNAC) by some authors to differentiate it from SLAC.

Other post-traumatic causes

Intra-articular radius malunions

Osteoarthritis depends on the initial fracture location and reduction and magnitude of step-off in the distal radius contour. It results in OA and stiffness in the long run. Associated fibrosis is secondary to intra-articular haematoma.

Other causes of stiffness are due to embedment of the first carpal row in the distal radius, sequelae of comminuted fractures, irregular articular contour, and when external fixation is maintained for too long.

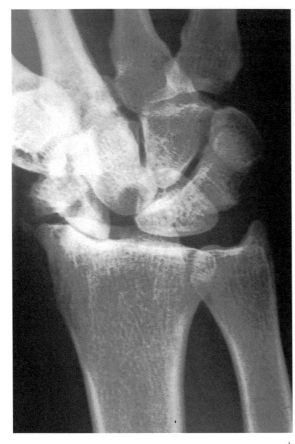

a)

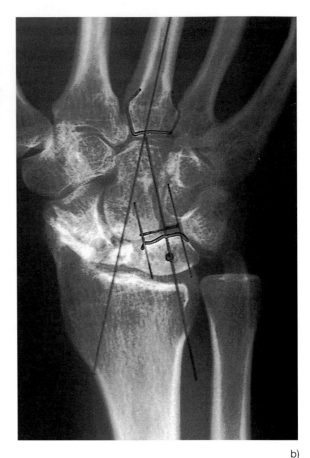

b)

Figure 20

(a) SLAC. (b) SNAC.

Carpal dislocations

Even well reduced, these combine ligament tears, chip fractures, osteochondral defects and ischaemia, sometimes aggravated by the surgical treatment. Articular stiffness is frequent. In cases with no or insufficiently reduced carpal dislocations, wrist stiffness is the rule.

Kienböck's disease (idiopathic necrosis of the lunate)

At stage III with radioscaphoid osteoarthritis, this results in reduced wrist motion. At stage IV, the lunate fossa is devoid of cartilage and stiffness is present (Fig. 22).

Sequelae of complex wrist trauma

Even without significant fractures, these may result in capsuloligamentous retraction or intra-articular fibrosis, and this may be combined with NSD.

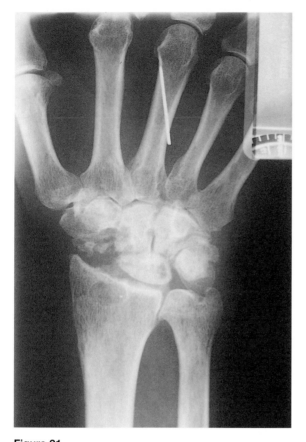

Figure 21

Osteonecrosis of the scaphoid proximal pole.

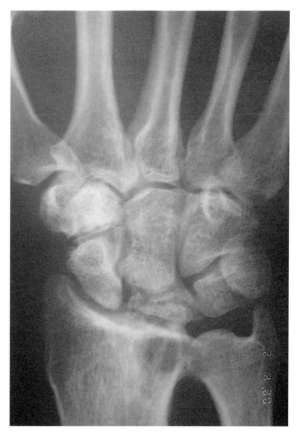

Figure 22

Kienböck's disease stage IV.

Inflammatory diseases

Rheumatoid arthritis is a special entity. Bone and joint destruction is caused by a disease initiated in the synovial tissue. Different types of evolution exist, some largely destructive and some resulting in wrist ankylosis (Fig. 23). Adapted medical and surgical treatments should be used to prevent stiffness and deformities in the wrist and the hand. The cause of impairment is usually complex and may be not confined to wrist stiffness. This will not be discussed here due to the complexity of the problem.

Other inflammatory diseases may cause wrist stiffness.

Infections

Stiffness after infection is now mainly due to post-traumatic open wounds or post-surgical sepsis which results in fibrosis, bone and joint destruction and stiffness.

Tuberculosis is rare nowadays but it may be evoked in presence of total carpal coalition (Fig. 24).

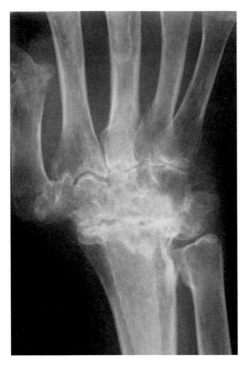

Figure 23

Ankylosis of a wrist with RA.

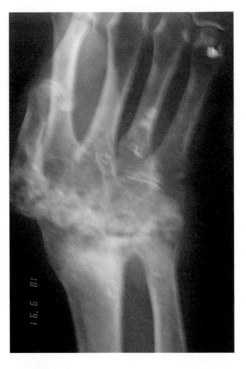

a)

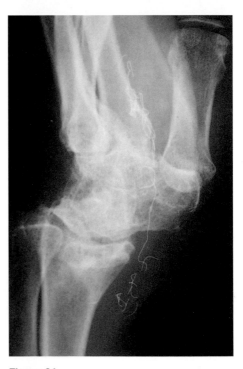

b)

Figure 24

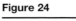

(a), (b) Wrist tuberculosis.

Idiopathic arthritis

Found in less than 5% of all arthroses, they are consequences of precipitation diseases: chondro-calcinosis, gout, hydroxyapatite deposition disease and others. Bone, ligaments and joint spaces are affected and the X-rays are very specific (Fig. 25). They are present in elderly people, more than 75 years of age and result in a very small number of stiffnesses. They usually do not require treatment.

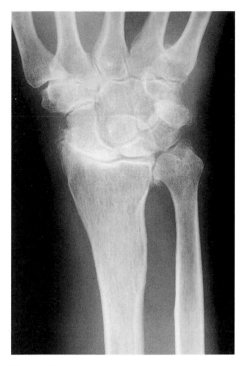

Figure 25

Wrist chondrocalcinosis.

References

Natrass GR, King GJ, McMurtry RY, Brait RF (1994). An alternative method for determination of the carpal height ratio, *J Bone Joint Surg* **76A**:88–94.

Nelson DL (1990) The functional range of motion of the wrist. *American Society for Surgery of the Hand, 45th Annual Meeting*. Toronto.

Palmer AK, Werner FW, Murphy D, Glisson R (1985) Functional wrist motion: a biomechanical study, *J Hand Surg* **10A**:39–46.

Ryu J, Cooney WP III, Askew IJ, An KN, Chao EYS (1991) Functional ranges of motion of the wrist joint, *J Hand Surg* **16A**:409–19.

Watson HK, Ballet FL (1984) The SLAC wrist: scapholuate advanced collapse pattern of degenerative arthritis, *J Hand Surg* **9A**:358–65.

Youm Y, McMurtry RY, Flatt AE, Gillespie TE (1978) Kinematics of the wrist. I. An experimental study of radial–ulnar deviation and flexion–extension, *J Bone Joint Surg* **60A**:423–31.

26
General causes of radiocarpal stiffness

Marc Garcia-Elias

Stiffness of the radiocarpal joint is frequently the consequence of lack of motion and/or swelling as a result of trauma, infection, vascular disease, tumour or other localized problems. There are other forms of stiffness, however, in which there is no local cause, but rather the consequence of a systemic disease. Several mechanisms may be involved: activation of a chronic inflammatory process of the synovial structures, induction of global cartilage deterioration, alteration of the necessary muscle balance, etc. Three groups of diseases have been found to be specially prone to producing carpal stiffness: 1, systemic inflammatory processes; 2, infectious diseases; and 3, degenerative processes. This chapter will review the mechanisms by which these conditions alter the normal function of the wrist and how this may eventually result in stiffness, if not a complete ankylosis.

Systemic inflammatory arthropathies

Several systemic diseases may induce an inflammatory arthropathy of the wrist resulting in a lack of motion. All of them have in common a targeting of the synovial cell, thus inducing the release of collagen and/or cartilage deteriorating enzymes which are responsible for the progressive articular deteriorating process. The most common arthritides leading to wrist stiffness are: rheumatoid arthritis, juvenile rheumatoid arthritis, ankylosing spondylitis, psoriasis, and crystal-induced arthritis.

Rheumatoid arthritis

Rheumatoid arthritis (RA) is a chronic, inflammatory disease, responsible for episodic pain, swelling and impairment of function usually affecting several joints and their periarticular tissues, causing tenosynovitis and arthrosynovitis. The inflammatory reaction may also involve other structures causing vasculitis, myositis, neuropathies, etc. (Nalebuff and Austin 1991). The initiating cause of RA is not known, although there is evidence about the existence of a genetic predisposition as a factor in the development of the autoimmune response characteristic of the disease. Both cellular and chemical articular changes occur from altered antigen-antibody reactions resulting in the release of hydrolytic enzymes (metalloproteases), oxygen radicals and arachidonic acid metabolites (prostaglandins, thromboxanes, etc.) which promote the inflammatory reaction (Harris 1990). During this process, several destructive enzymes are released and are responsible for the cartilage, tendon, ligaments and/or bone damage. If the concentration of collagen deteriorating enzymes (collagenases) predominates over other types of metabolites, there will be more capsuloligamentous destruction (joint destabilization) than cartilage wear. Conversely, if the predominant degradative enzymes released during the inflammatory process target the cartilage (proteoglycanases), the joint will remain stable throughout the process of progressive joint narrowing, leading to stiffness.

The wrist is a common target of RA (Nalebuff and Austin 1991). When affected by the disease, the joint becomes deformed and stiff either as a result of primary joint involvement or as the consequence of the disease affecting adjacent joints or tendons. According to different authors, the incidence of wrist involvement varies from 64 to 85%, most of

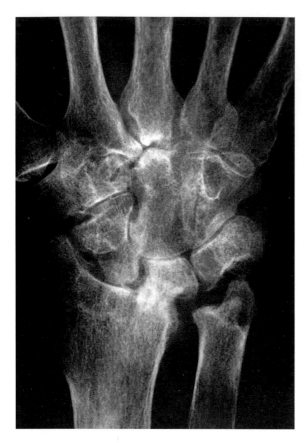

Figure 1

Spontaneous fusion of the radiolunate joint in a 60-year-old woman with rheumatoid arthritis. Despite the joint changes no substantial instability appeared. In these type of rheumatoid patients (Simmen type I) joint stiffness progresses to a complete ankylosis so no stabilizing surgery is necessary.

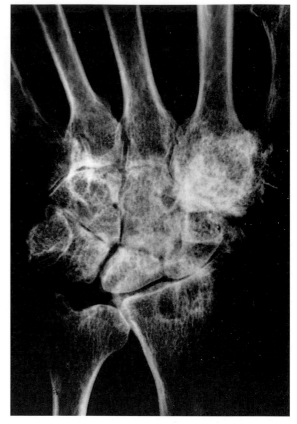

Figure 2

A 70-year-old woman with rheumatoid arthritis, presenting a Simmen type II (secondary arthrosis) of her wrists. The cartilage loss progressed slowly, allowing the joint to react by forming osteophytes, subchondral sclerosis and capsular fibrosis, all of which contributed to the development of wrist stiffness.

them with a bilateral involvement (Thirupathi et al 1983, Simmen 1996). The most frequent presentation involves inflammation of the synovium of both joint and extensor tendon sheaths, with pain, swelling and functional impairment. If the synovitis is not controlled in the early stages of the disease, there is proliferation of a typical granulation tissue (pannus) formed by fibroblasts, small vessels and inflammatory cells. This process, however, is very seldom homogeneous in all areas of the joint, but predominates at specific well-vascularized areas from where it releases collagen and proteoglycane

degradative enzymes. Depending upon which enzymes prevail, the cartilage and bone will be more involved in the disease than the ligaments, or vice versa. Consequently, there will be different patterns of joint degeneration.

According to Simmen (1996), three different patterns of carpal deterioration exist depending upon which structures have been destroyed first (tendons, ligaments or cartilage): the ankylotic, the osteoarthritic and the destructive patterns. In the first, there is a rapid destruction of the cartilages leading to a spontaneous ankylosis of an otherwise stable joint (Fig. 1). In a second group of patients, the destructive process is also concentrated on the cartilage, but at a much slower pace. The subchondral bone in these cases reacts as if the process was degenerative with sclerosis, preservation of wrist alignment, and a slow development of wrist stiffness (Fig. 2). In the third group (destructive group) there is a predominant destruction of ligamentous structures, rapidly losing both alignment and stability.

Among the ligament destructive group, there are also different patterns of wrist involvement, depending upon which group of ligaments have been disrupted first. The most frequent locations of pannus proliferation are: 1, the synovial layer around the radioscapholunate ligament; 2, the basistyloid fovea of the head of the ulna; and 3, the synovial sheath of the fourth, fifth and sixth extensor compartments. When the collagen destructive process predominates around the scapholunate interval, the ligaments mostly involved are the extrinsic radiocarpal ligaments (radioscaphocapitate, long radiolunate, dorsal radiotriquetral) and the intrinsic scapholunate ligaments. This tends to evolve into a typical wrist instability pattern which associates a scapholunate dissociation and an ulnar translocation of the lunate and triquetrum (Taleisnik 1985). By contrast, if the pannus formation predominates around the basistyloid fovea of the ulna, there is a tendency for a destabilization of the distal radioulnar joint through rupture of the triangular fibrocartilage complex. Finally, if the synovitic proliferation prevails in the extensor compartments, tendon ruptures may occur, with the subsequent alteration of the muscle balance around the wrist. These ruptures are not only the result of the action of collagen deteriorating enzymes released by the inflammed tenosynovium, but are also secondary to the mechanical damage produced by friction of these tendons over the edges of ostephytes typically appearing at the rheumatoid radioulnar joint. All these cartilage, ligament and tendon ruptures promote specific wrist deformities which are further maximized by the action of the forces normally acting over these joints (Garcia-Elias 1996). These will progressively disorganize the adjacent joints, inducing cartilage degeneration and ligament insufficiency, thus further contributing to stiffness.

In general, three different clinical courses of the disease have been recognized. In about one-third of the patients there is one single episode of inflammation, causing some joint deterioration, lasting about 2 years, followed by a permanent arrest of the disease. These are the so-called monocyclic patients (Flatt 1995). In others, probably half of all patients, there is a polycyclic course in which the disease appears and disappears in repeated episodes between periods of relative calm. Finally, there are about 15% of the patients with a progressive form of the disease leading to a complete destruction of the joints without any substantial period of remission.

Staging of the disease is important for planning a correct treatment regime. The more widely used staging system was proposed by the American Rheumatism Association (Steinbrocker et al 1949). In stage I, there is only a persistent synovitis without obvious radiographic changes except for mild periarticular osteoporosis. In stage II, there is limitation of motion, muscle atrophy and signs of persistent synovitis. Radiologically, some erosive changes and cartilage destruction can be observed, although the joint architecture is mostly preserved. In stage III, the deformities have progressed as well as the adjacent muscle atrophy. In this stage the joints are already subluxed, the cartilages severely destroyed and stiffness is substantial. Stage IV is the terminal stage, where the joint is already completely dislocated or fused by means of a bony or fibrous ankylosis.

Juvenile rheumatoid arthritis

Rheumatoid arthritis in young prepubertal patients has different characteristics compared to adults. Also of an unknown origin, this clinical condition frequently initiates as a painless swelling of the joints and extensor tendon sheaths of the hand. The condition may evolve in the form of systemic multiarticular involvement (56% of cases), or only affect a few joints (oligoarthritis 11%), or in the form of a monoarticular affectation (33%) (Mathies 1977). In the adolescent, the disease may evolve in the form of severe systemic illness with cachexia, high fever without bacteraemia, lymphadenopathy and leucocytosis (Still's disease). In all these forms of juvenile RA, the wrist is one of the most frequently involved joints and tends to develop a rapid deterioration of the cartilages, with substantial osteopenia, leading to spontaneous fusion. The reason for such a localized and severe destructive tendency is unknown.

Ankylosing spondylitis

Ankylosing spondylitis is a systemic inflammatory disease which affects mainly the sacroiliac and spine articulations, but which may also have multiple peripheral musculoskeletal manifestations. Assymetrical abnormalities of the small joints of the hand and wrist appear in approximately one-third of the patients with a long duration of the disease (Resnick and Niwayama 1988). All joint compartments can be affected, but the midcarpal joint is the one most frequently involved. Except for the juxtaarticular osteoporosis, which in these patients is

minimal, synovitis resembles that of RA (Soren 1978), with periarticular swelling, bone erosions, and a rapid joint space narrowing due to chondritis. On many occasions ankylosis is the final stage of the disease occurring over a relatively short time (Fig. 3). Less frequently, there is an ulnar and palmar subluxation of the carpal condyle relative to the radius and ulna due to failure of the radiocarpal ligaments.

Psoriatic arthritis

Psoriatic arthritis is an inflammatory osteoarthritic process, included in the generic group of spondyloarthropathies, which affects patients with a past history of psoriatic skin lesions (Moll and Wright 1973). The synovitic process is undistinguishable from that of RA except for having a negative rheumatoid factor. Finger joint involvement is more frequent than wrist involvement, and usually follows a unilateral pattern with a tendency to affect articulations of a single ray. When the wrist is altered by the disease, all the intracarpal joints appear to be equally affected by extensive and rapidly progressing articular erosions with separation of the subchondral margins of adjacent bones and absence of osteoporosis. Soft tissue swelling is minimal and yet very painful. The joint frequently evolves towards a complete ankylosis of the joint.

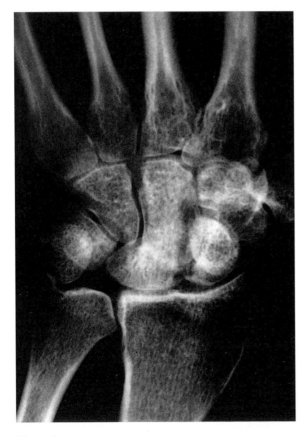

Figure 3

Midcarpal joint stiffness in a 52-year-old man with ankylosing spondylitis. The lunocapitate joint narrowing is associated with a degenerative lunotriquetral dissociation. As a result there is pain and loss of motion.

Crystal-induced arthritis

Two types of crystal-induced arthritis can develop significant wrist stiffness: gout and calcium pyrophosphate dihydrate (CPPD) crystal deposition disease. Gout is a metabolic problem that results from deposition of monosodium urate in the articular soft tissues, usually associated with sustained hyperuricaemia. In the hand, gout has a wide spectrum of clinical presentations, from acute, inflammatory, very painful arthritis, resembling an acute septic problem, to a chronic presentation with similar features to those of RA. Usually the acute presentation of the disease involves only one joint, although polyarticular episodes have been described. When the wrist is affected by the disease, usually it is in the form of acute attacks of gout. These are caused by the release of lysosomal enzymes, products of the damaging effects of intra-articular tophi (aggregates of sodium urate crystals). In chronic cases there is synovitis with collagenase and proteoglycanase release, inducing cartilage and ligament deterioration and consequent stiffness. These cases may have a typical radiographic appearance consisting of both erosive bone lesions and radiodense soft-tissue masses which represent calcification of tophi.

Calcium pyrophosphate dihydrate crystal deposition disease, also known as 'pseudogout', is another crystal-induced polyarticular disease eventually resulting in carpal stiffness. It may remain asymptomatic over a long period, to be discovered incidentally on a routine radiographic study. On the other hand, it can also appear as a very disabling and destructive arthropathy responsible for episodes of acute arthritis resembling those of gout, with the exception of having normal serum levels of uric acid. Of an unknown origin, the disease is associated with the deposition of CPPD crystals in the hyaline cartilage, fibrocartilaginous structures, ligaments and tendon sheaths. When accumulation of crystals is sufficiently high, there will be a typical radiological appearance for which the descriptive term of 'chondrocalcinosis' has been used. In the wrist the disease has a particular predilection for the radiocarpal compartment causing a fairly typical radioscaphoid joint space narrowing, with subchondral sclerosis, virtually identical to alterations secondary to old scapholunate dissociations or SLAC (scapholunate advanced collapse) wrists (Fig. 4). The scaphoid migrates proximally into the radius, while the lunate remains normally aligned with the rest of the carpus, thus creating a 'stepladder' appearance, very suggestive of the disease. Also frequently found among these patients are mineral deposits on both the proximal and distal surfaces of the triangular fibrocartilage (Berger and Buckwalter 1990). These calcifications, however, are only seen in about 65% of patients with CPPD crystal deposition disease (Resnick et al 1983). This indicates that the primary alteration in these patients is cartilage degeneration, the calcification being just a secondary feature. Stiffness is, therefore, the consequence of a mechanically altered articular capsulosynovial disease.

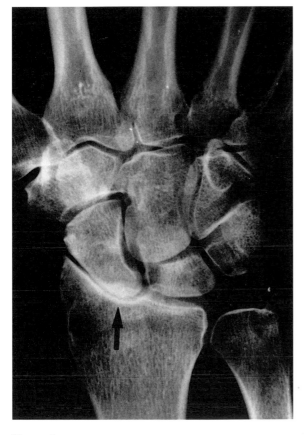

Figure 4

Typical degenerative appearance of a wrist with calcium pyrophosphate dihydrate crystal deposition disease. The radioscaphoid articular surfaces are completely eroded (arrow), the scapholunate joint is dissociated while the radiolunate Interval appears undisturbed. In this case no calcifications of the triangular fibrocartilage were present and the disease was diagnosed by aspiration of the joint and observation of CPPD crystals under the polarizing microscope.

Wrist infections

Although fortunately not very frequent, deep articular infections of the wrist may induce permanent disability with stiffness in a very high percentage of cases (Nagy 1996). They may be caused by a wide variety of microorganisms (bacteria, viruses, mycoplasma, yeast and fungi) which may have been inoculated into the joint through penetrating wounds, by intra-articular injections, during surgery, or by haematogenous transmission. In the latter case, the joint infection may be the initial manifestation of a life-threatening systemic infection or become the only focus of the organism proliferation.

Post-traumatic or post-surgical infections

The most frequent microorganism isolated in post-traumatic septic wrists is *Staphylococcus aureus*, accounting for 66% of the cases reported (Rashkoff

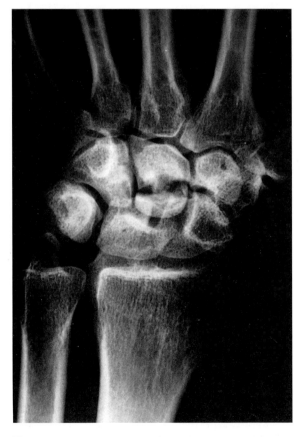

Figure 5

Osteomyelitis of the capitate bone as a complication of a surgical excision of an intraosseous ganglion. The bone appears fractured and collapsed. A sequestrum within the septic pseudoarthrosis can be seen. In this case, stiffness is not only caused by the soft-tissue involvement but also by the secondary midcarpal instability.

et al 1983). Infections incurred after surgery may have a variety of pathogens, and unfortunately in most cases multiresistant microorganisms are involved (Fig. 5). An altered immunologic status (i.e. diabetes mellitus, HIV infection) may reduce the capability of the host to fight the infection, resulting in a higher incidence of morbidity and final disability. Wrist pyarthrosis induces synovitis, cartilage damage and weakening of the capsuloligamentous structures, all of which are likely to result in a severe alteration of carpal kinematics with subsequent stiffness of the joint. The extent and nature of cartilage and ligament damage will depend upon the virulence of the infection, the host reaction, the effectiveness of treatment and the healing potential of damaged structures (Nagy 1996). Unlike RA, septic arthritis tends to involve homogeneously all the intracarpal joints and the articulating bones, with a special predominance at the midcarpal level which typically undergoes extensive joint narrowing with subsequent ankylosis.

Wrist tuberculosis

Skeletal infection with *Mycobacterium tuberculosis*, once a devastating widespread disease, has decreased considerably to become a rarity today. The incidence of wrist tuberculosis has also been reduced significantly (Bush and Schneider 1984). The bacillus usually enters the body through the lungs, where it causes the initial infection, and from there it is transferred by the bloodstream to the bones and joints. Wrist infection may occur in the form of a primary synovitis or secondary to an adjacent osteomyelitis which has progressed to the point of communicating with the joint. The infected synovial pannus spreads out over the empty articular joint spaces, except for the weight-bearing cartilage areas which are typically spared from the initial deterioration process. At the same time, infected granulomatous tissue enters the subchondral bone, eroding underneath the cartilages and cortical insertions of ligaments (Gunther 1991). Subsequently, the subchondral support to the cartilage decreases and the mechanical performance of the stabilizing ligaments diminish until the carpus collapses under the influence of the forces normally acting over these joints. In the early stages of the disease, wrist tuberculosis is characterized by soft-tissue swelling, marked local osteoporosis, loss of subchondral plates and preservation of the joint spaces. In later stages, after bone collapse, there is a complete loss of joint congruity leading to stiffness and eventually to a complete ankylosis once the infection has healed.

Degenerative osteoarthropathies

Osteoarthritis has long been understood as a degenerative process without inflammation, for which the alternative terms of 'degenerative joint disease' or 'osteoarthrosis' have often been used. Recently, however, evidence has been collected suggesting that most of these patients have indeed concurrent synovitis, although benign and slowly progressive (Soren 1978, Flatt 1995). When the process affects a joint not known to have been previously damaged nor with a predisposing congenital anomaly, the case is designated as a primary or idiopathic osteoarthritis. Secondary osteoarthritis appears more commonly related to an old traumatism, although it can be the result of systemic diseases, such as haemophilia, neuropathy (Charcot joints), metabolic disorders (acromegaly, hypothyroidism, hyperparathyroidism), or evolve from an unstable congenital disease (Altman 1990).

Primary osteoarthritis of the wrist resulting in carpal stiffness is very rare except for those involving the scaphoid-trapezium-trapezoid (STT) joint (Carstam et al 1968). It usually has a bilateral distribution, frequently combined with degenerative changes at the trapeziometacarpal joint. As an isolated condition it is quite uncommon (Fig. 6). According to North and Eaton (1983), only 6% of 68 dissected wrists from patients over 50 years old had an STT osteoarthritis in the absence of a trapezometacarpal degeneration. Pain and tenderness at the base of the thumb are typical findings, and may be associated with restricted motion and adjacent soft tissue swelling. Radiographic features include joint space narrowing and sclerosis of the apposing articular surfaces. In advanced cases, significant osteophyte formation invading the flexor carpi radialis compartment is relatively common. In such instances, recurrent tendonitis, ganglia formation or even tendon ruptures may be found. STT osteoarthritis frequently coexists with a moderate to severe carpal malalignment: the whole proximal carpal row is found abnormally extended in a non-dissociative dorsal intercalated segment instability

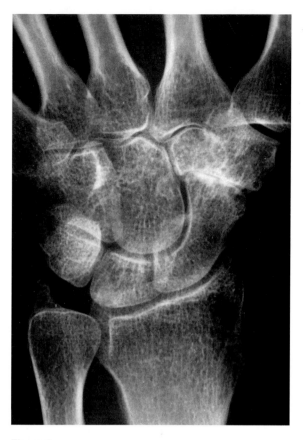

Figure 6

Isolated idiopathic osteoarthritis of the scaphotrapezial–trapezoidal joint. Stiffness in these patients appears in the later stages of the disease.

(DISI) fashion (Crosby et al 1978). Whether or not this is the consequence or the cause of the degenerative process is controversial. In a cadaver study, Viegas et al (1993) found a high correlation between the existence of an STT osteoarthritis and the presence of tears of the scapholunate interosseous membrane. As a result, it is uncertain whether this type of degenerative process should be listed as primary or secondary to an underlying chronic, dynamic carpal instability problem.

Secondary osteoarthritis eventually resulting in wrist reduction of motion is quite common. Joint space narrowing, sclerosis, osteophytes and subchondral cysts around the radioscaphoid and capitolunate articulations, combined with a scapholunate separation are typical abnormalities occurring after a long unsolved scapholunate dissociation injury (Fig. 7). Such radiographic changes are termed the scapholunate advanced collapse, or SLAC wrist (Watson and Ryu 1984). Other similar post-injury degenerative patterns are seen following old, unstable scaphoid non-unions. All these problems are the consequence of both altered joint motion and abnormal transmission of loads, and are incompatible with a normal range of wrist motion. Stiffness, in these cases, appears slowly but progressively, and often remains asymptomatic until it reaches an advanced stage of joint destruction.

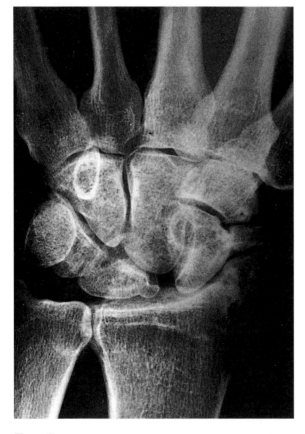

Figure 7

A 56-year-old man who sustained a motorcycle accident more than 30 years before this X-ray was taken. The wrist is now painful and stiff. Both the scapholunate gap and the extensive cartilage wear at the radioscaphoid joint (SLAC wrist) confirm the existence of an old scapholunate dissociation in this case, the osteophytes between radius and scaphoid probably prevented the complete collapse of the latter.

References

Altman RD (1990) Classification of disease: osteoarthritis, *Semin Arthritis Rheum* **6**(suppl 2):40–7.

Berger RA, Buckwalter JA (1990) Calcium pyrophosphate dihydrate crystal deposition patterns in the triangular fibrocartilage complex, *Orthopedics* **13**:75–80.

Bush DC, Schneider LH (1984) Tuberculosis of the hand and wrist, *J Hand Surg* **9A**:391–8.

Carstam N, Eiken O, Andrew L (1968) Osteoarthritis of the trapezio-scaphoid joint, *Acta Orthop Scand* **39**:354–8.

Crosby EB, Linscheid RL, Dobyns JH (1978) Scaphotrapezial–trapezoidal arthrosis, *J Hand Surg* **3**:223–34.

Flatt AE (1995) *The Care of the Arthritic Hand.* Quality Medical Publishing: St Louis: 153–88.

Garcia-Elias M (1996) Carpal kinetics. In: Büchler U, ed. *Wrist Instability.* Martin Dunitz: London: 9–13.

Gunther SF (1991) Tuberculosis of the hand and wrist. In: Jupiter JB, ed. *Flynn's Hand Surgery*, 4th edn. Williams & Wilkins: Baltimore: 785–91.

Harris ED (1990) Rheumatoid arthritis. Pathophysiology and implications for therapy, *N Engl J Med* **322**:1277–89.

Mathies H (1977) *Characteristic Features of the Most Important Rheumatic Diseases.* Eular: Basle: 18–24.

Moll JMH, Wright V (1973) Psoriatic arthritis, *Semin Arthritis Rheum* **3**:55–78.

Nagy L (1996) Wrist instability following acute and chronic infection. In: Büchler U, ed. *Wrist Instability*. Martin Dunitz: London: 205–12.

Nalebuff EA, Austin GJ (1991) Rheumatoid hand surgery. In: Jupiter JB, ed. *Flynn's Hand Surgery*, 4th edn. Williams & Wilkins: Baltimore: 387–406.

North ET, Eaton RG (1983) Degenerative joint disease of the trapezium: a comparative radiographic and anatomic study, *J Hand Surg* **8**:160–7.

Rashkoff ES, Burkhalter WE, Mann RJ (1983) Septic arthritis of the wrist, *J Bone Joint Surg* **65A**:824–8.

Resnick CS, Miller BW, Gelberman RH, Resnick D (1983) Hand and wrist involvement in calcium pyrophosphate dihydrate deposition disease, *J Hand Surg* **8**:856–63

Resnick D, Niwayama G (1988) Ankylosing spondyltis. In: Resnick D, Niwayama G, eds. *Diagnosis of Bone and Joint Disorders*. WB Saunders: Philadelphia: 103–70.

Simmen BR (1996) Patterns of carpal collapse in rheumatoid arthritis: surgical implications. In: Büchler U, ed. *Wrist Instability*. Martin Dunitz: London: 193–204.

Soren A (1978) *Histodiagnosis and Clinical Correlation of Rheumatoid and Other Synovitis*. JB Lippincott: Philadelphia: 116–21.

Steinbrocker O, Traeger CH, Batterman RC (1949) Therapeutic criteria in rheumatoid arthritis, *JAMA* **140**:659–62.

Taleisnik J (1985) *The Wrist*. Churchill Livingstone: New York: 327–56.

Thirupathi RG, Ferlic DL, Clayton ML (1983) Dorsal wrist synovectomy in rheumatoid arthritis, *J Hand Surg* **6**:848–55.

Viegas SF, Patterson RM, Hokanson JA, Davis J (1993) Wrist anatomy: incidence, distribution, and correlation of anatomic variations, tears, and arthrosis. *J Hand Surg* **18A**:463–75.

Watson HK, Ryu J (1984) Degenerative disorders of the carpus, *Orthop Clin North Amer* **15**:337–53.

27
Flaps and tenolysis for radiocarpal joint stiffness

Guy Foucher

The anatomical structures contributing to extra-articular wrist stiffness are numerous. On the palmar aspect, the skin and musculotendinous structures are the most frequently responsible, but a median nerve repair under tension with a protective splint in flexion can induce a wrist flexion deformity with pain during active extension. Another mechanism, hopefully rare (three cases in our series), is secondary to an anastomosis of the median nerve with the flexor carpi radialis.

Palmar skin insufficiency is the more frequent aetiology. It could be due to a crush injury with progressive skin necrosis and retraction and is also frequent in deep burn injury.

The key to treatment is to provide supple and ample skin after excision of all scar tissue. Currently, the techniques have improved, and it is not a wise solution to use a distant pedicle flap, e.g. a groin flap (MacGregor 1987), which 'steals blood' after the pedicle is cut. In most cases, nerves and tendons need some associated surgery such as neurolysis, nerve graft, tenolysis or tendon graft. It is then more appropriate to provide a flap with independent and permanent vascularization which, at least, does not steal the blood of deep structures and can possibly even provide some 'trophic' help to the recipient nerves and tendons (Foucher 1984a, 1984b and 1987). A second prerequisite is to provide a 'sealed' recipient site to avoid any inflammatory reaction, often seen in 'semi-open' pedicle flaps, secondary to partial disunion of the tube (Foucher et al 1987). We favour using, in this area, some regional island forearm flaps, most having a retrograde flow. They share all the advantages of the free flaps without the incumbent risk of microsurgery and the necessity of a distant donor site. When the island forearm flaps are contraindicated (mainly for vascular reasons) or unavailable, a good alternative is the free lateral arm flap (Katsaros et al 1991) which could be harvested under the same tourniquet field. However, we found some drawbacks to this flap: it is quite bulky, its nutrient artery can be rather small and its donor site is conspicuous in an exposed area, not really superior to the cosmetic sequelae of the so-called 'Chinese' forearm flap (Fenton and Roberts 1985).

Numerous flaps are available, and here is not the place to give technical details, but besides the well-known radial forearm flaps (Yang et al 1981, Song et al 1982, Braun et al 1985) and the ulnar flap (Lovie et al 1984, Guimberteau et al 1988), many others have been described to avoid sacrifice of a major artery. Goffin et al (1992) raises a radial flap based on a constant side-branch of the radial artery found consistently 2 cm proximal to the radial styloid process; this flap can be reasonably large, easily reaching the anterior aspect of the wrist, but with a quite short pedicle. Becker (1990) has described an ulnar flap based on the ulnodorsal branch of the ulnar artery, 3 cm proximal to the pisiform bone. The ascending branch allows a 12 cm-long flap to be harvested in an easily concealed area. Unfortunately, again, the pedicle is rather short. More recently, Bakhach (1995) has described a smaller flap, harvested on the ulnar side of the hand (10 × 3 cm large), based on the descending branch of the same artery. Two interosseous flaps are also available, the classical posterior interosseous flap (Zancolli et al 1986, Masquelet and Penteado 1987) and the less well-known anterior interosseous flap (Hu et al 1994) taken from the dorsum of the distal third of the forearm, based on a posterior branch of the anterior interosseous artery. Finally, a muscular flap, the pronator quadratus island (Dellon 1984), isolated on the anterior interosseous artery, could be also useful; it provides a 'cushion' to protect, for example, a painful neuroma in continuity of the median nerve with acceptable functional results.

The quite large choice among forearm flaps explains the limited indications, at least in our experience, for free flap in this area.

To avoid sacrificing a major vessel, we have in some cases used the radial forearm flap as a bipedicled island flap, without interrupting the radial artery, by shifting it more medially (Foucher et al 1984b and 1987). Another advantage of this flap is the excellent fascia which can be harvested simultaneously and wrapped around a grafted median nerve to protect it from the surrounding tendon and which allows differential gliding of the structures (tendon from nerve and nerve from skin). We have also used forearm flaps as free flaps when the hand is devascularized with interruption of both the radial and ulnar arteries at the wrist level. For example, the free radial flap allows re-establishment of the flow in the ulnar artery. Another alternative that we have used only once in a deep wrist burn, treated initially with a simple skin graft put directly on the radius, is to transfer a compound ulnar flap including an ulnar vascularized nerve to re-establish simultaneously the flow through the radial artery and the continuity of the median nerve (inserting at the same stage silastic rods to prepare a secondary flexor tendon grafting).

Flexor tendons are also frequently involved in such stiff wrists in flexion, either at the tendon level (after primary repair followed by adhesions), or at the muscular level (with ischaemic retraction). Adhesions of flexor tendons are frequent after prolonged immobilization of the wrist in flexion. The flexor tendons remain stuck to the forearm skeleton (when not trapped in a fracture site). Examination is the key to diagnosis, and splinting is the solution, at least in cases seen early. Tenodesis effects unveil the diagnosis; by increasing flexion of the wrist, better finger extension is noted. Differential diagnosis with Volkmann's syndrome, besides the history, is the usual palpation of a forearm 'mass'. However, although rare, some muscle retraction can happen in long-standing deformity without ischaemia of the muscle.

Splinting the fingers in extension is useful for stabilizing the wrist (Ehrler et al 1983) to really pull on the adhesions (Fig. 1a). If some limitation of extension remains at the wrist level after recovery of the flexor tendons course, another type of dynamic splint is necessary (Fig. 1b). If splinting is unsuccessful, a formal tenolysis is performed. It is not a complicated procedure at this level, and we have described our postoperative regimen (Foucher et al

1993). The wrist is splinted in neutral (or slight extension), and the fingers are maintained in flexion at the end of the operation. Two catheters are inserted close to the median and ulnar nerves to allow injection of bupivacaine at first dressing. At 48–72 hours, after injection in the catheter, the patient is allowed to extend and flex the fingers. Due to pain, fear, muscle weakness, and early postoperative adhesions, this manoeuvre is frequently difficult; but with adhesions in flexion, the surgeon can break them by gentle passive extension of the fingers. The splinting in slight flexion of the fingers remains for 3 weeks, being only removed hourly for short sessions of active motion. This splint has not caused any final lack of extension, and had decreased the rate of flexor tendon ruptures (the patient cannot use his hand during the 3 weeks of protection).

In the case of moderate muscle retraction noted at surgery, after extensive freeing of the flexor tendons, we proceed with an intramuscular tendon step lengthening, which does not preclude early postoperative active motion. However, we rely more on wrist tenodesis manoeuvres which means that full extension of the fingers is allowed in wrist flexion, and full flexion of the fingers is accompanied by wrist extension. After a moderate lengthening, flexor strength takes a year to recover.

We use the same operation in moderate Volkmann ischaemic retraction combined, if necessary, to a median nerve neurolysis. When the nerve seems devascularized on a quite long segment, we wrap it in an island bipedicle forearm fascia flap. This means that we isolate a forearm fascia flap bipedicled on the non-interrupted radial artery and simply shift this flap more ulnarly to surround the ischaemic median nerve. In more accentuated retraction, we perform classical operations as described by Scaglietti (1957) and Zancolli (1968). It is not the place here to discuss the role of first row carpectomy in difficult cases of long-standing fixed wrist in flexion, but we found it useful in rare situations.

In conclusion, wrist flexion stiffness is frequently secondary to multiple factors, and a combination of the aforementioned procedures is frequently necessary. The worst prognosis comes when a reflex sympathetic dystrophy is indicated, rendering the splinting painful and delaying any attempt at surgical correction.

This is also true for wrist extension stiffness where the two main structures involved are the skin

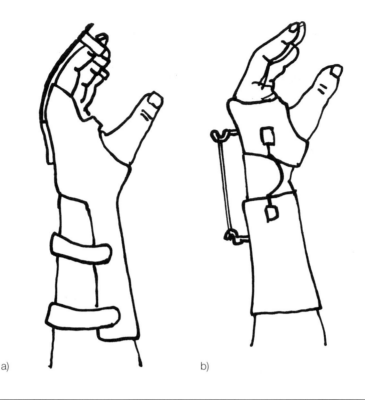

a) b)

Figure 1

(a) Splinting the fingers in extension. (b) A dynamic splint.

and the extensor mechanism in zone 6 to 8 (Verdan 1975).

Insufficiently treated, deep dorsal burn can be followed by the classical deformity associating dorsiflexion of the wrist, hyperextension of the MP (metacarpophalangeal) joint, flexion of the proximal interphalangeal joint, and thumb adduction. Crush injuries are less frequently complicated by this type of deformation, except when wrist extensor tendon losses are treated by simple suture under tension with prolonged immobilization in wrist extension.

An insufficient skin cover is frequently associated with an extensor tendon loss. The two possibilities are a staged repair with a first step of skin cover, with (Engel et al 1977) or without insertion of silastic rods, followed by extensor tendon grafting. The second option is a one-stage replacement with either conventional tendon grafts plus a flap or a compound free or island flap composed of skin and

vascularized tendons. Among the flaps available for such reconstruction, the dorsalis pedis plus extensor (Taylor and Townsend 1979, Reid and Moss 1983, Lee et al 1994) and the tensor fasciae latae flaps are the more classical. We have described the technique of the compound radial forearm flap transferred *en bloc* with the vascularized brachioradialis tendon (which could be divided in three strips) and the palmaris longus (Foucher et al 1984b and 1987). In fact, we have not been able to find any functional difference between vascularized and non-vascularized tendons in zone 6. With the combined problem of wrist extension stiffness, we favour a two-stages repair with initial insertion of a flap, followed by a dynamic wrist splinting (Fig. 1b) to increase the range of flexion. A dynamic MP flexion splint is also frequently needed. The flaps that we favour are again the island forearm, relying on free flaps only in case of contraindications. Fascia flaps have been disappointing in our experience, and we prefer skin flaps. The extensors are repaired at a second stage by conventional bridge grafts. The dorsal retinacular ligament frequently injured is not repaired to avoid adhesion and the bow stringing is usually limited in such a stiff wrist.

After a heavy crush extending proximally, the muscles are sometimes in bad condition, and it is more logical to perform a tendon transfer, using the classic flexor superficialis transfer of the third and fourth fingers through the membrane (Boyes 1960). Extensor tendon injury in zone 7 is also a frequent cause of wrist and finger flexion restriction due to adhesions underneath the strong dorsal retinacular ligament. The tenodesis effect is obvious at examination, showing a more restricted range of flexion of the MP and IP during maximum flexion of the wrist. Again, dynamic splinting stabilizing the wrist initially in extension and progressively in flexion, combined with MP (and IP) dynamic flexion, is efficient in cases seen early after repair. Otherwise, tenolysis of the extensor with partial excision of the retinacular is performed followed by an active range of motion and dynamic splinting of finger and wrist.

In conclusion, these limitations of extension or flexion are frequent. The skin and musculotendinous units are the most frequently involved structures and a capsular wrist contraction is seldom associated (Watson and Dhillon 1993). Emphasis has to be put on early motion and splinting to avoid or correct this problem. Later, surgery is frequently necessary, encompassing complex operations.

References

Bakhach J, Saint Cast Y, Gazarian A, Martin D, Comtet JJ, Baudet J (1995) Ulnar parametacarpal flap. Anatomical study and clinical application, *Ann Chir Plast* **40**:136–47.

Becker C (1990) Lambeau antébrachial des branches distales de l'artère cubitale. Gilbert A, Masquelet AC, Hertz VR, eds. *Les lambeaux artériels pédiculés du membre supérieur.* Expansion Scientifique Français: Paris: 102–6.

Boyes JH (1960) Tendon transfer for radial palsy, *Bull Hosp Joint Dis* **21**:97–105.

Braun F, Hoang P, Merle M, Van Genechten F, Foucher G (1985) Technique et indications du lambeau antébrachial en chirurgie de la main: a propos de 33 cas, *Ann Chir Main* **4**:85–97.

Dellon AL (1984) The pronator quadratus muscle flap, *J Hand Surg* **9**:423–7.

Ehrler S, Braun F, Foucher G, Xenard J (1983) Rôle de la stabilisation du poignet dans la conception de l'orthèse de la main, *Rev Réadapt Fonct Prof Soc* **10**:20–3.

Engel J, Stur C, Horoshowsky H (1977) Dorsal silicone rods in the primary care of war injuries, *Hand* **9**:153–6.

Fenton OM, Roberts JO (1985) Improving the donor site of the radial forearm flap. *Br J Plast Surg* **38**:504–5.

Foucher G (1994) Extensor loss and hood reconstruction. 'Casle' flap in extensor tenolysis. In: Kasdan L, Amadio PC, Bowers WH, eds. *Technical Tips for Hand Surgery.* Mosby: St Louis: 245–8.

Foucher G, Gilbert A, Merle M, Jacob Y (1984a) Lambeau radial 'chinois'. In: Tubiana R, ed. *Traité de Chirurgie de la Main*, Vol. 2. Masson: Paris: 244–9.

Foucher G, Van Genechten F, Merle M, Michon J (1984b) A compound radial artery forearm flap in hand surgery: an original modification of the Chinese forearm flap, *Br J Plast Surg* **37**:139–48.

Foucher G, Citron N, Hoang P (1987) Technique and applications of the forearm flap in surgery of the hand. In: Urbaniak J, ed. *Microsurgery for Major Limb Reconstruction.* Mosby: St Louis: 256–63.

Foucher G, Lenoble E, Ben Youssef K, Sammut D (1993) A postoperative regime after digital flexor tenolysis. A series of 72 patients, *J Hand Surg* **18B**:35–40.

Goffin D, Brunelli F, Galbiatti A, Sammut D, Gilbert A (1992) A new flap based on the distal branches of the radial artery, *Ann Hand Surg* **11**:217–25.

Guimberteau JC, Goin JL, Panconi B, Schumacher B (1988) The reverse ulnar artery forearm island flap in hand surgery: 54 cases, *Plast Reconstr Surg* **81**:925–32.

Hu W, Martin D, Foucher G, Baudet J (1994) Le lambeau interosseux antérieur. *Ann Chir Plast Esth* **39**:3, 288–300.

Katsaros J, Tan E, Zoltie N, Venkataramakrishnan (1991) The use of the lateral arm flap, *J Hand Surg* **16A**:598–604.

Lee KS, Park SW, Kim HY (1994) Tendocutaneous free flap transfer from the dorsum of the foot, *Microsurgery* **15**:12, 882–5.

Lovie MJ, Duncan GM, Glasson DW (1984) The ulnar artery forearm free flap, *Br J Plast Surg* **37**:486–92.

MacGregor AD (1987) The free radial forearm flap – the management of the secondary defect, *Br J Plast Surg* **40**:83–5.

Masquelet AC, Penteado CV (1987) Le lambeau interosseux postérieur, *Ann Chir Main* **6**:131–9.

Reid CD, Moss ALH (1983). One stage flap repair with vascularized tendon grafts in dorsal hand injury using the 'Chinese' forearm flap, *Br J Plast Surg* **36**:473–9.

Scaglietti O (1957) Sindromi cliniche immidiate e tardive da lesioni vascolari nelle fratture degli arti, *Riforma Med* **71**:749–55.

Song RY, Gad YZ, Song YG, Yu YS, Song YL (1982) The forearm flap, *Clin Plast Surg* **9**:21–6.

Taylor GI, Townsend P (1979) Composite free flap and tendon transfer: an anatomical study and a clinical technique, *Brit J Plast Surg* **32**:170–83.

Verdan C (1975) Primary and secondary repair of flexor and extensor tendon injuries. In: Flynn E, ed. *Flynn's Hand Surgery,* 2nd ed. Williams & Wilkins: Baltimore: 144–76.

Watson HK, Dhillon H (1993) Stiff joints. In: Green D, ed. *Operative Hand Surgery*, Vol. 2. Churchill Livingstone: New York: 549–62.

Yang G, Chen B, Gao Y (1981) Forearm free skin flap transplantation, *Nat Med J China* **61**:139.

Zancolli EA, Angrigiani C (1986) Colgajo dorsal de antebrazo en 'isla'. *Rev Assoc Argentine Ortho Trauma* **51**:161–8.

Zancolli E (1968) *Structural and Dynamic Bases of Hand Surgery.* JB Lippincott: Philadelphia.

28

Limited arthrodesis and scapholunate advanced collapse treatment for radiocarpal joint stiffness

Philippe Saffar

Numerous treatments have been proposed depending on the OA localization and extent, patient age and occupation and the number of previous procedures:

- radiolunate arthrodesis
- proximal row carpectomy
- denervation
- limited wrist arthrodesis
- total wrist arthrodesis
- prostheses.

The current practice is to avoid total wrist arthrodesis. There is almost always an area where the cartilage is preserved and the radioulnate joint space is usually in good shape. The scapholunate advanced collapse (SLAC) treatment proposed by Watson and Ballet (1984) is the standard.

It consists of a lunocapitate arthrodesis associated with a scaphoidectomy. In the beginning, the scaphoid was replaced by a Silastic scaphoid prosthesis. The drawbacks created by Silastic implants led to their abandonment and a scaphoidectomy is now performed without replacement.

A four-bone (four-corner) arthrodesis uniting the lunate, triquetrum, capitate and hamate bones is currently preferred to lunocapitate arthrodesis because healing is easier, but ROM is not as good as for lunocapitate arthrodesis.

Capitolunate arthrodesis

A dorsal longitudinal approach between dorsal compartments III and IV leads to the wrist joint at the level of the scapholunate joint. If the proximal lunate cartilage is in good shape, this type of arthrodesis is recommended (Fig. 1). The scaphoid bone is first removed and the bone is preserved to be used as a graft (Fig. 2). The remaining cartilages of the distal lunate and proximal head of the capitate are then removed as well as the subchondral bone. It is necessary to be at the cancellous bone level.

The difficulty of this procedure is regaining carpal height, reducing the lunate on top of the capitate. Reduction is sometimes easy, but distraction forces may be present in long-standing cases, making it difficult to restore the normal position of the lunate. Removal of intra-articular fibrous tissue may help.

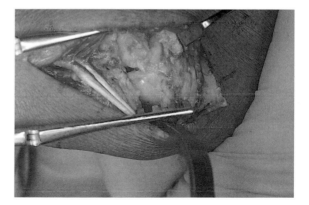

Figure 1

Posterior approach: there is cartilage wear at the proximal pole of the scaphoid. The cartilage of the capitate head is intact.

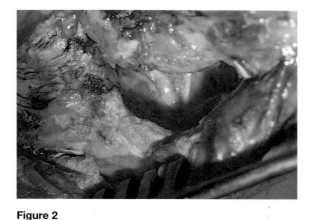

Figure 2

The scaphoid bone has been removed.

Provisional fixation is performed after reduction using a K-wire introduced along the lunate and capitate axis (Fig. 3). Cancellous graft (harvested from the scaphoid bone) is introduced between the two bones to regain normal carpal height and fixation is then completed using crossed K-wires plus staples (Fig. 4). 'Shape memory' staples provide a better healing rate and should be used whenever possible (Fig. 5).

Compression screws should not be used because they may cause carpal collapse.

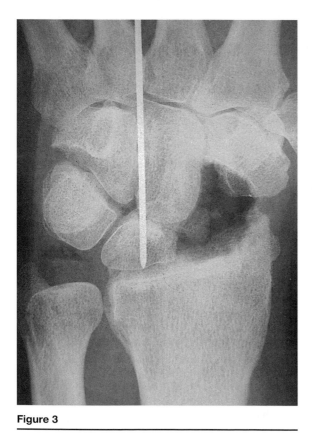

Figure 3

Scaphoid removed; a provisional K-wire has been inserted.

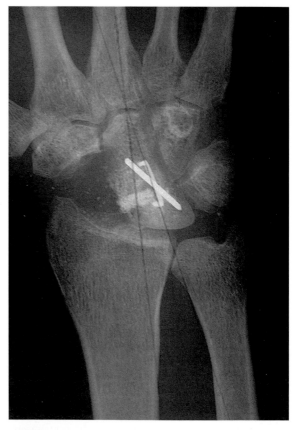

Figure 4

Capitolunate arthrodesis with graft plus scaphoidectomy.

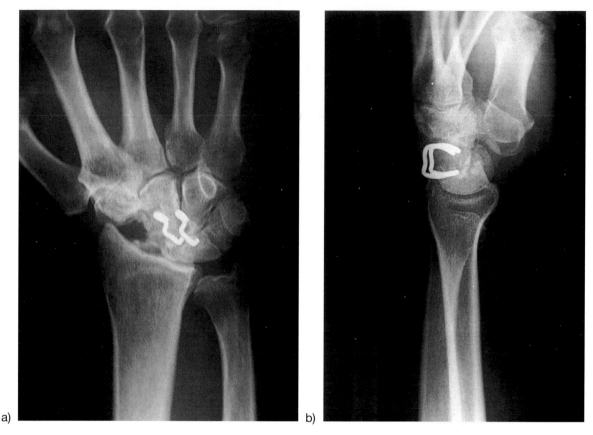

a)   b)

Figure 5

Capitolunate arthrodesis with memory staples (a, AP; and b, lateral).

Four-corner arthrodesis

A dorsal longitudinal incision is made at the level of compartment IV. The dorsal retinaculum is opened and the extensor tendons retracted ulnarly. Inspection of carpal cartilage and ligaments confirm that this is a SLAC stage III. Scaphoid resection is completed. After retracting the extensor tendons radially, the four medial carpal bones are prepared for arthrodesis by resection of adjacent carpal bone cartilage. Reduction of the lunate on the capitate bone is mandatory to try to restore carpal height and prevent dorsal impingement of the carpal block with the distal dorsal radius. Fixation with K-wires and/or shape memory staples is the usual technique (Fig. 6). After undermining, so that a graft applied at the dorsal aspect of the four bones will be at the level of the dorsal aspect of the carpus, the graft may be fixed by screws. Sandow et al (1992) have described a dowel graft uniting the four bones after removing a round piece of bone at the conjunction of the four bones.

At the end of the limited arthrodeses procedures, the wrist should be placed in maximum extension to check the possibility of impingement of the carpus with the radius distal end. If this is the case, removal of the distal radius opposed to the carpus block should be performed until no impingement is present.

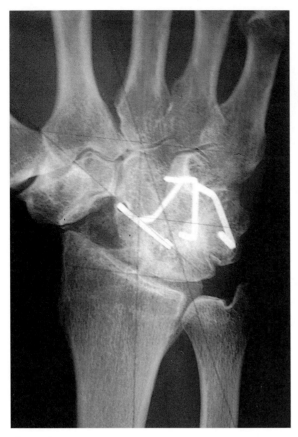

Figure 6

Four-corner arthrodesis.

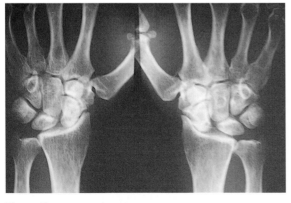

Figure 7

Bilateral 'SLAC' at different stages in the same patient.

Discussion

The term 'SLAC treatment' was also used for arthritis secondary to scaphoid non-unions and other aetiologies. The term 'SNAC' (Fig. 8) (scaphoid non-union advanced collapse) has been proposed for these cases and seems more convenient. Four-corner arthrodesis results in less non-union than capitolunate arthrodesis. Scaphoid implants have been completely abandoned because of numerous complications such as dislocation or subluxation, and synovitis. Results are as good without scaphoid implants and the wrist radial deviation mentioned by Watson and Ballet (1984) have not been a concern for other authors.

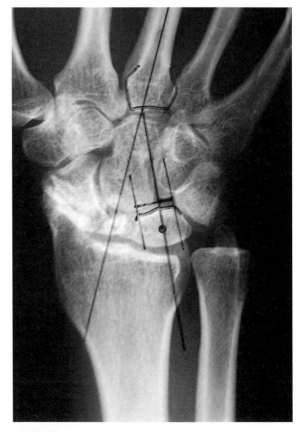

Figure 8

'SNAC': scaphoid non-union advanced collapse.

Pain relief is effective, but few patients are completely painless. Residual pain may impede the return to a hard work.

Complications include NSD in 7% of the cases. Total wrist arthrodesis was necessary in a small number of cases.

Dorsal impingement was seen in some cases. On lateral X-rays, contact between the radius's dorsal rim and the capitolunate block is present in wrist extension in 50% of the patients. Narrowing of the posterior part of the joint space and osteophytes on radius and lunate are visible. The difference of pain between the two groups was statistically significant (1.61/0.83). This indicates a preventive treatment of this impingement.

Contraindications of limited carpal arthrodeses are:

- a carpal ulnar shift
- radiolunate cartilage changes.

Radiolunate arthrodesis

A dorsal approach is used. After assessing the status of the cartilage, particularly of the head of the capitate and interosseous ligaments, the remnants of the articular cartilage of the proximal lunate and lunate fossa are excised. Manual distraction is applied to regain the normal carpal height, thus allowing the scaphoid to restore its normal alignment.

A corticocancellous graft is harvested from the iliac crest or from the proximal end of the ulna. A trough is made in the dorsomedial and distal part of the radius and in the dorsal part of the lunate (Fig. 9). The corticocancellous bone graft is interposed to restore the normal carpal height, and to disimpact the carpus from the radius. The dorsal aspect of the graft must be at the level of the dorsal radius, and thus avoid impeding the normal gliding of extensor tendons. The graft may be harvested from the dorsal part of the radius, and slide distally to cover the lunate (Fig. 10). Surplus cancellous bone is packed between radius and lunate.

Internal fixation may be obtained using two screws, one going through the graft and the volar cortex of the radius and the second through the graft and the volar cortex of the lunate. A small plate may also be used.

A volar splint is applied for 4 days, and then

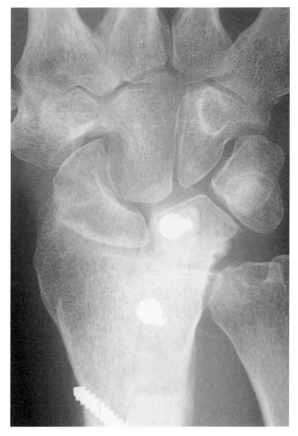

Figure 9

Radiolunate arthrodesis.

replaced by a cast until union is achieved. Rehabilitation on a daily basis is necessary to regain a good ROM.

Associated procedures may be necessary. A distal radial osteotomy performed for an associated distal radial malunion, a carpal tunnel release or a Darrach procedure.

Denervation

Wrist denervation was first described by Wilhelm (1966). It may be considered as an associated procedure or as a salvage procedure.

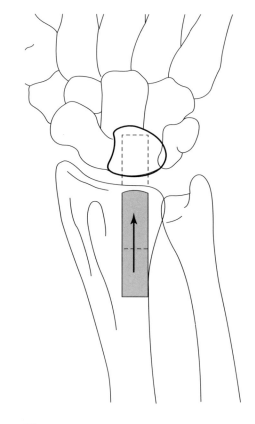

Figure 10

Sliding graft for radiolunate arthrodesis.

An anatomical description of the articular branches emerging from the surrounding nerves was made by Wilhelm (1966), Foucher (1989), Zarcolli and Cozzi (1991), and recently by Dubert et al (1990) and Fukumoto et al (1993). It appears possible to relieve pain by cutting all the articular branches: the anterior and posterior interosseous nerve, the superficial branch of the radial nerve, branches of the musculocutaneous nerve, the palmar branch of the median nerve, and branches of the ulnar nerve. The technique of denervation has been thoroughly described by Foucher (1989) and Buck-Gramcko (1993), and both complete and incomplete denervations have been performed. To cut all branches, several approaches are necessary: a curved palmar radial incision, a mid-dorsal longi-tudinal, and three small incisions at the dorsal aspect of the second, third and fourth interosseous spaces. It is a relatively simple and fast procedure with a short time out of work for recovery. Buck-Gramcko (1993) recommends a preoperative block-age by local anaesthesia to try to predict the result of the procedure; other authors do not, however, think this is predictive. The procedure has been combined with other surgical procedures in a great number of cases. Results reported for the personal series of Buck-Gramcko (1993) indicate 60% of patients pain-free or with a slight pain, 30% improved and 10% not improved. Best results are obtained for scaphoid non-union or arthritis; less good are the results for Kienböck's disease and intra-articular distal radial fractures. There is no improvement on strength and range of motion. Osteoarthritis increased in 20% of the cases and in some cases, pain increased after some months.

The best indication is a middle-aged man with a global OA and a good ROM after a scaphoid non-union. In wrist stiffness, it is not the best indication but it may be associated with other procedures.

Total wrist arthrodesis

This was the standard procedure used for wrist OA with stiffness. Many orthopaedic surgeons tend to overuse this technique because they are not aware of all the surgical possibilities which allow motion to be regained. The rationale is: it is already stiff, so why hesitate? Furthermore, wrist arthrodesis had the reputation of giving a strong pain-free wrist. Series published demonstrate, however, that the complication rate is high (Abbott et al 1942, Clendenin and Green 1981, Gaisne et al 1991, Zachary and Stern 1995) and that the results are not as good as it was supposed. Residual pain may be present in 10–20% of cases. The tenodesis effect of the wrist on finger flexion is suppressed and this decreases grip strength. Loss of grip strength is reported as 30–50% of the opposite side in the different series after radiocarpal arthrodesis. Complications are frequent: non-union, fracture of the graft or plate, extensor tendon problems. These complications are related to the number of previous procedures. If a wrist arthrodesis has to be performed, it should not be preceded by several other procedures. It is still the gold standard for some surgeons.

Technique

Numerous techniques have been described, the main difference being whether a plate is or is not inserted. Position of the wrist is usually in 25° of extension and ulnar deviation, except for rheumatoid arthritis (RA).

Wrist arthrodesis without plate

A dorsal incision is performed longitudinally in the middle axis of the radius. The dorsal retinaculum is opened and extensor tendons retracted. One may routinely cut the distal end of the posterior interosseous nerve. A trough 2 cm long is made at the dorsal aspect of the radius and carpus ending at the second and third metacarpal (this last feature is disputed and some surgeons stop the trough at the level of the carpus). Cartilages of all the radiocarpal and intercarpal joint spaces are removed. A corticocancellous graft is harvested at the iliac crest, taking care to obtain a slightly curved graft which will be applied in the trough, the wrist being in a 30° extension position. The graft is then fixed by two screws to the radius and the carpus (Fig. 11). The joint spaces are packed with cancellous grafts. Care should be taken that the corticocancellous graft should be at the level of the normal radius to prevent extensor tendons rubbing. After closure of the dorsal retinaculum and the skin, a bulky bandage is applied with a splint and replaced by a cast for 6 weeks.

Wrist arthrodesis using a plate

To obtain better rigidity during healing, a plate was proposed (Müller et al 1969). This does not prevent preparation of the joint spaces and cancellous or corticocancellous graft packing. The healing rate seems better with this technique, although some plate ruptures have been observed due to arthrodesis non-union.

Indications of wrist arthrodesis still exist, such as complete destruction of radiocarpal cartilages in the scaphoid and lunate fossa (usually after comminutive intra-articular fractures, after spontaneous or postoperative infections, or in some palsies when tendon transfers are not possible).

Mannerfelt technique of wrist arthrodeses

This uses a Rush pin which is inserted in the third metacarpal through the radius associated with two staples and is used in rheumatoid disease and provides a good result. Fusion is easier in RA than in post-traumatic cases. The position is neutral for one wrist and in slight flexion for the second wrist.

Wrist prostheses

For more than 30 years, different type of prostheses have been tried. Until now, the only indications are for treatment of RA. When used for post-traumatic

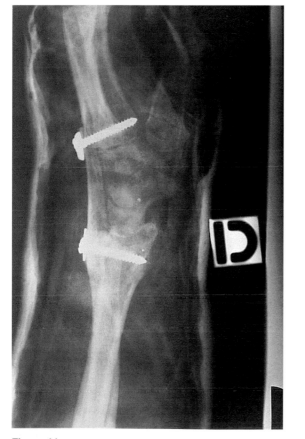

Figure 11

Total wrist arthrodesis with graft.

cases, prostheses have always been failures and this currently continues to be the case. For RA, series have been reported. Swanson Silastic implants are not real prostheses but merely 'spacers' maintaining the space between radius and metacarpals. Results are good in about 50% of the cases with a six to eight follow-up depending on the authors. Implant fracture occurs in approximately 50% of the cases: it results in wrist deviation but not always in pain, and patient satisfaction is around 60–70% (Swanson 1973). Swanson stated that to obtain good results, ROM in flexion–extension should not be more than 50°. Meuli (1975) and Volz (1978) were the first to promote real prostheses of a ball-and-socket type for the first and an anteroposterior movement for the second. Complications were imbalance because the axis of insertion were not physiological; ulnar deviation occurred most frequently. These devices have been modified. The real problem is related to stem fixation. Cement was not sufficient to prevent loosening at the distal stems, which are inserted in one or two metacarpals, and stress-shielding occurring at the proximal implantation. Infection and dislocation are other complications which may occur. Cementless prosthesis are now in use, but problems do not seem to be resolved. Hamas, Beckenbaugh, and Guepar prostheses (Alnot 1982) are other devices currently implanted.

Wrist prostheses seem reserved for the moment to very low-demanding patients with a good bone stock.

References

Abbott LC, Saunders JB, Bost FC (1942) Arthrodesis of the wrist with the use of grafts of cancellous bone, *J Bone Joint Surg* **24**:883–98.

Alnot JY (1982) Les arthroplasties du poignet, *Ann Radio* **25**:288–92.

Buck-Gramcko D (1993) Wrist denervation procedures in the treatment of Kilnböck's disease, *Hand Clin* **9**:517–20.

Clendenin MB, Green DP (1981) Arthrodesis of the wrist. Complications and their management, *J Hand Surg* **6A**:253–7.

Dubert T, Oberlin C, Alnot JY (1990) Anatomy of the articular nerves of the wrist. Implications for wrist denervation techniques [in French], *Ann Chir Main Meno Super* **9**:15–21.

Foucher G (1989) Technique de dénervation du poignet, *Ann Chir Main* **8**:84–7.

Fukumoto K, Kojima T, Kinoshita Y, Kodo M (1993) An anatomic study of the innervation of the wrist joint and Wilhelm's technique for denervation, *J Hand Surg* **18A**:484–9.

Gaisne E, Dap F, Bour C, Merle M (1991) Arthrodesis of the wrist in manual workers, *Rev Chir Orthop Reparatrice Appar Mot* **77**:537–44.

Meuli HC (1975) Arthroplastie du poignet, *Ann Chir* **27**:527–30.

Müller ME, Allgower M, Willenegger H (1969) *Manuel d'Osteosynthèse. Technique A.O.* Springer: Berlin.

Saidow MJ, Wai YL, Hayes MG (1992) Intercarpal athrodesis by dowel bone grafting, *J Hand Surg* **17B**:463–6.

Swanson AB (1973) Flexible implant arthroplasty for arthritic disabilities of the radiocarpal joint, *Orth Clin North Am* **4**:383–94.

Volz RG (1978) Total wrist arthroplasty, *Clin Orth* **128**:180–9.

Watson HK, Ballet FL (1984) The SLAC wrist: scapholunate advanced collapse pattern of degenerative arthritis, *J Hand Surg* **9A**:358–65.

Wilhelm A (1966) Die Gelenksdenervation und ihre anatomischen Gründlagen. Ein neues Belhandlungsprinzip in der Handchirurgie, *Hefte Unfallheilkunde* **86**:1–109.

Zachary SV, Stern PJ (1995) Complications following AO/ASIF wrist arthrodeses, *J Hand Surg* **20A**:339–44.

Zarcolli EA, Cozzi EP (1991) *An atlas of Surgical Anatomy of the Hand.* Churchill Livingstone: New York.

29

Arthroscopic wrist joint arthrolysis and proximal row carpectomy

John Stanley

Arthroscopic diagnosis of wrist problems, first proposed by Chen (1979), later investigated by Johnson and now a fairly widely accepted investigative tool, has the additional advantage of the therapeutic management of wrist pathology.

It is now widely accepted that debridement of degenerative joint disease or synovectomy, debridement of triangular fibrocartilaginous tears, repairs of triangular fibrocartilaginous tears and arthroscopic-assisted fracture reduction are procedures that should become standard procedures for those who practise wrist arthroscopy. However, the stiff joint remains a considerable challenge, both for the arthroscopist and as an open procedure. It is well recognized that the patient with a stiff joint who has an open surgical procedure has a very difficult and painful postoperative rehabilitation because of the damage to the capsule caused by the surgery itself. Therefore, there is a considerable advantage to performing arthroscopic surgery, in that the injury to the capsule is minimal, the rehabilitation time therefore much shorter, and the pain and discomfort for the patient much less.

Arthrolysis

To perform arthrolysis of the joint following significant wrist trauma in the form of distal radial fracture and intra-articular fracture is difficult and is made more difficult by the fact that there is often significant capsular scarring, which can on occasions make entry into the wrist joint impossible. Therefore, before surgery can be considered, it is essential to have access to at least two portals: normally, the 3–4 portal between the extensor pollicis longus and the extensor digitorum communis tendon is the viewing portal, and the 4–5 portals

between the extensor digitorum communis and the extensor digitorum quintus tendon, or the 6R portal between the extensor digitorum quintus and the extensor carpi ulnaris tendon, would be used as the working portal. However, in the post-traumatic stiff joint, whether it be from direct trauma or from algodystrophy or other causes, the joint capsule is often contracted; it is, therefore, often necessary to enter the joint through the 6R portal initially and to have a surgical portal through the 4–5, since it is often not possible to use the 3–4 portal as the primary entry-point without the risk of damage to the articular cartilage. The adhesions within the joint are often significant and require the use of a suction punch and a 2.9 mm radius blade to clean. It is time-consuming and the results of arthrolysis depend very much upon the proportion of stiffness caused either by the intra-articular adhesions in the radio-carpal and the midcarpal joints or by the capsular contracture caused by repair of capsular tears and avulsions. The midcarpal joint, if it is significantly scarred, is extremely difficult to enter without serious risk of damaging the surfaces; therefore, the success of arthrolysis of the joint is wholly dependent upon the ease with which it is possible to enter the joint with the arthroscope and the instrumentation.

Our results from arthrolysis, which are based upon small numbers only, have shown an increased range of motion; this has by no means reached even 80% of normal but the operation has increased the range to the functional minimum suggested by Ryu et al (1991), and there is no doubt that the postoperative management is much less often complicated by excessive pain, stiffness and recurrent algodystrophy. It is necessary for the patients to undergo a vigorous postoperative rehabilitation programme, and it is normal both to instil bupivacaine, a long-acting local anaesthetic, and to put a narcotic into the joint immediately after surgery in order to reduce postoperative pain and therefore improve the effectiveness of the therapy in the first few hours after surgery. If it seems possible to achieve a reasonable range of motion, then the therapy programme should persist on an intensive basis for between 6 and 8 weeks. As yet the absolute indications for arthroscopic arthrolysis are unclear and this, I believe, is a procedure best reserved for those who are significantly experienced in wrist arthroscopy.

Proximal row carpectomy

Proximal row carpectomy (PRC), first suggested by Stamm in 1939 and published in 1944, has been used for a wide variety of problems affecting the wrist, the most common of which is the old ununited fracture of the carpal scaphoid associated with secondary degenerative changes in the scaphoid fossa of the distal radius. The treatment for the stiff wrist joint, in particular those joints that have radiocarpal disease, has for some time been controversial: a number of options for treatment have been proposed and which one is chosen by a surgeon for a particular patient is generally dependent entirely upon his own – often very limited – experience of each of these options. As a result of this approach to the problem, the most commonly offered final solution is total arthrodesis of the wrist joint. This usually cures the pain at the price of losing any residual motion, and if this fails to solve the problem all that remains to do is to discharge the patient to the pain clinic or to someone else! The discussion in this chapter is of the treatment of stiffness of the joint and therefore arthrodesis cannot be considered.

Scapholunate advanced collapse (SLAC) as described by Ashmead et al (1994), fracture dislocation of the carpus, Kienböck's disease, and arthritis secondary to scaphoid non-union are well recognized as giving rise to significant problems of stiffness in the radiocarpal joint; PRC may, therefore, be indicated. Schernberg (1992), Saffar and Fakhoury (1992), Culp et al (1993), Neviaser (1993) and others have all published on this subject and have discussed the indications for PRC in the treatment of wrist disease. There is general agreement that it is necessary to have the lunate fossa unaffected by the arthritic process and, therefore, that

this procedure is absolutely contraindicated in rheumatoid arthritis and is to be performed with caution if there are early changes to the capitate head. The results published in the literature would support the view that PRC is a procedure carrying a reasonable chance of adequate function, although a prolonged rehabilitation is commonly seen: Taleisnik (1985), for example, is muted in his view about this procedure and comments upon the prolonged rehabilitation programme and the uncertainty of the long-term results.

The expected final outcome of PRC has been reported to be good to excellent in 82–95% of cases, with a range of flexion/extension arc up to 60–70% of normal and grip strengths up to 60–80% of normal. This would suggest that there is a firm place for PRC in wrist salvage. Inevitably, however, some discomfort remains and 33% of patients will continue to have moderate to severe pain after surgery as reported in Culp's series (1993). One not uncommon cause of persistent discomfort and pain is the late impingement of the radial styloid with the trapezium. Radial styloidectomy is often necessary as part of this procedure, particularly if elongation of the styloid following arthritis in the scaphoid fossa is present. However, Green (1993) indicates the importance of preservation of the radioscaphocapitate ligament anteriorly in order to preserve the stability of the distal row of the carpus on the radial surface, and therefore a posterolateral styloidectomy is recommended rather than the over-generous 1.5 cm of the styloid which will include both the anterior and posterior aspects of the scaphoid fossa and will inevitably detach the ligament from the distal radius. Significant reductions in range of motion and reduction of power of grasp are to be expected and radial deviation is commonly restricted.

However, despite the generally encouraging reports there remains a general reluctance on the part of surgeons to excise the whole proximal row, even though the surgery is straightforward and relatively undemanding. Perhaps the reason for this is the conception that this is a salvage procedure and only those wrists so bad as to require salvage are suitable; however, this conception is not strictly true and the criteria for the consideration of PRC include good surfaces on the lunate and capitate, which places the ideal wrist for PRC at a stage of the disease when the disease is not severe, but will cause increasing difficulty and will inevitably give rise to serious levels of symptoms, although the wrist has not yet deteriorated to a level when the joint is only suitable for arthrodesis or arthroplasty.

PRC is not a substitute for arthrodesis or arthroplasty but is a procedure to be used before these other alternatives become necessary. A particular example of this process is seen in Kienböck's disease at stage 3a, or 3b (Lichtman and Degnan 1993) when PRC is an important and successful option, and Gelberman (personal communication) most strongly recommends that PRC be considered as a reasonable option in these circumstances.

PRC is indicated in those patients with stiff painful wrists when joint surfaces are well preserved in the lunate fossa and on the capitate head: e.g., in the patient with gross flexion deformity after a hemiplegia or cerebral palsy or in scaphoid non-union Kienböck's disease and late fracture dislocation when it is felt that the penalty following capitohamotriquetolunate (four-corner) fusion is unacceptable.

References

Abrams RA, Petersen M, Botte MJ (1994) Arthroscopic portals of the wrist: an anatomic study, *J Hand Surg* **19A:**940–4.

Ashmead IV D, Watson HK, Damon C, Herber S, Paly W (1994) Scapho-lunate advanced collapse wrist salvage, *J Hand Surg Am* **19(5):**741–50.

Chen F (1979) Arthroscopy of the wrist and finger joints, *Orthrop Clin North Am* **10(3):**723–33.

Culp RW, McGuigan FX, Turner MA, Lichtman DM, Osterman AL, McCarroll HR (1993) Proximal row carpectomy: a multicenter study, *J Hand Surg Am* **181:**19–25.

Green DP (1993) *Operative Hand Surgery* 3rd edn. Churchill Livingstone: New York.

Imbriglia JE, Broudy AS, Hagberg WC, McKernan D (1990) Proximal row carpectomy: clinical evaluation, *J Hand Surg* **15A:**426.

Lichtman DM, Degnan GG (1993) Staging and its use in the determination of treatment modalities for Kienböck's disease, *Hand Clin* **9(3):**409–16.

Neviaser RJ (1983) Proximal row carpectomy for posttraumatic diseases of the carpus, *J Hand Surg* **8:**301.

Ryu JY, Cooney III WP, Askew LJ, An KN, Chao EY (1991) Functional ranges of motion of the wrist joint, *J Hand Surg Am* **Jan(202):**12–15.

Saffar P, Fakhoury B (1992) [Resection of the proximal carpal bones versus partial arthrodesis in carpal instability]. *Ann Chir Main Memb Super* **11(4):**276–80.

Schernberg F (1992) [Operative technique of arthroplastic resection of the three proximal bones]. *Ann Chir Main Memb Super* **11(4):**264–8.

Stamm TT (1944) Excision of the proximal row of the carpus, *Proc R Soc Med* **38:**74.

Taleisnik J (1985) *The Wrist*. Churchill Livingstone: New York.

30
Rehabilitation for radiocarpal joint stiffness

Jean-Luc Roux, Jean-Claude Rouzaud, Jean Goubau and Yves Allieu

Introduction

The decrease in range of motion between radius and first carpal row is probably underestimated. In a study of wrist rehabilitation after distal radial fractures (Vidal and Allieu 1972), normal wrist mobility was found in only 22% of cases. Despite this, few patients complained of isolated wrist joint stiffness. This good tolerance of wrist stiffness could be because the wrist is a complex joint with two levels of mobility: radiocarpal and mediocarpal. Only one of these two joints can provide functional mobility as defined by Palmer (1985) or Brumfield and Champoux (1984), which is less than half of the total range of motion of the wrist. At least Nelson et al (1993) has shown the rapid adaptation at a reduced range of motion for activities of daily living.

However, if the wrist is not essential to position the hand in space, it is indispensable for the tenodesis effect and for muscle synergy. The wrist improves the hand function. Tetraplegic patients have demonstrated this, for them: 'the wrist is already the hand'. So we therefore always try to preserve as much wrist motion as possible.

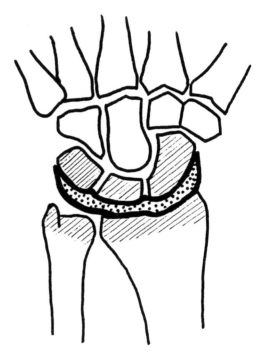

Figure 1

The radiocarpal joint is a single synovial space in the centre of an articular complex which can be called the 'radio scapho-luno-triquetro-ulnar joint.

Radiocarpal joint characteristics

Wrist rehabilitation has to take into account several characteristics of this joint. The radiocarpal joint can be defined arthrographically as a synovial space, but anatomically we can talk of the 'radio-scapho-luno-triquetro-ulnar joint (Fig. 1).

The first carpal row cannot be isolated as a single bone. Mobility between the scaphoid, lunate and pyramidal is very important for achieving complete inclination of the wrist. For example, flexion and rotation of the scaphoid is necessary for radial deviation. Each bone of the first carpal row needs a specific motion. To restore this automatic motion between the bones, the ligaments must be preserved without forgetting the necessity of direct mobilization.

During active motion, the muscles mobilizing the wrist act distally and not directly on the bones of the radiocarpal joint. The flexor carpi radialis, palmaris longus, extensor carpi ulnaris, extensor carpi radialis brevis and longus, insert distally on the metacarpus. Only the flexor carpi ulnaris acts directly on the carpus by pisiform insertion.

During passive motion, the therapist holds the forearm in one hand and the hand of the patient in the other. In this way there is no direct mobilization of the bones of the first carpal row. The conditions of mobilization of the radiocarpal joint are very different from a simple joint between two long bones.

A difficult direct mobilization is necessary to avoid the natural tendency of an adhesional phenomenon of the first carpal row, due to its intercalated position (Fig. 2).

We have demonstrated the importance of the passive longitudinal rotation between the distal radius and the metacarpal basis (Roux 1992). It will be interesting to exercise this movement by active pronation–supination using resisting movements or by passive motion. This is the best way to stretch the radiocarpal ligaments (Fig. 3).

It should not be forgotten that all displaced fractures of the distal radius are articular, shortening of the radius causes an ulnocarpal abutment, a deviated radius in the sagittal plan which leads to a first row desaxation – DISI (dorsal instability of the segment intercalated) or VISI (volar instability of the segment intercalated) – and an 'adaptative carpus instability'. We must, therefore, always try to restore normal anatomy to give a better range of motion Fig. 4).

Rehabilitation

The best way to treat stiffness is to avoid it. Preventive care must not be limited to early motion, but should include a correct position of immobilization and minimalization of pain and oedema.

When assessing a stiff wrist, one should have an aetiologic diagnosis before commencing treatment.

Preventive care

To avoid stiffness, general preventive care for oedema and pain are necessary:

- elevation of the hand, arm sling
- active motion of the digits (note: when you ask your patient to move the fingers that a synergic muscle effect can induce a secondary displacement of Colles' fractures by simultaneous contraction of the wrist extensor and digital flexor muscles)
- massage
- pain control (ice, medication, local anaesthesia, etc.)
- early motion to decrease oedema (decreased oedema increases motion).

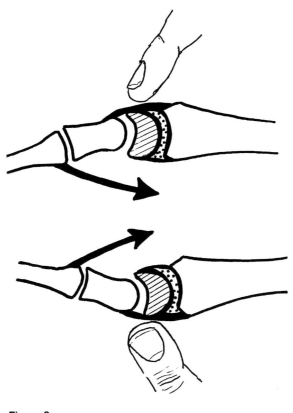

Figure 2

Active and passive mobilization have no direct action on the first carpal row. This intercalated segment needs direct mobilization.

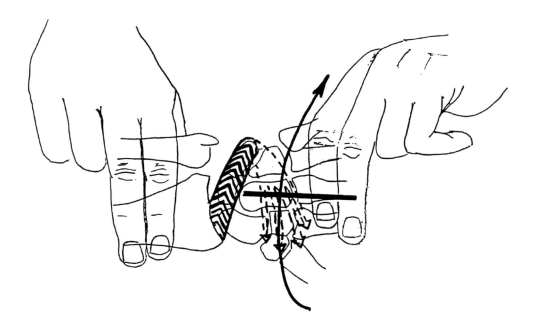

a)

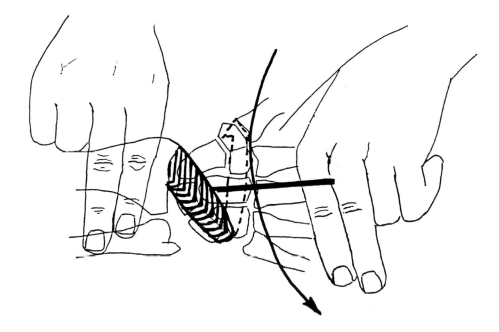

b)

Figure 3

The longitudinal rotation between the radius and the metacarpal basis stretching the radiocarpal ligaments can improve motion of the first carpal row. (a) Supination way: stretching the posterior radiocarpal ligaments (posterior view). (b) Pronation way: stretching the anterior radiocarpal ligaments (anterior view).

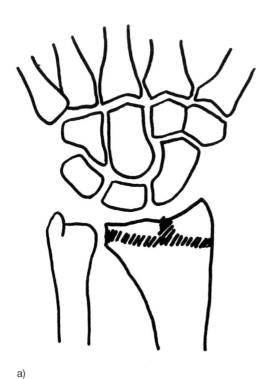 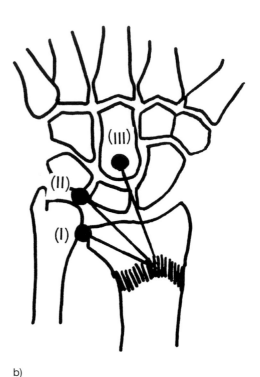

a)   b)

Figure 4

(a) Non-displaced fractures of the distal radius can be articular. (b) Each displaced fracture of the distal radius must be considered as an articular fracture for the radiocarpal joint: (I) distal radioulnar incongruency, (II) ulnocarpal impingement, (III) 'adaptative carpus'.

After surgery, early motion improves healing of bone, cartilage and soft tissues (Buckwalter 1966). Considering this a stable osteosynthesis must be the goal of surgical treatment.

At the level of the wrist, osteosynthesis is not always stable enough to allow early motion, and early motion is not always necessary to restore normal motion. For example, after conservative treatment for non-displaced scaphoid fracture and despite long immobilization of 3 months, patients generally recover a complete range of motion. So the debate between 'movers' and 'resters' is not closed (Salter 1996).

Cast immobilization retains many indications and it is very important to take care of the position of the wrist. It is usual to place the wrist in neutral or slight extension in the sagittal plane, or in neutral inclina-

tion in the frontal plane. However, in the horizontal plane it is only the position of radius relative to the ulnar which is defined by pronosupination and not the position of carpus relative to radius. This position can vary more than 40° in the horizontal plane and can put the radiocarpal ligaments under tension (Roux 1992, Roux and Allieu 1996). For example, putting the carpus in supination under the radius to treat a dorsal radiotriquetral ligament tear is like immobilizing an ankle external ligament tear in a varus cast. Therefore, care must be taken when making a cast, taking into account the radiocarpal position, not only in the sagittal and frontal planes, but also in the horizontal plane. This precaution can decrease stiffness, and also pain and reflex sympathetic dystrophy (Fig. 5).

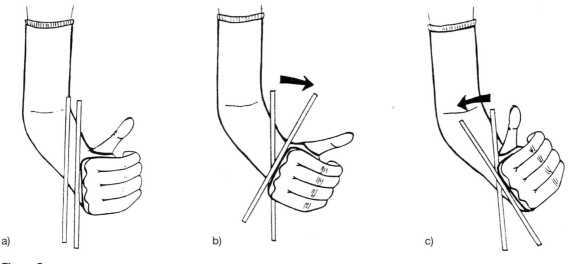

a)   b)   c)

Figure 5

When making a long cast with the forearm in neutral prono-supilnation, the wrist can be placed (a) in the neutral position, (b) in pronation, or (c) in supilnation

Stiffness treatment

The surgeon and therapist must form a team and work together on a rehabilitation programme. This organization is very important for delivering a single, clear message to the patient, and not two interpretations of the same message.

Except in the case of very rare congenital synostosis, a stiff wrist has a 'history': trauma, rheumatism, osteonecrosis. The initial approach should include a physical examination and basic roentgenography.

Extra-articular stiffness must be eliminated at the physical examination:

- at skin level: retractile scar, adhesions
- at tendon level: adhesion with the skin, bone or both
- at muscle level: retraction as in a Volkmann syndrome.

These extra-articular causes frequently need a specific extra-articular surgical procedure: skin flaps, tenolysis, tenotomy. Sometimes an articular surgical procedure is used for an extra-articular stiffness such as proximal row carpectomy in muscle retraction.

Articular stiffness can be isolated or associated with extra-articular stiffness. Roentgenography with a dynamic lateral view are necessary to demonstrate bone injuries, carpal instability and precise stiffness level (mediocarpal or radiocarpal).

Normal X-rays

The 'team' of therapist and surgeon establishes the programme and ensures the follow-up.

Reflex sympathetic dystrophy is a very frequent cause of stiffness. If we suspect this pathology in spite of a normal X-ray, we must eliminate it by a scintigraphy.

Non-surgical procedures
Passive mobilization is used: gentle manual mobilization can be used to initiate movement, but aggressive mobilization should be avoided to prevent further trauma and pain. Application of heated paraffin before exercise can relax the tissues and increase comfort. Slight traction is applied to

open the joint and allow surfaces to glide. To improve radiocarpal joint motion, radiometacarpal rotation is applied holding the radius in one hand and the metacarpal bases in the other. These movements stretch the radiocarpal ligaments. At least a direct mobilization of each bone of the first carpal row is necessary to replace the lack of direct action from ligaments and the absence of tendinous insertion.

Continuous passive motion is very advantageous for this kind of wrist stiffness and can be used first to initiate mobilization. Different devices are suitable, but we prefer a system which combines not only rehabilitation in the sagittal and frontal planes, but also in the horizontal plane. The prono-supination couple acts distally on the hand and produces radiometacarpal rotation movements to loosen the adhesional phenomenon between the radial articular plateau and the proximal carpal row.

Active mobilization is mandatory to increase muscle strength and tendon gliding.

Splinting: dynamic and static progressive, prefabricated or custom made, can be associated.

Surgical procedures

If physiotherapy fails, surgery is indicated if the range of motion is less than 25° in extension and 25° in flexion, depending, on the patient's motivation and desires, and in the case of a negative CT (computed tomography) scan (Voche and Merle 1993). Postoperative care with early mobilization is essential following the operation.

The type of stiffness is the guide to the type of surgical approach. Sometimes arthroscopy can be used.

Abnormal X-ray

Usually, the surgeon intervenes before the therapist, but the surgical indication is a 'team' decision.

Patient complaints are more often of chronic wrist pain, rather than a lack of range of motion. Progressive stiffness is often well tolerated.

Acute injuries are excluded here, and we consider only wrist arthrosis or arthritis requiring palliative surgery to preserve some range of motion. Standard roentgenography and dynamic lateral series assess which is the better indication.

In all the cases of wrist stiffness, the surgeon and therapist must thoroughly assess the range of motion the patient needs in daily activities including work and leisure. The patient's motivations are very important. A rehabilitation programme is elaborated and together the therapist and surgeon must form a team using a single language.

References

Allieu Y (1984) Instabilité du carpe. Instabilités ligamentaires et désaxations intracarpiennes. Démembrement du concept d'instabilité du carpe, *Ann Chir Main* **3**:317–21.

Brumfield RH, Champoux SA (1984) A biomechanical study of normal functional wrist, *Clin Orthop Rel Res* **187**:23–5.

Buckwalter JA (1966) Effects of early motion on healing of musculoskeletal tissues, *Hand Clinics* **12**:13–24.

Nelson D, Manske P, Mitchell M, Khan A, Hymes R (1993) Functional range of motion of the wrist, *Communication, 1st Congress of the FESSH, Brussels.*

Palmer AK (1985) Functional wrist motion: biomechanical study, *J Hand Surg* **10A**:39.

Roux JL (1992) La rotation longitudinale radio-métacarpienne (etude biomécanique et applications cliniques). Thesis: Montpellier University 1992.

Roux JL, Allieu Y (1996) Immobilisation du poignet, un positionnement vicieux insoupçonné, *J Traumatol Sport* **13**:50–62.

Salter RB (1996) History of rest and motion and the scientific basis for early continuous passive motion. *Hand Clinics* **12**:1–11.

Thompson ST, Wehbe MA (1966) Early motion after wrist surgery, *Hand Clinics* **12**:87–96.

Tubiana R, Kulhman JN (1984) Raideurs du poignet. In: Tubiana R, ed. *Traité de Chirurgie de la Main*, Vol. 2. Masson: Paris: 965–75.

Vidal J, Allieu Y (1972) Fractures de l'extrémité inférieure de l'avant-bras. In: *Encycl. Méd. Chir.* Appareils locomoteurs. Paris: **6**:14042A10–20.

Voche P, Merle M (1993) Arthrolyse du poignet. Indications et Techniques, *Rev Chir Orthop* **79**:135–9.

31
Causes of stiffness of the distal radioulnar joint

John Stanley

The ability to place the hand accurately in space is a function of the shoulder, elbow and wrist joints, and placing the hand in supination or pronation increases the sophistication of that motion and positioning. There are a number of anatomical factors important to the normal function of the forearm and hand and one should not concentrate attention solely upon the distal radioulnar joint (DRUJ), when it is crucial to appreciate that the forearm as a whole is a functional unit dependent upon the correct alignment of the bones to afford the correct axis of motion, upon supple gliding tissues to allow that motion, and upon structurally sound ligaments and membranes which place constraints upon the motion, keeping it within the normal range.

Osteology

The ulnar head articulates with the sigmoid notch of the radius distally (Fig. 1) and the radial head articulates with the radial notch of the ulnar proximally; this arrangement allows the radius to rotate about

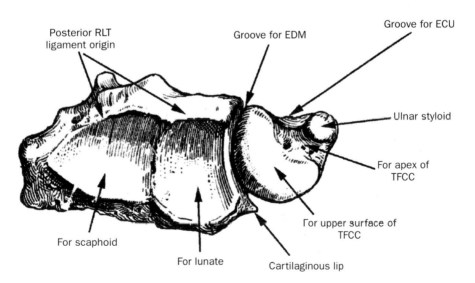

Distal Radius and Ulna in pronation

Figure 1

Distal radius and ulna in pronation: ECU, extensor carpi ulnaris; EDM, extensor digiti minimi; RLT, radiolunotriquetral; TFCC, triangular fibrocartilaginous complex

a

b

c

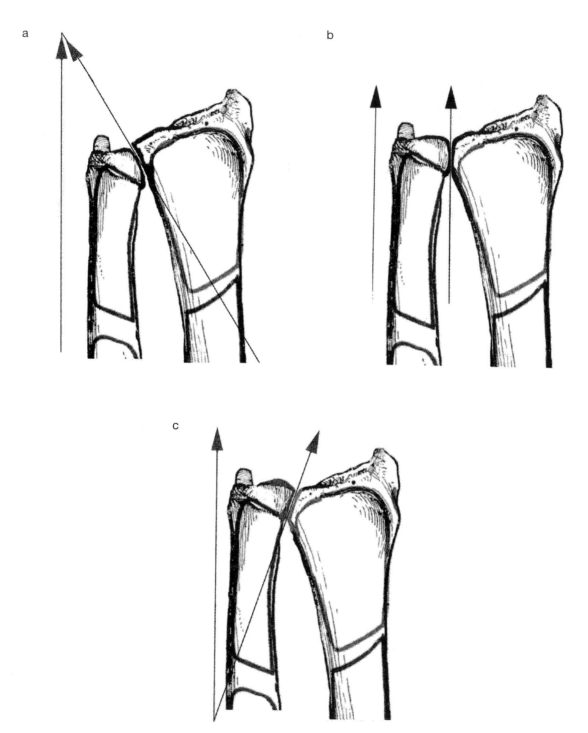

Figure 2

(a,b,c) The three different types of configuration of the distal radioulnar joint

the ulna, which in turn is seen as forearm pronation (palm down) and supination (palm up). The longitudinal axis of rotation for this motion passes through the ulnar head distally and the radial head proximally and therefore lies at an oblique angle to the centre line of the forearm. The alignment of the proximal joint is constant; the alignment of the distal joint varies from individual to individual but may be categorized into three basic types which appear to be related to ulnar variance (Fig. 2). The longitudinal alignment is of particular interest when joint levelling procedures are proposed. The ulnar head has a radius of curvature which is less than the sigmoid notch seat and therefore there is a considerable incongruity between the radius and ulnar components of the DRUJ; there are a number of variants (Fig. 3). There is no such incongruity at the proximal radioulnar joint.

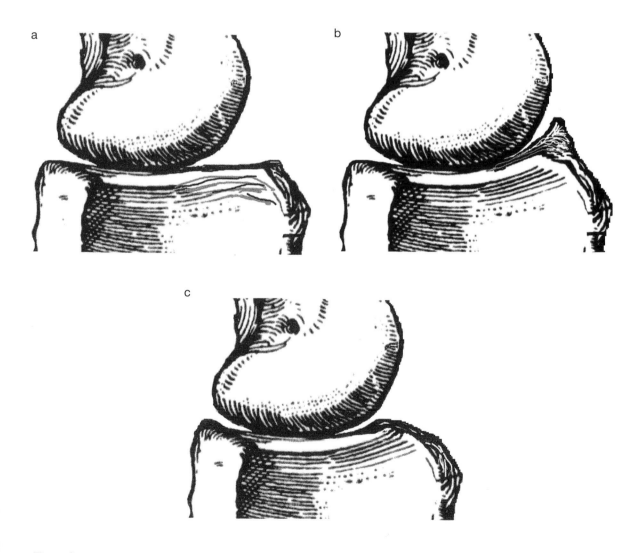

Figure 3

The three separate types of sigmoid notch: (a) the flat surface; (b) the ski slope; (c) the sigmoid shape

The distal surface of the ulnar head articulates with the triangular fibrocartilage which is attached to the edge of the sigmoid notch and to the fovea at the base of the styloid process of the ulna and to the styloid itself.

The radius

The radius is by far the larger of the two bones distally since it carries the articular surface for the scaphoid and lunate, and therefore a disproportionate degree of attention tends to be paid to this part of the wrist with consequent lesser attention paid to the ulna.

The longitudinal axis of rotation of the forearm passes from the radial head proximally across the interosseous membrane to the ulnar head distally (Fig. 4). This axis ensures that pronation and supination can occur but it is essential to appreciate that the ulna remains fixed throughout rotation of the forearm and that it is the radius which rotates around the fixed ulna and not the other way round. This has significant implications when considering the biomechanics of the DRUJ. Perhaps the most significant fact to appreciate is that the radius describes an arc of motion in the longitudinal plane, resulting in a relative shortening of the radius (or apparent lengthening of the ulna) when the forearm is fully pronated since, of course, in this position the two bones cross, whereas in full supination the bones are parallel (Fig. 5). This change in relative lengths can only be accommodated at the distal joint as the capitulum prevents any proximal movement of the radius and the trochleo-olecranon articulation any proximal migration of the ulna. This is particularly important in the understanding of ulna–carpal impaction syndrome.

The soft tissues

The attachment of the radius to the ulna is by way of the annular ligament and capsule proximally, the interosseous membrane in the forearm and distally the capsular ligaments and triangular fibrocartilaginous complex. Each area has a particular function, the disturbance of which always interferes with the normal motion of the forearm rotation.

The interosseous membrane

Studies of the interosseous membrane have shown the special nature of this structure and have defined its particular function. The load transmission from the hand to the wrist results in approximately 80% of the force being applied to the radius and 20% to the ulna (although this will vary according to the ulnar variance). A positive ulnar variance (Fig. 6) would suggest a higher proportion of force through the ulna, and conversely an ulna-minus variance would suggest the reverse. The changes are, however, not proportional to the variance since the triangular fibrocartilage fills the space between the

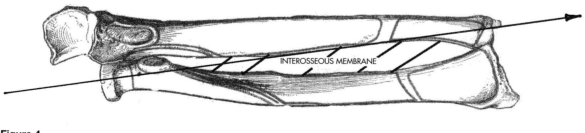

Figure 4

The line of rotation of the forearm with the fibres of the interosseous membrane

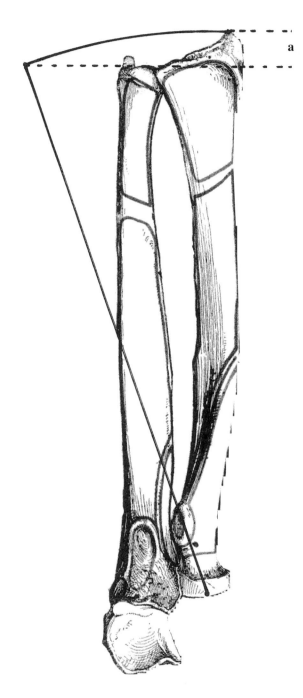

Figure 5

The apparent lengthening of the ulna in full pronation (a) is due to the arc of motion of the radius around the ulna

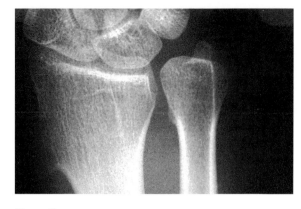

Figure 6

Ulnar-plus variance

ulnar head and the proximal carpus. Since at the elbow the force transmission is much greater through the ulna than the radius, this change from distal to proximal is occasioned by the alignment of the fibres of the interosseous membrane, which by nature of the alignment resists radial longitudinal shift by the method of transmitting the forces through the membrane to the ulnar shaft. The effect of this is to compress the proximal joint and the DRUJ (Fig. 7), as does the pronator quadratus muscle at the wrist. Injury to the interosseous membrane results in either restricted rotation or longitudinal instability of the forearm, as seen in the Essex–Lopresti lesion. The stability and motion of the DRUJ also requires a competent interosseous membrane in addition to the normal capsular, muscular and musculotendinous stabilizing factors.

The ligaments and the triangular fibrocartilaginous complex

The ligaments of the DRUJ are required to allow the radius to rotate around the ulna through an arc of motion of at least 160° while maintaining stability. In order to achieve this, it is necessary for the ulnar head to translate from anterior to posterior, a motion permitted by the joint incongruence between the head and the radial sigmoid notch but limited by the capsular ligaments and the ulnocarpal

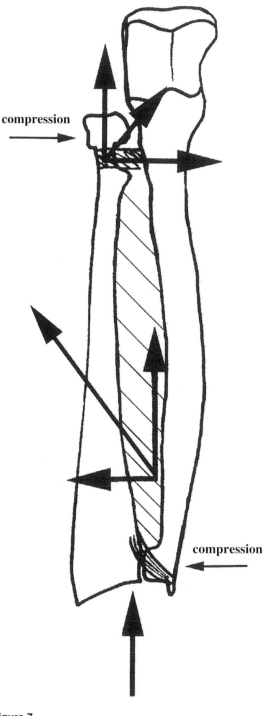

compression

compression

Figure 7

The mechanism by which the DRUJ and proximal radioulnar joint are compressed when axial loading is applied

ligament attachments to the triangular fibrocartilaginous complex (TFCC). The ligaments are discrete condensations in the capsule and dorsally are blended with the interosseous membrane. The ligaments fuse with the deep surface of the ulnocarpal ligaments and with the proximal edge of the radiotriquetral ligaments, both volar and dorsal (Fig. 8). There is a cartilaginous lip on the volar surface of the sigmoid notch, and into this the volar ligament is inserted.

The TFCC includes the meniscal homologe which lies on the deep surface of the ulnar collateral ligament running from the styloid process of the ulna to triquetrum. The attachments of the TFCC maintain the relationship of the structures which contribute to the stability of the DRUJ during the action of prono-supination. There are four principal attachments of the TFCC to the surrounding tissues. These are as follows:

- to the radius
- to the volar, radioulnar and ulnocarpal ligaments
- to the dorsal extension of the interosseous membrane and dorsal ulnocarpal and radiotriquetral ligaments, including the base of the fifth and sixth extensor compartments
- to the ulna collateral ligament.

Additional stability is maintained through the arc of motion by the compression generated by the interosseous membrane mechanism described above, and by the action of the pronator quadratus muscle.

The extensor retinaculum

The role of the extensor retinaculum in the stabilization of the DRUJ is secondary to the more direct ligament and muscular restraints; however, the relationship of the extensor retinaculum and the extensor carpi ulnaris tendon to the ulnar head, as it lies in its groove on the dorsum of the ulnar head, is as a stabilizer of the joint. The medial prolongation of the extensor retinaculum to the fascia and sheath of the flexor carpi ulnaris tendon likewise is a factor in stability, and with the extensor carpi ulnaris it clasps the lower ulnar shaft. The two tendons are closely related during movement and maintain a fixed relationship during forearm rotation.

Perhaps the most important and difficult concept to appreciate is the fact that the ulna is the fixed

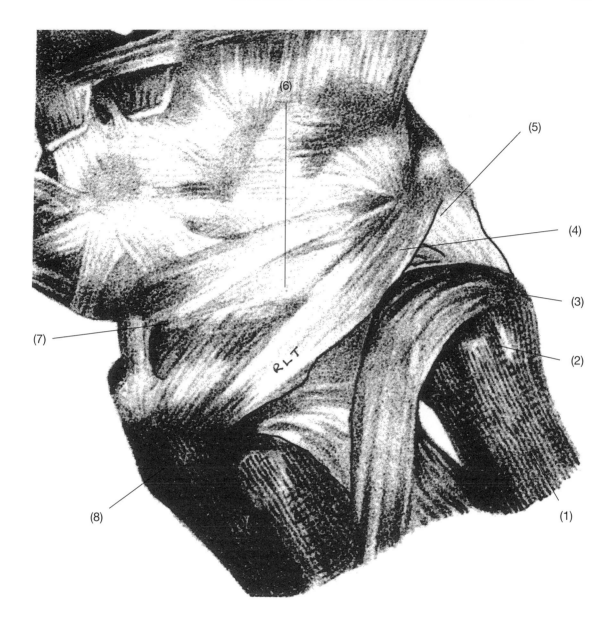

Figure 8

The complex posterior ligament system of the DRUJ; in particular, the relationship with the radiolunotriquetral ligament (RLT)
1, Ulna; 2, Dorsal radioulnar ligament; 3, TFCC; 4, Dorsal radiolunotriquetral ligament; 5, Triquetrum; 6, Lunate; 7, Scaphoid; 8, Radius

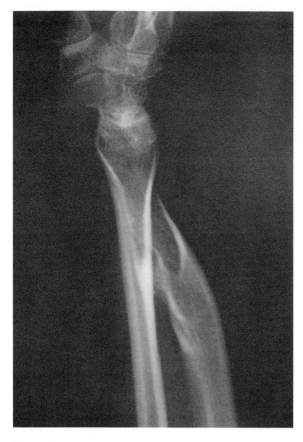

Figure 9

The distortion of the ulna with the multiple exostoses is apparent and it is clear that forearm rotation is limited by the abnormal shape of the distal ulna and the proximal distortion

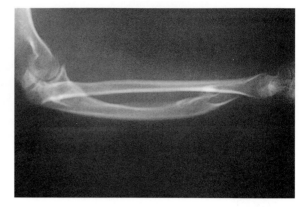

Figure 10

This is more apparent when one examines the full forearm and identifies dislocation of the radial head and bowing of the ulna which will give rise to absent pronosupination

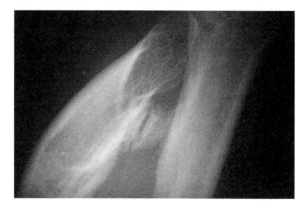

Figure 11

In addition to distortion of the shaft, synostosis between the radius and ulna occurs in a number of cases

reference point and the radius and hand are merely suspended from the ulnar shaft and head. This concept has important implications when surgery is considered for restricted pronosupination.

Congenital stiffness

For adequate forearm rotation, it is essential that the radius is able to rotate around the axis of the forearm which runs through from the radial head to the ulnar head; as described above, this requires a rotation

and translational motion at the DRUJ. Disturbances of development of the forearm bones which disturb this alignment will have a direct effect on the ability to rotate the forearm and will give rise to stiffness in pronosupination. It is very important when examining patients with restricted pronosupination due to congenital abnormalities to appreciate that the pathology may be at any level in the forearm, up to and including the elbow. Congenital radiohumeral synostosis precludes any pronosupination at all. The forearm bones are essentially normal, as is the DRUJ. In cases with radioulnar synostosis, where there is failure of differentiation of the forearm bones proximally, again there would be no pronosupination possible.

However, the causes of the problem at the DRUJ are related to various degrees of hypoplasia or dysplasia. The hyperplastic problems of radial club hand or ulnar club hand are well recognized and have varying degrees of expression, from almost complete absence of the radius or ulna to hypoplasia of the DRUJ only. In these situations, the treatment of stiffness of the DRUJ is extremely difficult, and it has to be very carefully considered whether surgery will actually fundamentally improve the patient sufficiently to make the surgical procedure worthwhile. This is true particularly since children will often be able to accommodate for the lack of pronosupination sufficiently well to be able to live comfortable lives with reasonable function, although the awkwardness with which they perform tasks is sometimes disturbing to the parents and to the doctor. The child often is unaware of the problem and many authors suggest that minimal surgical intervention is necessary and that it is really a matter of placing the hand in the most favourable position; in gross stiffness of the forearm due to other deficiencies, a rotation osteotomy may be the only treatment worthwhile to bring the hand into a pronated position allowing for functional activity. The most important aspect of treatment is the centralization of the hand at birth or shortly thereafter, in order to allow for adequate development of the hand as a functional unit, rather than waiting for several years to correct the very ulnar-deviated hand that can occur in these cases. If there is progressive deterioration of ulnar deviation, the ulnar 'anlage' (the distal cartilaginous portion) requires excision and the carpus to be centralized upon the radius.

In the second group of patients, those with dysplasia, there are a number of well recognized conditions – diaphyseal aclasia is one (Fig. 9) – where disturbance of epiphyseal cartilage allows cartilage 'rests' to remain within the shaft, producing significant and progressive exostoses which can mechanically interfere with the rotation of the forearm. These characteristically occur in the ulna; there is a short ulna and bowing of the forearm (Fig. 10), and as these exostoses continue growing, at least up until the time of fusion of the epiphyses, repeated surgery to remove the exostoses is necessary (Fig. 11). These patients with bowing of both the radius and the ulna present a considerable difficulty, (Fig. 12) and at the end of growth, it is technically possible to do a 'compound' osteotomy of the radius and ulna. However, this is a major procedure and is unlikely to increase pronosupination significantly, since the disturbance of the interosseous membrane is usually sufficient to negate any gains that are made by osteotomy.

There are other dysplastic conditions, such as the Madelung deformity with disturbance of the development of the ulnar head, translation of the carpus and the articulation of the lunate in the interval between the radius and ulna. Although there is restriction of pronosupination often in these cases, there is little indication for surgery; most of the complaints by the patients are of cosmetic disturbances at the wrist rather than of the functional impairment. Late degenerative changes can occur, although they are uncommon. In these cases a complex series of wedge osteotomies on the radius with appropriate surgery to the ulna is very hazardous and the patients may not be wholly satisfied with the functional improvement; furthermore, the scars may become hypertrophic in young patients and destroy any advantage that may be gained on the cosmetic aspects of these cases.

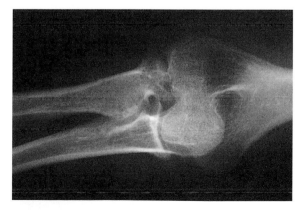

Figure 12

The distortion of the proximal radioulnar joint must be identified in order to prevent unnecessary surgery to the DRUJ for poor pronosupination

Finally, there are conditions such as arthrogryposis multiplex congenita in which there is a distinct restriction of pronosupination due to lack of differentiation of tissues; these patients have significant functional disturbances, of which the DRUJ is only a very small part.

In summary, the precise diagnosis of the congenital condition causing the problem with the DRUJ needs to be assessed; careful evaluation of the proximal radioulnar joint (Fig. 4) and the proximal radius and ulna is essential to avoid misunderstanding the mechanisms, since congenital problems due to hypoplasia and aplasia often require late excision of the 'anlage' and centralization of the forearm bone without any hope of pronosupination. In those conditions that develop as a dysplasia, repeated surgery may be required along with osteotomy in order to align the long axes of the bones of the forearm. The Madelung deformity rarely, if ever, requires surgery; if it does, it has to be considered extremely carefully with the patient fully aware of the difficulties that might arise and the scarring that inevitably does ensue.

Post-traumatic stiffness

Restriction in motion of the forearm rotation of pronation and supination gives rise to a significant functional impairment and disability. The hand is usually used in the pronated position and for most of the activities of daily living loss of this motion has a serious impact upon the individual; supination itself is a less frequently used movement but restriction of this motion gives rise to the most complaints by patients. The reason for this is related to the ability to compromise and adapt to the impairment: loss of pronation can be more easily overcome by the simple method of lifting the elbow by abducting the shoulder, thus bringing the hand more parallel to the horizontal plane; although this is awkward and unsightly, it is nevertheless effective. The loss of supination prevents the palm being placed upward (as when accepting money in a shop or holding a tray of food with one hand) and has no effective adaptation, in that it is not possible to bring the elbow any closer than the trunk. Therefore it is often the latter that is particularly complained of, but the loss of either or both ranges of motion requires careful evaluation and, if possible, appropriate treatment.

The diagnosis of any condition should include the nature of the problem, its extent, the pathology and the prognosis, and therefore a logical approach to the evaluation of the patient and the institution of appropriate investigations are essential components of any diagnostic process.

A history of trauma associated with a fracture or dislocation of the wrist, forearm or elbow would alert the examining physician to the possibility of either malunion, with or without significant soft tissue scarring, or the late effects of algodystrophy. Distal radial fractures with disturbance of the ulnar–radial seat should be considered important aetiological factors, in particular those distal radial fractures that remain significantly angulated and/or involve disturbance of the sigmoid notch (Fig. 13).

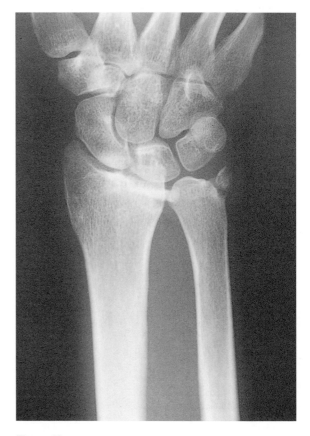

Figure 13

Injury to the styloid process of the ulna, type II, with detachment of the TFCC and injury to the radial sigmoid notch

There are particular fractures and fracture dislocation patterns which may involve the proximal radius joint and the DRUJ singly or in combination. Injuries involving the radial head or proximal ulna should be considered as possible causes of stiffness in rotation, as should a history of previous forearm bone fractures. The Monteggia fracture of the proximal half of the ulna shaft with anterior dislocation of the radial head is one such fracture; another example is seen in the reverse fracture pattern seen in the Galeazzi fracture of the radial shaft and dislocation of the DRUJ with the attendant soft tissue injury to the interosseous membrane and the capsular ligaments of the DRUJ. A rare but complete lesion is seen in the Essex–Lopresti injury where there is a longitudinal compression of the forearm with a comminuted fracture of the radial head, a full longitudinal tear of the interosseous membrane and a late axial subluxation of the DRUJ (Fig. 14).

The development of scarring in the interosseous membrane must also be considered as a possible effect following forearm bone fractures, in addition to any malalignment of the fractures with loss of the normal axis of rotation. Rarely a cross-union between radius and ulna occurs with a complete lack of any rotation. Therefore it is useful when examining patients for stiffness of the DRUJ to have

a clear idea of the potential causes which may lie outside the joint, so that efforts to improve range of motion and function are targeted at the appropriate mechanical problems.

The local causes of restricted motion of the DRUJ are to be found in the alignment of the joint, the joint surfaces and the soft tissue envelope of the joint. The aetiology of the stiffness is rarely due to one cause alone; although there may be a principal cause, the subordinate elements may reduce the potential for a good or excellent result.

The history, examination and investigations will give an indication of the problem and, it is necessary to have a diagnostic and management algorithm in mind when examining patients with stiffness of the DRUJ.

Stiffness following trauma would suggest the causes outlined above; an absence of a history of trauma would suggest that the problems are more likely to be associated with either very late post-traumatic degenerative disease or inflammatory joint disease, and therefore different investigation and treatment options may be indicated.

Degenerative joint disease may present with an increasing discomfort on use, tending to settle with rest. Osteoarthrosis of the DRUJ is not uncommon and may represent an old injury but may be secondary to other disease such as synovial chondro-

(a)

(b)

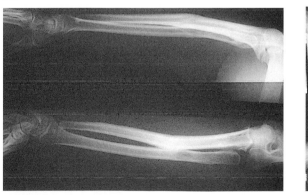 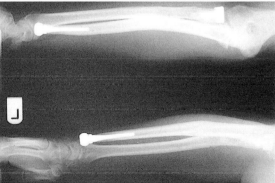

Figure 14

A classic Essex–Lopresti lesion does not include fracture of the shaft of the ulna but does include rupture of the interosseous membrane and disruption of the DRUJ. This gives an Essex–Lopresti lesion and a fracture shaft of ulna. The radial and ulna heads have been previously removed (a) and have been replaced (b) with considerable improved in pronosupination

matosis. Loose bodies may result from previous mild trauma and may represent an osteochondral injury; both the former and the latter tend to present with a history of catching and locking but the osteochondral defect will give a classical painful arc when the DRUJ is examined in forced compression and rotation.

The differential diagnosis of DRUJ disease must include ulnar abutment or ulnocarpal impaction syndrome as well as tears of the TFCC. There is a consistency of complaint about these conditions in that there is pain when the patient grasps or lifts with the wrist in ulnar deviation and investigations; plain radiographs, arthrography and arthroscopy usually identify the cause.

Within the joint itself a number of potential causes of restricted motion are seen and they may be classified into disturbance of joint congruity, disturbance of joint alignment, damage to the articular surfaces, capsular contracture and ulnocarpal impaction syndrome.

Disturbance of joint congruity

This is extremely common following distal radial fractures; the fractures that do involve significant comminution of the DRUJ disturb the ulnar seat on the radius, either by displacement or by angulation or by both (Fig. 15).

The treatment, of course, ideally is to create a good alignment of the joint at the time of the initial fracture and reduction, but the late presentation of these problems requires some form of arthroplasty, and in the presence of an intact TFCC and the absence of stylotriquetral abutment, a Bowers' hemi-interpositional tendon arthroplasty (Fig. 16) or a matched ulnar procedure is effective, although a Darrach excisional arthroplasty can be performed.

Disturbance of joint alignment

Marked angulation of distal radial fractures or malunion of shaft fractures of both ulna and radius can

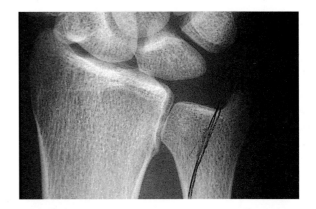

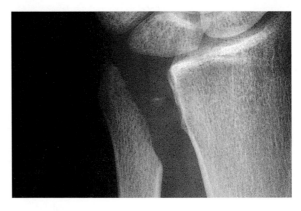

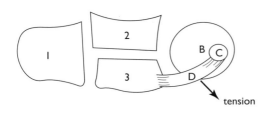

Figure 15

Diagrammatic representation of the damage to the DRUJ from a Frykman VII or VIII

Figure 16

(a) Before Bowers' hemi-interpositional tendon arthroplasty; (b) after Bowers' hemi-interpositional tendon arthroplasty

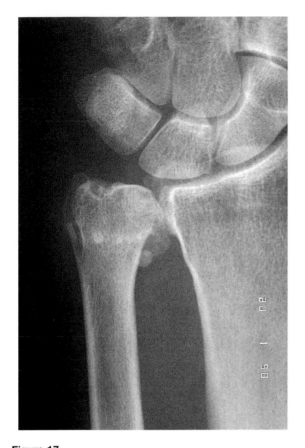

Figure 17

Late degenerative changes at the DRUJ following fracture

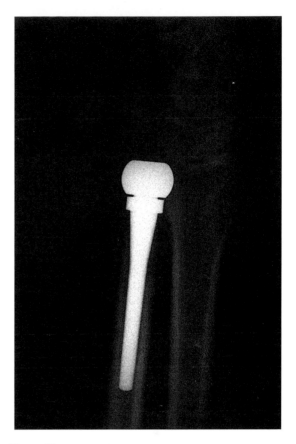

Figure 18

A titanium ulnar replacement

give rise to significant alignment problems at the DRUJ, leading to stiffness. CT imaging of the wrist in the transverse plane in pronation and supination will identify abnormal axial motion; almost invariably the treatment requires radial osteotomy with an opening wedge and grafting to bring the radius into alignment with the ulna. Excision of the ulnar head in these circumstances always leads to instability, which is difficult and sometimes impossible to correct.

Damage to the articular surfaces

Secondary degenerative changes following chondrolysis or cartilage injury give rise to degenerative

arthrosis, in these circumstances, since this is a late presentation, consideration should be given to one of the various excisional arthroplasties (Fig. 17) or to joint replacement (Fig. 18).

Capsular contracture

Recent work by Kleinmann (personal communication) shows that selective capsulectomy of the DRUJ can give rise to significant improvement in range of motion where the alignment, the congruity and the joint surfaces are normal. The restriction of supination requires an anterior capsulectomy with preservation of the TFCC and its attachment to the ulnocarpal ligament. Difficulty in pronation requires a dorsal capsulectomy deep to the extensor reti-naculum, again with preservation of the attachment of the TFCC to the proximal edge of the radio-lunotriquetral ligament.

Ulnocarpal impaction syndrome

Almost invariably, distal radial fracture in patients over 45 years of age results in some radial shorten-ing with apparent ulnar lengthening. With every mil-limetre of ulnar lengthening, forces acting on the ulnar side of the wrist increase by 40%. Therefore, in the presence of radial shortening which is often seen after distal radial fracture, formal shortening of the ulna may be necessary. The success of this pro-cedure is very high and the complication rate very low.

Algodystrophy

Algodystrophy is a problem which occurs in approximately 3–4% of injuries around the wrist. The net effect is to cause capsule tightness and the treatment after resolution of the algodystrophy is to consider capsulectomy rather than any bony proce-dure, unless there is sufficient malalignment of the fractures. Rarely, chondrolysis occurs as a result of trauma, giving rise to an acute loss of cartilage and a very stiff DRUJ, the treatment of which is some form of excisional arthroplasty or Sauvé–Kapandji DRUJ arthrodesis with a proximal ulnar pseudarthrosis.

Rheumatoid arthritis

Rheumatoid arthritis and the other inflammatory arthroplasties generate recurrent synovitis due to immune complexes produced in reaction to colla-gen. This is a systemic disease affecting the whole person with major effects upon the musculoskeletal system.

There are two particular effects that are seen as a result of this particular pathological process, one is an exuberant synovitis resulting in recurrent effu-sion, which gives rise to capsular stretching, dis-placement of the extensor carpi ulnaris tendon out

of its groove, erosions of the ulnar head, erosions of the sigmoid notch of the ulna, marked instability and a resulting supination of the hand due to failure of the ulnar carpal ligament (Fig. 19). There is usu-ally, however, in these situations a good range of motion, although the marked instability of the DRUJ often gives rise to attrition rupture of the extensor tendons (Fig. 20).

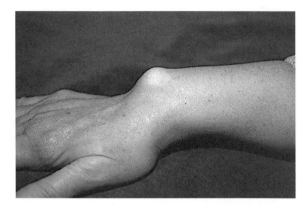

Figure 19

Supination of the hand is visible, with the prominence of the ulnar head and the so-called 'caput ulnae syndrome'

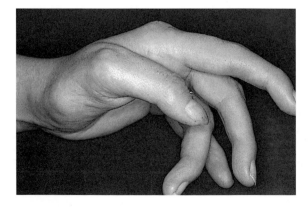

Figure 20

Rupture of the extensor tendons results from 'caput ulnae syndrome'

The second effect occurs in those patients whose disease involves them in low-grade synovitis without recurrent effusions but which causes significant cartilage damage, disruption of the TFCC, and some failure of the ulnar carpal ligament in supination of the hand, associated with significant impairment of pronosupination due to often secondary degenerative arthrosis superimposed upon the rheumatoid disease itself (Fig. 21). These patients have significant problems, in particular in achieving supination of the hands, although normally the functional position of the hand in pronation is maintained.

In all patients with polyarthropathy, careful evaluation of the whole wrist is essential. It is not possible to deal with the DRUJ in isolation: consideration has to be given to the radiocarpal joint, since translation of the carpus and volar subluxation of the carpus are common accompaniments in rheumatoid disease and the type of surgery proposed to the ulnar head has to be considered very carefully. Simple excisional arthroplasty, as described by Darrach in 1909, is sufficient to relieve pain and discomfort but in the presence of significant translation

of the carpus, there is always the risk that the carpus will further translate and instability ensue. It is, therefore, necessary to have a good radiographic evaluation of the wrist in order to classify the wrist and define whether there is translation of the carpus and, indeed, whether there is significant midcarpal and radiocarpal disease. In the situation where there is multiple disease, the surgery for the restoration of pronosupination has to be part of a more significant surgical programme.

Having defined the particular type of patient and having defined that the problem of pronosupination is indeed at the DRUJ, not the proximal radioulnar joint (which is a common problem in rheumatoid disease), the surgical options for the DRUJ are, in fact, quite simple. The Darrach procedure (the simple excision of the ulnar head) is an operation performed widely and successfully, and in the rheumatoid patient the results can be guaranteed to improve range and to improve pain. However, there is a penalty to be paid in some patients, in that once the ulnar head is excised (as described by Darrach and practised by most people) approximately 1 in 20 patients will have significant unremitting instability of the distal radius and ulna. It is important to remember that the ulna is the fixed point and the radius and hand are suspended from it by the interosseous membrane and the proximal and distal joints. By removing the distal joint in some patients there will be a significant increase in the instability, particularly if the interosseous mem-

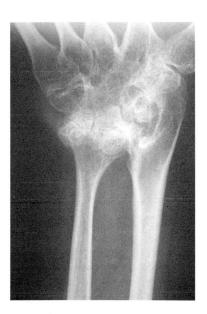

Figure 21

The secondary degenerative changes occurring in long-standing rheumatoid arthritis are apparent in this example of juvenile rheumatoid arthritis

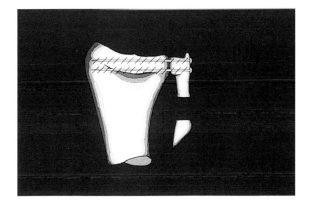

Figure 22

A diagrammatic representation of the Sauvé–Kapandji procedure

brane is attenuated. If this is the case at the time of surgery, then an alternative procedure should be considered: the matched ulna (as described by Kirk Watson), which preserves ulnar length out to the tip of the styloid process, is an appropriate procedure, providing there is no styloid triquetral abutment. The matched ulna is a more difficult procedure to perform and requires great care, and there is a risk that there will be new bone formation will occur and further impingement, and the patient may require further surgery; but if surgery is required, it is not required for instability but for further impingement.

The Bowers' procedure, which is a hemi-interpositional tendon arthroplasty, is quite inappropriate in the rheumatoid patient, particularly as the TFCC and the ulnar carpal ligaments are often damaged in rheumatoid disease and are essential for a successful Bowers' procedure.

The Sauvé–Kapandji procedure (distal radioulnar arthrodesis with a proximal excisional arthroplasty of the shaft of the ulna) (Fig. 22) is a very successful procedure. Indeed, if there is any suggestion of translation of the carpus or of instability of the DRUJ joint, then the procedure is, in my opinion, the operation of choice; good fixation can be obtained and excision of 1.2 cm is sufficient. The modification of this operation by Kapandji (the Kapandji II procedure) involves incorporating an ulna-shortening procedure where the head is recessed. This is a useful procedure and the further modification by Zachee and De Smet – in which the insertion of pronator quadratus into the excised segment is brought up between the stump of the ulna and the residual head and sutured to the extensor carpi ulnaris – stabilizes the segment; instability at the pseudarthrosis is much less common and in their (45) cases they had extremely good results.

The discussion of implant arthroplasty for the DRUJ remains. Designs are being tested at this time: the Herbert implant is under trial at the Wrightington Hospital and other centres and is a useful solution for the markedly unstable DRUJ which has had a previous excisional arthroplasty. The Swanson silicone implant does not stand the test of time and is not recommended (Fig. 23).

In summary, rheumatoid arthritis gives rise to significant instability in some patients, a combination of stiffness and instability in others and in still others just stiffness. The surgery has to be carefully thought through as part of an overall programme. Proximal joint disease has to be examined to ensure

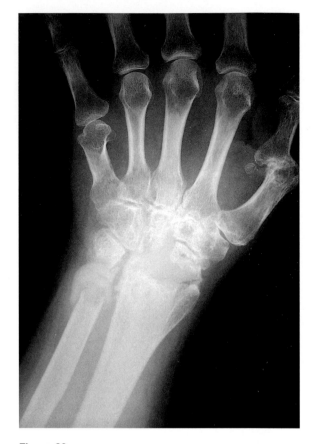

Figure 23

An example of an ulnar head replacement of the silicone elastomer type which gave good results in the first year or so but failed in 15–20% of patients thereafter

that there is no hidden cause for restriction of pronosupination. The Darrach procedure is sufficient for the majority of patients but those patients who have some instability may require either an implant arthroplasty or a Sauvé–Kapandji procedure. The matched ulna should be reserved for those cases in which there is a significant risk of the development of instability; the procedure does have a significant risk of reimpingement but may be the procedure of choice in patients with marked instability problems.

References

Adams BD (1993) Effects of radial deformity on distal radioulnar joint mechanics, *J Hand Surg* **18A:**492–8.

af Ekenstam F (1992) Anatomy of the distal radioulnar joint, *Clin Orthop* **275:**14–18.

Almquist EE (1992) Evolution of the distal radioulnar joint, *Clin Orthop* **275:**5–13.

Bowers WH (1992) Distal radioulnar joint arthroplasty. Current concepts, *Clin Orthop* **275:**104–9.

Connor J, Nalebuff EA (1995) Current recommendations for surgery of the rheumatoid hand and wrist, *Curr Opin Rheumatol* **7:**120–4.

Dell PC (1992) Traumatic disorders of the distal radioulnar joint, *Clin Sports Med*, **11:**141–59.

Drobner WS, Hausman MR (1992) The distal radioulnar joint, *Hand Clin* **8:**631–44.

Dumontier C (1992) [Distal radioulnar joint. Traumatic and degenerative diseases] *Ann Radiol Paris* **35:**384–95.

Dyer CR, Kischner SH, Brien WW (1994) The distal radioulnar joint following Galeazzi's fracture, *Orthop Rev* **23(7):**587–92.

Eglseder WA, Hay M (1993) Combined Essex–Lopresti and radial shaft fractures: case report, *J Trauma* **34:**311–12.

Friedman SL, Palmer AK (1991) The ulnar impaction syndrome, *Hand Clin* **7:**295–310.

Geel CW, Palmer AK (1992) Radial head fractures and their effect on the distal radioulnar joint. A rationale for treatment, *Clin Orthop* **275:**79–83.

Hagert CG (1992) The distal radioulnar joint in relation to the whole forearm, *Clin Orthop* **275:**56–64.

Hagert CG (1994) Distal radius fracture and the distal radioulnar joint—anatomical considerations, *Handchir Mikrochir Plast Chir* **26:**22–6.

Kauer JM (1992) The distal radioulnar joint. Anatomic and functional considerations, *Clin Orthop* **275:**37–45.

Kihara H, Short WH, Werner FW, Fortino MD, Palmer AK (1995) The stabilizing mechanism of the distal radioulnar joint during pronation and supination, *J Hand Surg* **20A:**930–6.

Linscheid RL (1992) Biomechanics of the distal radioulnar joint, *Clin Orthop* **275:**Σ46–55.

Lovett RJ (1991) The treatment of longitudinal ulnar deficiency, *Prosthet Orthot Int* **15:**104–5.

Macule Beneyto F, Arandes Renu JM, Ferreres Claramunt A, Ramon Soler R (1994) Treatment of Galeazzi fracture-dislocations, *J Trauma* **36(3):**352–5.

Nathan R, Schneider LH (1991) Classification of the distal radioulnar joint disorders, *Hand Clin* **7:**239–47.

Okuda Y, Morito T, Tamai K, Hirasawa Y (1994) Familial positive ulnar variance with secondary radioulnar joint arthritis, *J Hand Surg* **19A:**405–9.

Posner MA, Ambrose L (1991) Excision of the distal ulna in rheumatoid arthritis, *Hand Clin* **7:**383–90.

Rayhack JM, Gasser SI, Latta LL, Ouellette EA, Milne EL (1993) Precision oblique osteotomy for shortening of the ulna, *J Hand Surg* **18A:**908–18.

Schneiderman G, Meldrum RD, Bloebaum RD, Tarr R, Sarmiento A (1993) The interosseous membrane of the forearm: structure and its role in Galeazzi fractures, *J Trauma* **35:**879–85.

Stanton RP, Hansen MO (1996) Function of the upper extremities in hereditary multiple exostoses, *J Bone Joint Surg* **78A:**568–73.

Staron RB, Feldman F, Haramati N, Singson RD, Rosenwasser M, Esser PD (1994) Abnormal geometry of the distal radioulnar joint: MR findings, *Skeletal Radiol* **23:**369–72.

Taleisnik J (1992) The Sauvé–Kapandji procedure, *Clin Orthop* **275:**110–23.

Tsukazaki T, Iwasaki K (1993) Ulnar wrist pain after Colles' fracture. 109 fractures followed for 4 years, *Acta Orthop Scand* **64:**462–4.

Villa A, Paley D, Catagni MA, Bell D, Cattaneo R (1990) Lengthening of the forearm by the Ilizarov technique, *Clin Orthop* 125–37.

Vincent KA, Szabo RM, Agee JM (1993) The Sauvé–Kapandji procedure for reconstruction of the rheumatoid distal radioulnar joint, *J Hand Surg* **18:**978–83.

Waizenegger M, Schranz P, Barton NJ (1993) The Kapandji procedure for post-traumatic problems, *Injury.* **24:**662–6.

Watson HK, Gabuzda GM (1992) Matched distal ulna resection for posttraumatic disorders of the distal radioulnar joint, *J Hand Surg* **17A:**724–30.

Werner FW, Palmer AK, Fortino MD, Short WH (1992) Force transmission through the distal ulna: effect of ulnar variance, lunate fossa angulation, and radial and palmar tilt of the distal radius, *J Hand Surg* **17A:**423–4.

Williams CS, Jupiter JB (1993) [The painful ulnocarpal joint. Diagnosis and therapy], *Orthopäde*, **22:**36–45.

32
Treatment of stiffness of the distal radioulnar joint

Philippe Saffar

Distal radioulnar joint (DRUJ) incongruency is one of the complications which may lead to painful limitation of forearm motion. Loss of supination is more bothersome than loss of pronation where shoulder compensation of the motion is possible. Several procedures have been suggested to restore a painless rotation of the forearm:

- Some procedures resect the distal ulna:
  - (a) the Darrach procedure (Fig. 1) (Darrach 1913, Dingman 1952) has been so far the usual method, but several papers have stressed its disadvantages: 1, loss of grip strength; 2, loss of support of the ulnar carpus; and 3, instability of the distal ulnar stump

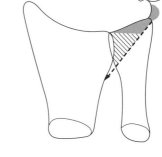

Figure 2

Bowers procedure.

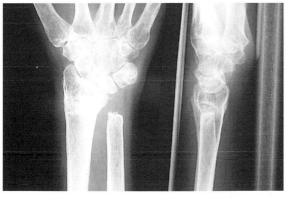

Figure 1

Darrach procedure associated with treatment of the distal radial malunion.

  - (b) more recently, in 1985, Bowers (Fig. 2) suggested a hemiresection–interposition technique (Fernandez 1988, Bowers 1990)

  - (c) In 1986 Watson et al (Fig. 3) proposed a matched distal ulnar resection (Watson and Gabzuda 1992).
- Conversely, other procedures maintain the distal ulna:
  - (a) the Sauvé-Kapandji procedure (Sauvé and Kapandji 1936, Baciu et al 1965, Kapandji 1986, Sanders et al 1991, Condamine et al 1992, Nakamura et al 1992, Minami et al 1995) (Fig. 4a, b) preserves the ulnar support of the wrist and results in more grip strength
  - (b) distal ulnar recession (Cantero 1977, Darrow et al 1985) consists of shortening the ulna at the level of the shaft (Fig. 5)
  - (c) the wafer procedure described by Feldon et al (1992) (Fig. 6) is a limited distal ulnar head resection preserving the DRUJ.

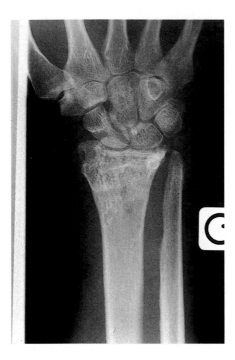

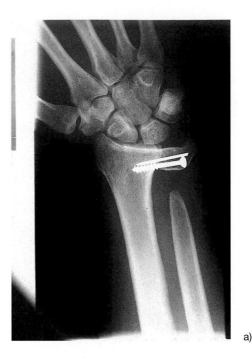

a)

Figure 3

Watson procedure.

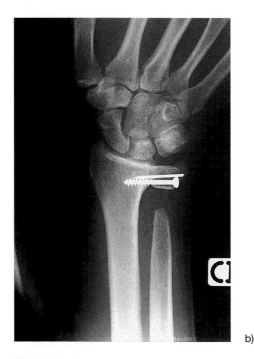

b)

Each of these procedures have been suggested in the treatment of chronic post-traumatic disorders of the DRUJ which may result from conditions such as DRUJ dislocation, malunited distal forearm fractures, osteoarthritis, rheumatoid arthritis, and congenital deformities such as Madelung's deformity.

The following techniques for resecting or maintaining the distal ulnar head will be described and compared: the Darrach procedure, Bowers' hemiresection arthroplasty, Watson's matched distal arthroplasty, Sauvé-Kapandji's technique, the wafer procedure and ulnar recession for treatment of chronic and mainly post-traumatic disorders of the DRUJ.

Figure 4

Sauvé-Kapandji procedure: (a) Radial and (b) ulnar deviation.

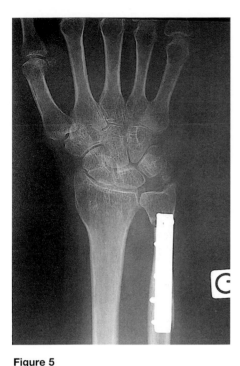

Figure 5

Distal ulnar recession.

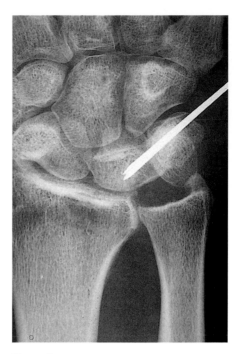

Figure 6

The wafer procedure (Feldon et al 1992).

Operative techniques

Resecting the DRUJ

Darrach's technique

A longitudinal posterior approach between the fourth and fifth compartment is performed; the dorsal superficial branch of the ulnar nerve is dissected and retracted. Then 12 mm of the distal ulna are resected without elevating the periosteum. It is very important to use all the soft tissues to carefully close the space and have an interposition between the triangular ligament and the distal ulnar stump. Dorsalization of the extensor carpi ulnaris (ECU) should stabilize the stump as will be explained later.

Watson's technique

The distal ulna is cut with an electric saw obliquely, parallel to the medial border of the radius and the distal ulna is stabilized at its distal end.

Bowers' technique

The distal ulna is cut obliquely, beginning at the level of the proximal border of the DRUJ, resecting only the joint. An interposition with a rolled tendon will be interposed between the distal ulna and the radius to prevent impingement.

Sauvé-Kapandji's technique

This is an arthrodesis between the distal ulna and the sigmoid notch of the radius. A bone cylinder of 1 cm with its periosteum is then resected proximal to the DRUJ creating an intentional pseudarthrosis where the pronosupination motion will take place.

Retaining the DRUJ

Ulnar recession

A transverse or step osteotomy is performed at the distal third of the ulnar shaft. The ulna is shortened removing a cylinder or two bone segments. The

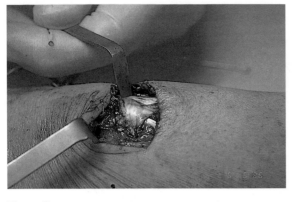

Figure 7

Stabilization of the extensor carpi ulnaris (ECU) (Spinner and Kaplan 1970).

magnitude of bone resection is calculated to level the distal ulna and the radius. Usually, less than 1 cm is removed. The bone is usually fixed using a plate.

Wafer procedure

The DRUJ joint is opened and only the convex part of the ulnar head is resected.

The two last procedures are less used because stiffness is usually less significant when the DRUJ is conserved.

When the ECU tendon was found to be unstable during the procedure, it was stabilized using an extensor retinaculum flap as proposed by Spinner and Kaplan (1970) (Fig. 7).

A radial corrective osteotomy using a volar opening-wedge osteotomy for increased volar tilt malunions or a dorsal opening-wedge osteotomy for increased dorsal tilt malunions may be performed in the same procedure. They tend to obtain a better congruency between the two bones.

Postoperative complications

Neurosympathetic dystrophy or extensor tendon problems are not frequent. Secondary reossification is possible after Sauvé-Kapandji procedures; iterative bone excision achieves a good range of motion.

The Darrach procedure may be used after a Watson or Bowers procedure has failed. Persistent pain is usually due to impingement of the ulnar distal end or shaft on the radial shaft.

Painful ulnar stump may be a problem after a too significant distal ulnar resection or a Sauvé-Kapandji procedure. Stabilization of this stump is a difficult problem.

Results of our series

Pain

The best results on pain in our comparative series were observed in the Sauvé-Kapandji group; the smallest improvement was in the Watson group.

Stabilization is defined as the delay after operation after which there is no further evolution. The Watson procedure seems to have a longer stabilization delay (average 7 months), than Darrach and Sauvé-Kapandji procedures (average of 3.5 and 4 months, respectively). A return to previous occupation was obtained in 58% of the patients who underwent a Watson procedure and in 70% of Sauvé-Kapandji procedure patients. No significant difference was observed for patients with workman's compensation.

Range of motion

The loss of range of motion was maximum in pronation and ulnar deviation. Pronation averaged $52 \pm 28°$ and supination $55°$ preoperatively and postoperatively pronation $77 \pm 28°$ and supination $80°$.

The best pronation–supination results were obtained with the Sauvé-Kapandji technique; the worst with the Bowers procedure.

Grip strength

Best results were obtained with the Sauvé-Kapandji procedure, grip strength averaging 93% of the contralateral side. The Watson procedure averaged

72% of the contralateral side, Bowers 61% and Darrach 60%.

Ulnar stump instability was studied, noting if the ulnar stump was passively unstable, and if it was painful.

Moderate pain was present in four Sauvé-Kapandji patients associated with ulnar stump instability. Ulnar stump instability was present in 40% of patients after the Sauvé-Kapandji procedure, but this did not impair overall results and function. It was also present in some cases of Darrach or Watson procedures. None of these patients underwent a stabilization procedure.

Discussion

The Sauvé-Kapandji procedure keeps the normal force transmission through hand and forearm. It preserves distal stabilization of ECU in the 6th extensor compartment or allows near anatomical repair using a Spinner procedure. We believe this has an important dynamic stabilizing effect on the ulnar stump. The somewhat shorter stump resulting from the Sauvé-Kapandji procedure is less dangerous for extensor tendons than the Darrach procedure ulnar stump; an eventual conflict would occur in an area where these tendons are not as fixed (proximal to the extensor retinaculum) explaining why there were no complications with the extensor tendons in our patients.

In all cases, painful stump problems are predictable when preoperative X-rays demonstrate a loss of parallelism of the diaphyses of radius and ulna, and this is particularly true for distal radial malunions in flexion after Smith's fractures (Fig. 8)

We share Hagert's opinion (Hagert 1992) concerning the DRUJ in relation to the whole forearm. He stated that the DRUJ is one of the points where forces pass from the hand to the elbow, and this creates an important transversal pressure through the DRUJ. The DRUJ is the only structure that keeps the two forearm bones apart.

If the DRUJ is a weight-bearing articulation, resection arthroplasties are doomed to failure, and interposition is not going to be of much help. Indeed, we observed progressive narrowing of the neo-DRUJ space in all our Watson and Bowers procedures.

Corrective osteotomy of distal radial malunion, when performed at the same time as the DRUJ

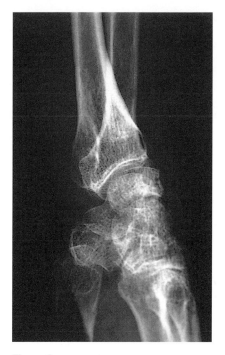

Figure 8

Loss of parallelism of the radius and ulna shafts.

procedure, has provided a faster outcome and better overall results, although it is a more significant procedure.

Ulnar carpal shift was never observed in our patients, as we had expected to happen after Darrach procedures. Actually, this has only been described after the Darrach procedure in rheumatoid patients (Bieber et al 1988). In post-traumatic patients (Rayhack et al 1987), early ulnar translation occurred as a consequence of undiagnosed radiocarpal dislocations. We believe such a translation cannot occur in non-rheumatoid patients, at least not until some years have lapsed. We have been disappointed by the ulnar translation indexes.

The Bowers procedure obtains good results for rheumatoid wrist, but not for post-traumatic wrist.

Ulnar recession is indicated when there is an ulnoradial discrepancy in length (long ulna after distal radial fracture or congenital) and if the cartilage of the DRUJ is in good shape. Congruency should be obtained and this depends also on the DRUJ joint shape.

References

Baciu C, Zgabura I, Roventa N, Chicli E (1965) Résultats éloignés a l'opération de Sauvé-Kapandji pour le traitement des fractures Pouteau-Colles vicieusement consolidées, *Acta Orthop Belg* **31**:920–35.

Bieber EJ, Linscheid RL, Dobyns JH, Beckenbaugh RD (1988) Failed distal ulnar resections, *J Hand Surg* **13A**:193–200.

Bowers WH (1985) Distal radioulnar joint arthroplasty: the hemiresection–interposition technique, *J Hand Surg* **10A**:169–78.

Bowers WH (1990) Instability of the distal radioulnar articulation, *Hand Clin* **7**:311–25.

Cantero J (1977) Raccourcissement du cubitus dans les séquelles de fracture de l'extrémité distale du radius, *Ann Chir* **31**:330–4.

Condamine JL, Lebreton L, Aubriot JH (1992) L'intervention de Sauvé-Kapandji. Analyse et résultats de 69 cas, *Ann Chir Main* **1**:27–39.

Darrach W (1913) Partial excision of the distal end of the ulna for deformity following Colles' fracture, *Ann Surg* **57**:764–5.

Darrow JC Jr, Linscheid RL, Dobyns JH, Mann JM, Wood M, Beckenbaugh B (1985) Distal ulnar recession for disorders of the distal radioulnar joint, *J Hand Surg* **10A**:482–91.

Dingman PVC (1952) Resection of the distal end of the ulna (Darrach's operation). An end-result study of twenty four cases, *J Bone Joint Surg* **34A**:893–900.

Feldon P, Terrono AL, Belsky MR (1992) The 'wafer' procedure. Partial distal ulnar resection, *Clin Orthop* **275**:124–9.

Fernandez DL (1988) Radial osteotomy and Bowers arthroplasty for malunited fractures of the distal end of the radius, *J Bone Joint Surg* **70A**:1538–51.

Hagert CG (1992) The distal radioulnar joint in relation to the wrist and forearm, *Clin Orthop* **275**:56–64.

Kapandji IA (1986) L'opération de Sauvé-Kapandji. Techniques et indications dans les affections non rhumatismales, *Ann Chir Main* **5**:181–93.

Minami A, Suzuki K, Suenaga N, Ishikawa J (1995) The Sauvé-Kapandji procedure for osteoarthritis of the distal radioulnar joint, *J Hand Surg* **20A**:602–8.

Nakamura R, Tsunoda K, Watanabe K, Horii E, Miura T (1992) The Sauvé-Kapandji procedure for chronic dislocations of the distal radioulnar joint with destruction of the articular surface, *J Hand Surg* **17B**:127–32.

Rayhack JM, Linscheid RL, Dobyns JH, Smith JH (1987) Posttraumatic ulnar translation of the carpus, *J Hand Surg* **12A**:180–9.

Sanders RA, Frederick HA, Hontas RB (1991) The Sauvé-Kapandji procedure: a salvage operation for the distal radioulnar joint, *J Hand Surg* **16A**:1125–9.

Sauvé L, Kapandji M (1936) Nouvelle technique de traitement chirurgicale des luxations récidivantes isolées de l'extrémité inférieure du cubitus. *J Chir* **47**:589–94.

Spinner M, Kaplan EB (1970) Extensor carpi ulnaris: its relationship to the stability of the distal radioulnar joint, *Clin Orthop* **68**:124–9.

Watson HK, Gabuzda GM (1992) Matched distal ulnar resection for posttraumatic disorders of the distal radioulnar joint, *J Hand Surg* **17A**:724–30.

Watson HK, Ryu J, Burgess RC (1986) Matched distal ulnar resection, *J Hand Surg* **11A**:812–17.

33

Rehabilitation of the distal radioulnar joint

Lynda Gwilliam

The treatment of the stiff distal radioulnar joint (DRUJ) is a challenge to many therapists. The reason why some patients respond to treatment and others do not is often ascribed to poor therapy or poor patient co-operation. This concept is now increasingly challenged as we acquire better knowledge about the anatomy and biomechanics of the DRUJ. Kapandji (1982) in *The Physiology of the Joints* explores the poorly understood and complex movement of rotation; he describes it as the movement of the forearm about its longitudinal axis. This movement involves two joints which are mechanically linked: the superior radioulnar joint (SRUJ) which anatomically belongs to the elbow joint, and the DRUJ which is anatomically separate from the wrist joint.

Although the DRUJ is anatomically separate from the wrist, the two are intimately linked. The movement of longitudinal rotation of the forearm introduces a third degree of movement to the wrist joint allowing it to be placed in any position to grasp or to support an object. Thus it is essential when studying functional capacity to integrate the physiology of the DRUJ with the physiology of the wrist since this 'functional coupling' of pronation–supination and wrist action allows the hand the freedom to be positioned for maximum functional impact. This is best illustrated by the relationship between wrist abduction–adduction and pronation–supination. In pronation the hand is usually tilted towards the ulna in an attempt to bring prehension grip into line with the axis of pronation–supination, but in supination the hand is tilted towards the radius favouring a more supportive grip. King et al (1986) have noted that clinically measured rotation averages 260° at the hand and 190° at the DRUJ. This gives an average of 4° of hand motion for 3° of joint movement and highlights how even the smallest loss of rotation can limit hand positioning and functional capacity quite considerably.

Functional problems associated with DRUJ stiffness are frequently encountered in the clinical setting, probably because the initial injury to the DRUJ is often overlooked or poorly treated. This is best illustrated by looking at fractures of the distal radius which are among the most common of all orthopaedic injuries. With a reported incidence of 1 in 500, they account for nearly one-sixth of all fractures seen in the emergency room. These distal radius fractures are not just confined to the elderly lady who slips on the ice; they have a bimodal age distribution with a peak occurrence in young adolescents and a second peak in the older population. Reviews of these injuries have documented that 50% or more involve either the radiocarpal joint or the DRUJ in addition to radial metaphyseal fractures (Alffram and Bauer 1962). This has far reaching consequences in terms of the demands placed on the rehabilitation services and the patient's functional capacity. Trying to improve range of motion following distal radial fractures which also include the DRUJ is very time consuming and limited in its success, so the patient has limited and often painful rotation which affects their occupation, social and daily life to varying degrees.

Initial therapeutic measures are best directed towards a detailed functional evaluation to establish the impact of a limited range of movement on the individual's lifestyle. This should also be accompanied by a detailed analysis of the movements necessary to perform these functional tasks so that it is clear to what degree the problems are associated with the DRUJ rather than the SRUJ or the wrist joint.

The results of this functional and anatomical assessment allow the therapist to formulate a treatment programme aimed at improving range of motion in specific joints and at minimizing functional disability and pain.

The therapy programme may include 'hands on' mobilization specific to the DRUJ and wrist joint, plus remedial activities that encourage and extend the functional use of these movements. One remedial activity that we have found to be particularly useful in increasing rotation is the MULE (myoelectric upper limb exerciser); by the application of different handles it is possible to encourage pronation–supination of the DRUJ and specific wrist movements in a way that is stimulating for the patient and that progressively increases movement and builds up muscle power and endurance prior to return to work.

It is often necessary to use splinting (Hunter et al 1990) as a means of maintaining/increasing the range of movements obtained by other therapy methods. These splints are worn between therapy sessions and/or at night. Splinting can be directed towards improving either pronation or supination (depending on which has the greatest loss of movement) or both (if both are equally stiff); in the latter case the patient would alternate splints as directed by the therapist. These splints, which can be either static or dynamic in their action, are designed to hold the soft tissues at the end point of their elastic limit so that the tissue accommodates and lengthens thus allowing an increase in range of movement (Brand 1952).

When stiffness of the DRUJ is mainly associated with soft tissue tightness and scarring, e.g. following either injury or prolonged immobilization of the wrist and DRUJ, then gains in range of movement can be made using splinting and other therapeutic measures; movement has a 'soft' end point feel to it and the therapist knows that treatment and time will resolve the situation. The therapist should question the biomechanics and the pathology of the injury in those patients with a 'hard' end feel to movement and where no progress is being made with therapy. At the time of initial injury, this group of patients had an undiagnosed or poorly treated injury to the DRUJ resulting in a mechanical block to rotation. Further surgery is required to resolve the mechanical problem and the therapist needs to recognize those patients who will improve and those who need to be referred back to the surgeon.

Surgery for the stiff DRUJ includes procedures such as ulnar shortening, Darrach's procedure, Bowers' procedure, matched ulnar, etc. Following such surgery the therapeutic dilemma is not to sacrifice the long-term stability of the DRUJ for an immediate improvement in movement. For this reason initial treatment should delay movement of the DRUJ thus preventing rotation and subsequent instability of the joint. This can be achieved by joint immobilization in an above-elbow plaster of Paris or in a thermoplastic splint. The latter has some advantages over plaster in that it is lighter and can be periodically released to allow flexion and extension of the elbow joint thus decreasing the risk of stiffness developing at this joint. The exact moment to begin mobilization following surgery to improve range of movement at the DRUJ still remains a matter of clinical judgement by the surgeon and therapist. Clinical guidelines include significant pain on movement or excessive movement, both indicators that immobilization should be continued and that instability may result if mobilization is commenced too soon or too vigorously.

Continued immobilization to allow the development and maturation of scar tissue is preferable to instability of the DRUJ since soft tissue tightness can be addressed by the therapeutic interventions previously described. Therapy is often prolonged and recovery incomplete. Functionally, loss of pronation is a greater problem than loss of supination. After a period of therapy without further improvement, surgical treatment should be considered if a significant functional deficit remains.

References

Alffram PA, Bauer GCH (1962) Epidemiology of fractures of the forearm: a biomechanical investigation of bone strength, *J Bone Joint Surg* **44A:**105–14.

Brand PW (1952) The reconstruction of the hand in leprosy, *Ann R Coll Surg Engl* **11:**350.

Hunter JM, Schneider LH, Mackin EM, Callahan AD, eds (1990) *Rehabilitation of the Hand, Part XV*, 3rd edn. CV Mosby: St Louis.

Kapandji IA (1982) *The Physiology of the Joints*. Churchill Livingstone: New York.

King GJ, McMurtry RY, Rubensten JD, Gertzbein SD (1986) Kinematics of the distal radioulnar joint, *J Hand Surg* **11A:**798–804.

Part IV
Finger stiffness

34

Causes of post-traumatic metacarpophalangeal joint stiffness

Jean-Yves Alnot and Emmanuel H Masmejean

Stiffness of a joint is defined as a limitation of its mobility, which may present in varying degrees (McCormack 1964, Mansat and Delprat 1980, Laseter 1983, de la Caffinière and Mansat 1987, Mansat et al 1990). As part of post-traumatic lesions, this limitation can be ascribed to two causes:

- an intra-articular cause with capsuloligamentous and/or articular surface lesions
- an extra-articular cause, specially due to adhesions which limit the sliding movement of flexor as well as extensor tendons (Alnot and Leroy 1981).

We must differentiate between limitation of motion due to pain and true stiffness, although pain may be associated with stiffness. We must also differentiate between true stiffness and a complete ankylosis with bony fusion.

Finally, when stiffness is induced by trauma (which has to be defined precisely), it will be essential to appreciate:

- active and passive range of motion, and define such a stiffness in extension, in flexion or in an intermediate position
- tendinous and cutaneous conditions
- radiological examination focused on the status of the articular surfaces.

At the level of the hand, trauma can involve a joint, a digital segment or the whole hand. Stiffness may involve an isolated joint, a digital segment with a staged lesion, which can pose some difficult problems, and finally, several digital segments, which will worsen the functional prognosis.

Initial lesions have to be precisely defined, along with previous orthopaedic and surgical treatments, physical therapy and previous immobilization positions.

Anatomical review

Articular surfaces

The metacarpophalangeal (MP) joint is a condyle with flexion–extension as well as some lateral and rotational motion.

The capsuloligamentous structures are the volar plate, the articular capsule and the collateral ligaments. These collateral ligaments consists of a metacarpophalangeal and a metacarpoglenoidal bundle. Tension of each bundle is variable with the joint position; it is stretched in flexion and relaxed in extension. The extension position allows some lateral and rotational movements.

Synovial tissue covers the internal aspect of the articular capsule with some culs-de-sac. The most important culs-de-sac are the dorsal one under the extensor apparatus and the volar one at the level of the volar plate (Evans et al 1968, Beltran 1975).

Tendinous apparatus

Flexor and extensor tendons systems, interosseous and lumbrical muscles determine the different displacements in the sagittal and coronal planes, as well as in axial rotation.

Other periarticular tissues

Among the periarticular tissues which can participate in joint stiffness, we must emphasize:

- skin status with existence of dorsal or volar lesions: there is a fundamental difference

between the thin dorsal skin and the thick palmar skin
- vasculonervous problems: these may cause lesions which may participate in stiffness and worsen the prognosis.

Aetiologies

For post-traumatic stiffness it is important to differentiate between stiffness involving the articular surface (cartilaginous or osteocartilaginous lesions) and stiffness without lesions of the articular surfaces.

Also, we need to define exactly the:

- capsuloligamentous retractions
- retractile scars and skin adhesions
- sequelae of injuries of flexor or extensor tendon (Alnot and Leroy 1981, Merle and Gibon 1981)
- existence of a distant fracture on the diaphysis of the proximal phalanx or the metacarpal (Smith and Peimer 1977, Thomine et al 1981)
- existence of peripheral neuromas, anaesthesias and paraesthesias which will further worsen the prognosis and modify the physical therapy possibilities due to the absence of an active mobility.

With all these elements in mind, it will be necessary to define the importance of the factors having favoured stiffness (Peacock 1966, Tubiana 1984):

- *Oedema:* post-traumatic inflammatory phenomena induce an oedematous infiltration which affects the structure of articular synovial tissue (synovitis) and tendon (peritendonitis) sliding movement. It leads to a spontaneous attitude of the oedematous hand with the interphalangeal joints in flexion and the MP joints in extension. The MP joint, which normally rests in flexion, positions itself in extension because of the tension on the dorsal skin
- A *haematoma* is regularly associated with traumatism with a secondary fibrous retraction
- An *infection* may have been a factor of severe sequelae on motion
- *Various traumas* may have had required conservative or surgical treatment thus directly influencing the functional result.

Incorrect immobilization of the joints may have induced a limitation of their motion. In most cases, this will result in MP joint stiffness in extension and

in interphalangeal joint stiffness in flexion (or more rarely in extension). It is essential to remember that prevention of such a stiffness is avoiding an unadapted immobilization and adhering to the notion of the intrinsic plus position, i.e. the wrist at zero slightly in extension, the MP joints in flexion and the interphalangeal joints in extension.

If a surgical procedure is performed using K-wires, a plate or an external fixator, it is important to underline the importance of a rigorous technique which will avoid an additional traumatism to the initial injury. The associated lesions are particularly important and the cutaneous and tendinous lesions have to be defined.

Finally, the patient's psychological characteristics play a certain part and have to be evaluated, and the emergence of reflex sympathetic dystrophy is always possible (Ravault and Durant 1961, Watson et al 1988).

Clinical aspects

On the functional or therapeutic level, it is essential to realize that the complete range of motion is not necessary in the movements of daily life. The full flexion–extension range of motion is not completely used.

So, we can define a useful range of motion, from 20° to 60–70°. Regarding this definition, we determine different types of stiffness in extension (0–30°) or in flexion (70–90°).

It is necessary to take into consideration the limitation of the articular movements and those due to soft tissue retraction. We need to differentiate the cases where there is a complete range of motion of the interphalangeal joints and the cases where there are some lesional associations.

Flexion or extension of the wrist will relax the teguments and tendinous apparatus, and will allow a more precise exploration of the mobility of the MP and interphalangeal joints. Centred plain X-rays also differentiate stiffness with or without lesions of the articular surfaces.

Stiffness in extension

This is the most frequent. The flexion can be limited by:

- cutaneous adhesions with sometimes a retraction of the dorsal skin
- lesions and adhesions of the extensor apparatus at the dorsal aspect of the joints of the wrist or the hand
- dorsal capsule retraction
- collateral ligament retraction
- and the osteoarticular lesions.

Knowledge of the anatomical lesions will allow the definition of a therapeutic scale of ascending gravity:

(a) Very simple cases which are induced by sequelae of the extensor tendons lesions and skin adhesions with normal mobility of the interphalangeal joints. A full range of motion will be obtained by a tenolysis without any procedure on the capsuloligamentous elements.
(b) An arthrolysis is mandatory when a capsuloligamentous retraction does exist (Fowler 1947, Tubiana and Dubousset 1971, Buch 1974, Vipin 1974, Gould and Nickolson 1979, Alnot 1982, Watson and Turkeltaub 1988).
(c) The most difficult cases are, of course, those involving osteoarticular lesions; there are only two therapeutic possibilities – beside abstention – arthroplasty or arthrodesis (Madden et al 1977, Young et al 1978).

Finally, certain cases are associated with various problems:

- stiffness in extension of all MP joints makes physical therapy, or surgical approach, difficult and affects the trophicity
- stiffness in extension of the MP joints associated with stiffness in flexion of the proximal interphalangeal joints; this possibility is not rare especially if the initial immobilization does not respect the principles of the intrinsic plus position.

Treatment of these two kinds of stiffness is possible in the same procedure. However, if there are complex problems due to cutaneous and trophic lesions, it will be better to begin by treating MP joint stiffness and then treat stiffness of the interphalangeal joint.

Stiffness in flexion

Stiffness in flexion is rare. The extension can be limited by:

- skin adhesions (sometimes retraction of the palmar skin)
- lesions and adhesions of the flexor tendons
- retraction with symphysis of the proximal cul-de-sac and the volar plate
- retractions or adhesions of the collateral capsuloligamentous apparatus and
- the bone and joint lesions.

Retractions can be found mainly on the volar plate, the skin and the flexor tendons. The problems are the choice of the surgical approach and of the physical therapy with an adapted splint (Weeks et al 1970, Gosset 1971).

Stiffness in flexion of the MP joints combined with stiffness in extension of the interphalangeal joints is a special case that needs to be mentioned. It is due to a retraction of the interosseous muscles (Bunnell et al 1948, Jackson and Brown 1970, Parkes 1971, Snow et al 1975).

The Bunnell test will evaluate the role of the retraction of the interosseous muscles. Maximal extension of the MP joints increases the limitation of the proximal interphalangeal joints flexion. MP joint flexion relaxes the interosseous muscles and allows a certain amount of proximal interphalangeal joint flexion.

Conclusion

As far as the prognosis is concerned, it is fundamental to differentiate between stiffness of one joint and stiffness of all the joints of a finger or the whole hand. The wrist, the first web and the thumb column have to be carefully examined to obtain a global view of the problem.

In pathology involving the digits, stiffness can be seen more often in extension at the MP level and in flexion at the proximal interphalangeal level.

Associations are frequent, as for other articular stiffness, and we should differentiate:

- monodigital stiffness, uni- or bi-articular, usually with an intact grasp
- complex stiffness, sequelae of pluridigital trauma, with loss of the pollicidigital and digitopalmar grasps.

Such a distinction emerges in parallel with the notion of articular and extra-articular stiffness:

- extra-articular stiffness, secondary to flexor and extensor tendon injuries, aponeurotic structures and cutaneous surfaces
- intra-articular stiffness due to lesions of the capsulo-ligamentous planes and/or articular surfaces.

Centred X-rays, showing the joint space, are essential for planning the treatment. This will result in differentiating between stiffness with and stiffness without articular surface lesions.

In fact, stiffness is often a combination of intra-articular and extra-articular lesions.

In planning treatment, we have to remember that surgical treatment in most cases must be preceded by a period of physical therapy followed with adapted splints for a long period (Wynn Parry 1971, Brand 1978, Week et al, 1978, Cambridge 1990).

Isolated stiffness will not be a problem, and surgical treatment may be performed without hesitation.

In complex stiffness, the patient needs to be advised what is at stake, and that a partial result will improve the overall functional recovery.

Therapeutic abstention may be a wise solution, when stiffness is moderate within a useful range of motion, and in cases of severe stiffness, results from sequelae of repeated procedures with an approximately functional position. In both cases, radical procedures can also be proposed, such as an arthrodesis or, eventually, an amputation of the digit segment.

Digital stiffness, particularly of the MP joints, represents a frequent problem in hand surgery. Surgical indications must remain restricted with the necessity of careful surgery followed by postoperative physical therapy (Bruner 1953, Evans et al 1968, Fitzerald 1977, Delprat and Mansat 1981).

In conclusion, we must insist on the preventive treatment of such stiffness. In the literature, such stiffness is most frequently the result of inadequate treatment of a diaphyseal fracture or a tendon injury. This confirms the importance of a correct conservative and surgical treatment with adequate immobilization and therapy.

References

Alnot JY, Leroy P (1981) Raideurs des doigts et lésions des tendons extenseurs, Rev Chir Orthop 67:539–40.

Alnot JY (1982) Arthrolyse des articulations métacarpophalangiennes des doigts longs dans les raideurs post-traumatiques en extension, Ann Chir Main 1:358–60.

Beltran JE (1975) The abnormal and pathological mobility of the metacarpo-phalangeal joint, Acta Orthop Scand 46:52–60.

Brand PW (1978) Hand rehabilitation management by objectives. In: Hunter JM, Schneider LH, Mackin EJ, Bell J, eds. Rehabilitation of the Hand. CV Mosby: St Louis: 3–5.

Bruner JM (1953) Problems of post-operative position and motion in surgery of the hand, J Bone Joint Surg 35A:355–66.

Buch VI (1974) Clinical and functional assessment of the hand after metacarpophalangeal capsulotomy, Plast Reconstr Surg 53:452–7.

Bunnell S, Doherty EW, Curtis RM (1948) Ischemic contracture local in the hand, Plast Reconstr Surg 3:424–33.

Cambridge CA (1990) Range of Motion Measurements of the Hand. Rehabilitation of the Hand: Surgery and Therapy. CV Mosby: St Louis: 82–91.

De la Caffinière JY, Mansat M (1987) Raideurs post-traumatiques des doigts longs, Rev Chir Orthop 67:520–33; 542–51.

Delprat J, Mansat M (1981) Rééducation des raideurs post-traumatiques des doigts longs, J Réadapt Méd 1:5–16.

Delseny JC (1976) A propos de l'anatomie fonctionnelle des articulations métacarpophalangiennes, Thesis: Toulouse.

Evans EB, Larson DL, Yates S (1968) Preservation and restoration of joint function in patients with severe burns, JAMA 204:843–8.

Fitzerald JA (1977) Management of the injured and post-operative hand, Physiotherapy 63:282–4.

Fowler SB (1947) Mobilization of metacarpophalangeal joint arthroplasty and capsulotomy, J Bone Joint Surg 29:193–202.

Gosset J (1971) La capsulotomie par voie palmaire dans les enraidissements métacarpophalangiens. In: Vilain R ed. Les Traumatismes ostéo-articulaires de la main. Expansion Scientifique Française: Paris: 97–100.

Gould JS, Nickolson RG (1979) Capsulotomy of the metacarpophalangeal and proximal interphalangeal joints, J Hand Surg 4:482–6.

Jackson IT, Brown GED (1970) A method of treating chronic flexion contractures of the fingers, Br J Plast Surg 23:373.

Laseter GF (1983) Management of the stiff hand: a practical approach, Orthop Clin North Amer 14:749–65.

Madden JW, de Vore G, Arem AJ (1977) A rational post-operative management program for metacarpophalangeal joint implant arthroplasty, *J Hand Surg* **2**:358–66.

Mansat M, Delprat J (1980) Raideurs post-traumatiques de l'interphalangienne proximale. In: *Actualités en Rééducation Fonctionnelle et Réadaptation, no. 5*. Masson: Paris: 183–91.

Mansat M, Delprat J, Chaffai MA (1990) Raideurs post-traumatiques des doigts. *Edit. Techniques. Encycl. Med. Chir. Techniques chirurgicales orthopédie*, 4470, 4.

McCormack RM (1964) Stiffness of the injured hand analyses, prevention and treatment, *J Trauma* **4**:581–91.

Merle M, Gibon Y (1981) Les raideurs des doigts après la chirurgie des tendons fléchisseurs, *Rev Chir Orthop* **67**:537–8.

Parkes AP (1971) The 'lumbrical plus' finger, *J Bone Joint Surg* **53B**:26.

Peacock EE (1966) Some biochemical and biophysical aspects of joint stiffness: role of collagen synthesis as opposed to altered molecular bonding, *Ann Surg* **164/1**:1–12.

Ravault P. Durant J (1961) Le rhumatisme neurotrophique du membre supérieur (nouvelle statistique de 520 cas), *Rev Lyon Méd* **10**:3–32.

Smith RJ, Peimer CA (1977) Injuries to the metacarpal bones and joints, *Adv Surg* **11**:341–74.

Snow JW, Pohl RO, Obi LJ (1975) Flexion contractures of the hand, *J Fla Med Assoc* **62**:19.

Thomine JM, Bendjeddou MS, Mole D (1981) Raideurs digitales et fractures diaphysaires, *Rev Chir Orthop* **67**:533–6.

Tubiana R (1984) Notions anatomo-pathologiques, étiologiques et cliniques sur les raideurs des doigts. In: *Traité de Chirurgie de la Main*, vol. 2. Masson: Paris: 903–11.

Tubiana R, Dubousset J (1971) Traitement des raideurs post-traumatiques des articulations métacarpo-phalangiennes de doigts (sauf le pouce). In: Vilain R, ed. *Les Traumatismes ostéo-articulaires de la Main*. Expansion Scientifique Française: Paris: 83–92.

Vipin IB (1974) Clinical and functional assessment of the hand after metacarpophalangeal capsulectomy, *Plast Reconstr Surg* **53**:452–7.

Watson HK, Carlson L, Brenner LH (1986) The 'dystrophile' treatment of reflex dystrophy of the hand with an active stress loading program, *Orthop Trans* **10**:188.

Watson HK, Turkeltaub SH (1988) Stiff joints in operative. In: Green D, ed. *Hand Surgery*. Vol. 1, 2nd edn. Churchill Livingstone: New York: 537–52.

Weeks PM, Wray R, Kuxhaus M (1978) The results of non-operative management of stiff joints in the hand, *Plast Reconstr Surg* **62**:58–63.

Weeks PM (1970) Volar approach for metacarpophalangeal joint capsulectomy, *Plast Reconstr Surg* **46**:473–6.

Wynn Parry CB (1971) Management of the stiff joint, *The Hand* **3**:169–71.

Young VL, Wray RC, Weeks PM (1978) The surgical management of stiff joints in the hand, *Plast Reconstr Surg* **62**:835–41.

35

Flaps and tenolysis for metacarpophalangeal joint stiffness

Guy Foucher

The anatomy of the metacarpophalangeal (MP) joint explains the natural tendency of this joint to get stiff in extension. In flexion, the lateral ligaments are taut (contrary to the extension position which allows lateral movement of the fingers), and this is the 'safe' position of immobilization. This explains also why many cases of stiffness in extension at this level are secondary to a treatment mistake after crush, burn, or even simple fractures (metacarpal or phalangeal) (de la Caffinière 1981). Any trauma induces an oedema, which is a liquid rich in proteins, leading to adhesion of the tendon and retraction of the lateral ligament. If the hand is immobilized in MP joint extension during this period, the shortening of the lateral ligaments does not allow any more flexion. Such a complication can be seen even without prolonged immobilization; 3 weeks could be enough. Other frequently involved mechanisms are extensor tendon injury (in zones 5–7), dorsal hand skin loss, extravasation, infection, hand replantation, paralysis (like medioulnar palsy) and reflex sympathetic dystrophy (Ehrler et al 1987).

A good history and a careful examination are necessary. The first step is to establish that the problem is a real stiffness in extension and not just the result of a tenodesis effect of the extensor tendons. In lesions proximal to the MP joint (zones 6 and 7), adhesion of the extensor mechanism can limit MP and IP (interphalangeal) joint flexion when the wrist is in neutral; however, full MP joint flexion could be obtained with wrist extension, ruling out any 'stiffness' of the MP joint (Zancolli 1986). An X-ray is also mandatory to confirm the integrity of the joint space. In this chapter we do not discuss the place of the spacer, the prosthesis and the vascularized joint replacement in the case of joint destruction (Foucher et al 1990a and 1990b, Foucher 1991 and 1993).

The pliability of the skin is then checked. Littler

(1977) has demonstrated the need for 'extra-skin' by pinching a fold of skin on the dorsum of the extended hand. This extra skin entirely disappeared in MP flexion. In long-standing MP extension stiffness or in dorsal skin loss, this extra skin is missing. Treated sufficiently early, remodelling of the scar tissue can allow good recovery of flexion through dynamic splinting with a MP dorsal bar. A conventional 'global' roll up flexes the IP joint, loosing its action on the MP joint (Ehrler and Foucher 1994). When there is a tenodesis effect of the extensor tendons through mobilization of the wrist, a stabilization of this joint is necessary, combined with an MP bar (Ehrler et al 1983). It is frequently difficult to decide when splinting has to give way to surgery. Reviewing our experience (Foucher et al 1989), we found that the decision could be taken at 8 weeks. If the range of motion obtained at this date is functionally insufficient (around 45°, according to Tubiana 1971), surgery has to be contemplated. This does not mean that in cases of sufficient range the splint can be discarded at this stage, and prolonged splinting is necessary to avoid recurrence. Efficiency of this conservative treatment has been illustrated by Weeks et al (1978) who found that 87% of a series of 336 MP joints responded favourably. When the splinting is inefficient, or the MP joint blocked in hyperextension, rendering splinting impossible, surgery is necessary.

Many different approaches have been described for MP joint arthrolysis, either palmar (Young et al 1978) or dorsal, transverse or longitudinal, centred on the joint or in the valleys (Buch 1974, Gould and Nickolson 1979).

In fact, the operation is frequently a combined tenoarthrolysis, necessitating a dorsal approach. The skin problem is frequently overlooked, explaining some postoperative difficulties of positioning and the limited range of flexion due to skin

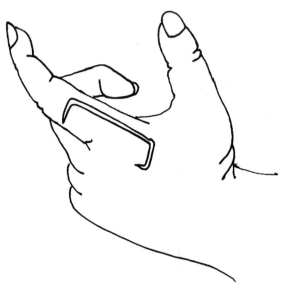

Figure 1

Dorsal square flap to approach a stiff metacarpophalangeal joint with retracted dorsal skin. The flap is either advanced or withdrawn according to the exposed structures.

tension and pain. When the skin has simply shrunk, a local flap can be used, but when the skin is scarred, as seen after burn or dorsal skin loss, a distant flap is necessary. We favour selecting a flap with independent vascularization; either an island forearm flap, or a free flap. These flaps are discussed in Chapter 27 and are not discussed further here. We will mention the Bakhach flap (Bakhach et al 1995) which is really helpful for this area, but distally based on an arterial anastomosis present at the neck of the fifth metacarpal. This flap can cover at least the three ulnar MP joints. A reverse flow metacarpal flap could only be used for very limited skin loss. When the skin is supple and simply retracted, we favour two types of local flaps which allow, at the same time, a good approach of the structure that needs to be free (namely joint and extensor mechanism) (Foucher 1994). When only one MP joint is involved, a rectangular dorsal flap is drawn, previously called a 'dorsal Hueston' (Fig. 1). This flap is only partially sutured, keeping open the proximal or distal border, according to the portion of the extensor tendon which has been denuded of its paratendon. The secondary defect is simply

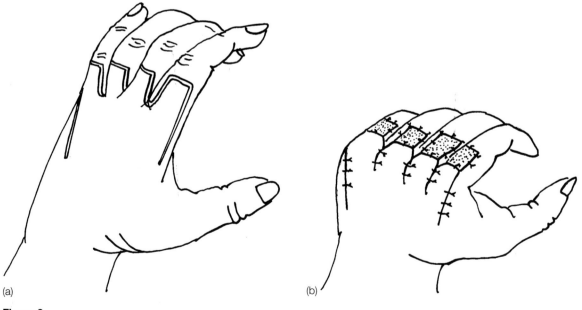

(a)   (b)

Figure 2

(a) 'Castle' flap which is elevated to expose multiple stiff metacarpophalangeal joint. (b) After having freed the joints, the flap is repositioned and the dorsum of the first phalanx grafted.

grafted. When more than one MP is involved, we use a so-called 'castle' flap (Foucher 1994), which means that we cut a square flap on the dorsum of each first phalanx (Fig. 2); then the proximally based flap is lifted to perform the dorsal tenoarthrolysis. When the procedure is completed, the flap is repositioned, covering the MP joint maintained in flexion, and the dorsum of the first phalanx is simply grafted on the paratendon.

The tenoarthrolysis begins with the extensor tenolysis starting in zone 6 and freeing the tendon distally to zone 5 without taking care of the controversial insertion of the extensor on the first phalanx. The extensor hood is also carefully freed. Any foreign material is removed at this time, for example a dorsal plate inserted for a metacarpal fracture; its mechanical check-rein effect on the flexion is obvious. In rare instances, a heavy fibrous tissue is found surrounding the extensor tendons which are, however, in good condition (this is sometimes called a Secretan's syndrome). In other instances, the extensor is in a very bad condition, as seen after iterative tenolysis. In such cases (eight cases in our series of 48 dorsal tenoarthrolysis), we simply excise the extensor tendon, postponing its reconstruction. If the junctura tendinum is preserved, it is frequently not necessary to perform this second stage (only once in our eight cases) due to a very limited lack of extension. The section of the extensor tendon makes arthrolysis easier, but it is mandatory in zone 5 to save the extensor hood due to the complexity of its reconstruction.

In three cases of deep dorsal burn, we have not been able to find any extensor mechanism in zone 5, and we have described a simple technique of reconstruction of the hood of the four fingers by harvesting a compound transfer of the radial forearm flap *en bloc* with a vascularized brachioradialis tendon (Fig. 3) (Foucher et al 1984). This tendon is then transposed transversally and secured distally and proximally to the remaining extensor mechanism (Foucher 1994). This avoids a complex reconstruction of the hood to prevent the sliding of the extensor tendons in the intermetacarpal valleys.

For the arthrolysis step, we use a technique compatible with early postoperative active motion and splinting, thus avoiding any splitting of the extensor tendons (Curtis 1975) or section of the hood (Buch 1974, Gould and Nickolson 1979). If the extensor has been cut in zone 6, it is simply lifted. Otherwise we do not cut any part of the hood, which is only proximally lifted to resect the dorsal capsule and

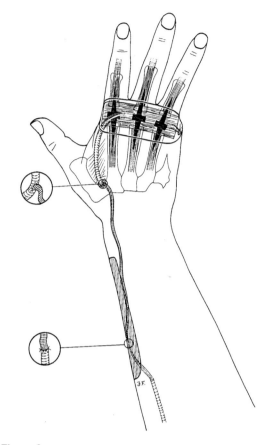

Figure 3

Compound island forearm flap to cover destroyed skin in zone 5, combined with absence of extensor mechanism and extensor hood. The vascularized tendon of the brachioradialis is interposed and sutured proximally and distally.

free the lateral ligament from the lateral part of the metacarpal head. This step is normally not sufficient to provide more than a few degrees of flexion. The next step is the partial disinsertion of the collateral ligament by cutting its most posterior fibres on the metacarpal head. This allows usually a good flexion but frequently with a 'cam effect' which means that the MP joint remains 'locked' in flexion, and when passively extended 'snaps' in extension like a trigger finger. This phenomenon disappeared after freeing the remaining lateral ligament from the metacarpal head. Usually, we avoid entirely disinserting the radial collateral ligament on the central rays thereby preventing an ulnar drift which is difficult to correct. If a total disinsertion is performed, a splint, similar to the one used for MP joint arthroplasty in rheumatoid arthritis, is worn for 3 weeks, allowing a full range of motion but restraining ulnar drift. Finally, a spatula is used to control the joint and free the volar plate adhesions.

When a skin flap has been transferred, we temporarily transfix the MP joint in flexion for 10 days. Early motion and prolonged splinting are always mandatory.

Results are predictable and our average gain in our series was 52° which compares favourably with the literature (40° for Mansat et al 1981, 21° for Gould and Nickolson 1979, 28° for Wisnicki et al 1987). As previously stressed, we think that relaxing the skin, and avoiding any suture on the extensor tendon or hood is responsible for an easier and more complete range of flexion.

Stiffness of the MP joint in flexion is less frequent (Weeks 1970) and usually related to periarticular structures. The main tissues involved are: the palmar skin (loss or retraction), the flexor tendon (adhesion), a Dupuytren disease or an intrinsic muscle tightness (ischaemic or spastic). A rare but easily corrected deformity in flexion is a locked MP joint, which could be due to many aetiologies; among our 11 cases, six were due to impingement of the accessory collateral ligament on an osteophyte which was clearly seen on a Brewerton X-ray view. Treatment is not always surgical, and injecting a local anaesthetic into the joint under pressure has freed the ligament in two of our cases.

Examination of the hand is an important step for assessing each structure and checking any tenodesis effect of a flexor tendon or Dupuytren band. After adhesion of a flexor tendon in the palm or wrist, a tenodesis effect is frequently found with better (if not total) extension of the MP in passive flexion of the wrist and IP joints.

We have not found any 'good flap' for the palm that is able to provide a supple and thin skin adherent to the superficial fascia. Only a full thickness skin graft fulfils all these requirements. Then we restricted the use of an island forearm skin or fascial flap (plus a graft) to the cases where major surgery is anticipated on nerves and/or flexor tendons. The bulky aspect of any skin flap needs very frequent secondary defatting.

When the skin is unscarred but simply retracted, as in long-standing intrinsic retraction due to ischaemia or spasticity (Smith 1993), we have used a volar 'castle flap' with success. The technique is similar to our description for the dorsum of the hand; the proximally based flap allows all restraining structures to be freed, and after extension is obtained, a full-thickness grafting of the secondary defect on the palmar aspect of the first phalanx is performed.

In trauma cases, it is mainly the flexor tendons which are responsible for secondary extension limitation, and in this area tenolysis is not a difficult procedure (see Chapter 27). In any long-standing MP joint flexion, it is necessary to check preoperatively, after releasing of all other structures, the intrinsic muscles by a Finochietto's manoeuvre (Finochietto 1920): when, the MP joint is maintained in extension, the passive range of flexion of the proximal IP joint remains limited; this limitation disappears when the MP is flexed. If incomplete MP joint extension is present and the muscle appears normal, we favour an intramuscular tendon step lengthening. The other alternative is the Bunnell 'sliding operation' (Bunnell 1953) to allow distal migration of the intrinsic muscles. Simple tenotomy is reserved to fibrotic non-functional muscles. The distal intrinsic release with triangular excision in the extensor hood, as performed by Littler (1977), does not correct the MP joint flexion, and is indicated only when full extension is obtained at MP joint level with a positive Finochietto test.

In conclusion, we stress again that most MP joint stiffness is in extension and could be avoided by careful postoperative immobilization in 'intrinsic plus' or 'functional' positions combined with a session of early active motion. Dynamic splinting in flexion with an MP bar needs to be adapted early if full range of MP joint flexion is not obtained after tissue healing.

References

Bakhach J, Saint Cast Y, Gazarian A, Martin D, Comtet JJ, Baudet J (1995) Ulnar parametacarpal flap. Anatomical study and clinical application, *Ann Chir Plast* **40**:136–47.

Buch VI (1974) Clinical and functional assessment of the hand after metacarpophalangeal capsulotomy, *Plast Reconstr Surg* **53**:452–7.

Bunnell S (1953) Ischaemic contracture local in the hand, *J Bone Joint Surg* **35A**:88–101.

Curtis RM (1975) *Joints of the hand.* In: Flynn EJ, ed. *Hand Surgery.* Williams and Wilkins: Baltimore: 222–39.

de la Caffinière JY (1981) Raideurs post-traumatiques des doigts longs, *Rev Chir Orthop* **67**:519–70.

Ehrler S, Braun F, Foucher G, Xenard J (1983) Rôle de la stabilisation du poignet dans la conception de l'orthèse de la main, *Rev Réadaptation Fonct Prof Soc* **10**:20–3.

Ehrler S, Foucher G, Braun F, Demangeat J, Constantinesco A, Brunot B (1987) Intérêt de la mise en place précoce d'une orthèse de la main dans l'algodystrophie. In: *Les Algodystrophies Sympathiques Reflexes*. Masson: Paris: 248–51.

Ehrler S, Foucher G (1994) Les orthèses de la main traumatique. *Main et Handicap, 7th Entretiens de l'Institut Garches, Paris*: 147–52.

Finochietto R (1920) Retraccion de Volkman de los musculos intrinsicos de las manos, *Bol Trab Soc Chir* **4**:31–5.

Foucher G, Van Genechten F, Merle M, Michon J (1984) A compound radial artery forearm flap in hand surgery: an original modification of the chinese forearm flap, *Br J Plast Surg* **37**:139–48.

Foucher G (1991) Le transfert articulaire vascularisé en ilôt composite en chirurgie de la main. A propos d'une série de 16 observations, *Rev Chir Orthop* **77**:34–41.

Foucher G (1993) Vascularized joint transfer. In: Green D, ed. *Operative Hand Surgery*, 3rd edn. Churchill Livingstone: New York: 1201–21.

Foucher G, Greant P, Ehrler S, Buch N, Michon J (1989) Le rôle de l'orthèse dans les raideurs de la main, *Chirurgie* **115**:100–5.

Foucher G, Lenoble E, Sammut D (1990a) Transfer of a composite island homodigital interphalangeal joint to replace the proximal interphalangeal joint, *Ann Hand Surg* **9**:369–75.

Foucher G, Sammut D, Citron N (1990b) Free vascularized toe joint transfer in hand reconstruction: a series of 25 patients, *J Reconstr Microsurg* **6**:201–7.

Foucher G (1994) Extensor loss and hood reconstruction. 'Castle' flap in extensor tenolysis. In: Kasdan ML, Bowers WH, Amadio PC, eds. *Technical Tips for Hand Surgery*. Mosby: St Louis: 245–8.

Gould JS. Nickolson BG (1979) Capsulotomy of the metacarpophalangeal and proximal interphalangeal joints, *J Hand Surg* **4**:482–6.

Littler JW (1977) The hand and upper extremity. In: Converse JM, ed. *Reconstructive Plastic Surgery* vol. 6. WB Saunders: Philadelphia: 3138–42.

Mansat M, de la Caffinière JY, Delprat J (1981) Arthrolyses et téno-arthrolyses, *Rev Chir Orthop* **67**:542–51.

Smith RJ (1993) Intrinsic contracture. In: Green D, ed. *Operative Hand Surgery*. Churchill Livingstone: New York: 607–26.

Tubiana R, Dubousset J (1971) Traitement des raideurs post-traumatiques des articulations métacarpo-phalangiennes des doigts. *Monographie du GEM, no. 4. Traumatismes osteo-articulaires*. Expansion Scientifique Française: Paris: 83–92.

Weeks PM (1970) Volar approach for metacarpophalangeal joint capsulotomy, *Plast Reconstr Surg* **46**:473–6.

Weeks PM, Wray RC, Kuxkaus M (1978) The results of non-operative management of stiff joints in the hand, *Plast Reconstr Surg* **61**:58–63.

Wisnicki JL, Leathers MW, Sangalang I, Kilgore ES (1987) Percutaneous desmotomy of digits for stiffness from fixed edema, *Plast Reconstr Surg* **80**:88–90.

Young VL, Wray RC, Weeks PM (1978) The surgical management of stiff joints in the hand, *Plast Reconstr Surg* **62**: 835–41.

Zancolli E (1968) *Structure and Dynamic Bases of Hand Surgery*. JB Lippincott: Philadelphia.

36

Treatment of metacarpophalangeal joint stiffness

Philippe Saffar

Metacarpophalangeal (MP) stiffness is a very disabling condition, especially for grasping objects. This chapter examines the surgical treatment of intra-articular stiffness.

MP approaches

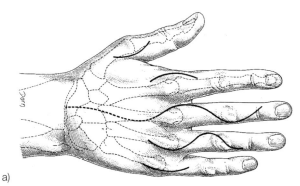

a)

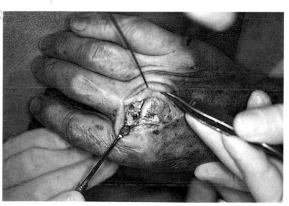

b)

Figure 1

(a) Longitudinal dorsal approach of the metacarpophalangeal joint (reproduced from Tubiana et al 1990, with permission).
(b) The approach demonstrated.

(a) A dorsal longitudinal curved incision may be performed between two adjacent MP joints. The extensor hood is cut near the extensor tendon at about 3 mm. The dorsal capsule is then opened and the joint exposed (Fig. 1a, b).

(b) A dorsal transversal slightly curved incision passing at the distal epiphysis of the metacarpal and through the intermetacarpal valleys is traced at the dorsal aspect of the MP joints. Approach of the MP is done also through the extensor hood (Fig. 2).

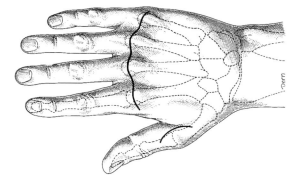

Figure 2

Transverse dorsal approach of the metacarpophalangeal joint (reproduced from Tubiana et al 1990, with permission).

(c) A volar approach is possible passing longitudinally between the two MP joints. The intermetacarpal ligament (IML) is cut and elevated in continuity with the volar plate of the MP joint and the periosteum of the metacarpal and P1. The joint is then visible and a procedure can be performed. At the end of the procedure, IML suture with overlapping allows realignment of the flexor apparatus in rheumatoid arthritis (RA).

Arthrodeses

Cartilages and subchondral bone of the distal metacarpal and proximal first phalanx are removed keeping a rounded contour to the bones. Reduction should approximate two surfaces, one concave and the other convex, with a maximum contact between each other. A flexion of 20–40° should be obtained from the second to the fifth MP joint to allow a pulp-to-pulp pinch with the thumb. Fixation may be performed using K-wires, screws or a tension-band system. Indications are post-infection, post-traumatic joint destruction or failed prostheses.

Arthroplasties

Without prosthesis

Various types of interposition for proximal interphalangeal (PIP) joints have been used:

- fascia lata, fascia and periosteum
- extensor tendons
- perichondrium: this technique has been regularly presented by Scandinavian authors (Engvist et al 1975, Skoog and Johansson 1976): rib perichondrium is harvested and applied on the resurfaced articular end of the MP joint, the germinative plane being on the joint side; a silastic sheet is interposed between the two phalangeal end and removed after 6 months
- a thin silastic sheet
- volar plate: Tupper (1989) has described an interposition of the volar plate; the volar plate was detached proximally and interposed after bone resection (Fig. 3a, b).

The use of external fixation without interposition was also reported.

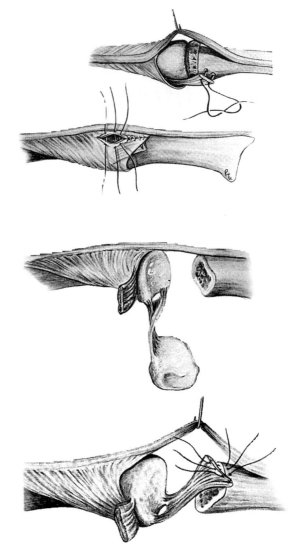

Figure 3

Tupper's volar plate interposition–arthroplasty technique.

With prosthesis

It is difficult to reproduce the mechanism of the MP joints with a prosthesis because metacarpal condyles are asymmetrical, there are strong collateral ligaments and a strong volar plate, and MP joints present two degrees of freedom: flexion–extension and laterality.

There is a close contact between bone, extensors and interosseous tendons, and, possibly more important, are the surrounding soft tissues and the balance of the finger tendons around the joint.

The aims of the digital prostheses are to obtain a good mobility, a longitudinal realignment, correction of the anterior subluxation when present, stability in the lateral plane, pain relief, good grasp and precise pinch.

Different types of implants have been tried. The most frequently used was proposed by Swanson in 1972. It is not a prosthesis but a spacer made of silicone. It is easy to implant, tolerant to slight malposition and provided good results when associated to soft tissue procedures obtaining a good tendon balance and a realignment, particularly for RA (Fig. 4).

Niebauer and Landy (1971), Nicolle and Calnan (1972), Sutter and Levack et al (1987) used the same type of material for their prostheses.

Usual results obtained for Swanson prostheses were a 30–50° range of motion (ROM) for the large series and a rupture rate of 50% in post-traumatic cases. The disadvantages are: frequent rupture, recurrence of malalignment and silicone synovitis. This last complication led to a less frequent use of this type of material.

Other types of prosthese were proposed: 1, constrained, semi-constrained or non-constrained; and 2, the stem being cemented, adjusted or free in the diaphysis.

Many new devices are presented in the market, but there are no published results for a large series with a long follow-up. By far the most used MP prosthesis is the silastic Swanson type. Used mainly for RA, this provides fair results.

Technique of insertion: after an adapted bone resection of the metacarpal condyles and base of the first phalanx, the two intramedullary canals are prepared with a burr in a rectangular fashion so that the implant may fit in the canal. Trial implants are used to choose the size of the prostheses needed. The prosthesis should flex without buckling (Fig. 5). Associated soft tissue procedures are often needed to rebalance the forces on the finger.

Each type of the other prostheses have their own technique of insertion and ancillary tools.

(a) Mechanical complications are common to all types of prostheses: rupture, metal or silicone particle wear, and debris, displacements and dislocations

(b) The postoperative course is also similar for all types of prostheses: initially a good ROM, realignment and pain relief. In the long term: the ROM decreases, deformity and pain recur. This course is partly explained by the 'sinking' of the prosthesis in the diaphysis, even with cemented stems. The joint space decreases and bone abutment leads to joint stiffness.

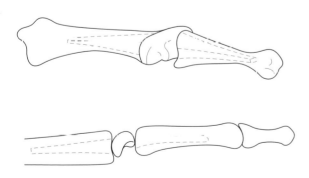

Figure 4

Swanson's silastic prosthesis.

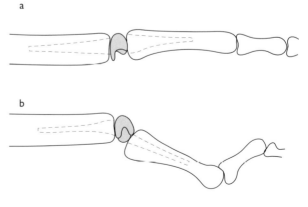

Figure 5

Buckling of the prosthesis.

References

Engvist O, Johansson SH, Skoog T (1975) Reconstruction of articular cartilage using autologous perichondrial grafts. A preliminary report, *Scand J Plast Reconstr Surg* **9**:203–6.

Levack B, Stewart HD, Flierenga H, Helal B (1987) Metacarpo-phalangeal joint replacement with a new prosthesis: description and preliminary results of treatment, *J Hand Surg* **12B**:377–81.

Nicolle FV, Calnan JS (1972) A new design of finger joint prosthesis for the rheumatoid hand, *Hand* **4**:135–46.

Niebauer JJ< Landy RM (1971) Dacron–Silicone prosthesis for the metacapophalangeal and interphalangeal joints, *Hand* **3**:55–61.

Skoog T, Johansson SH (1976) The formation of cartilage from free perichondrial grafts, *Plast Reconstr Surg* **57**:1–6.

Swanson AB (1972) Flexible implant arthroplasty for arthritic finger joints: rationale, technique and results of treatment, *J Bone Joint Surg* **53A**:435–55.

Tubiana R, McCullough CJ, Macquelet AC (1990) *An Atlas of Surgical Exposures of the Upper Extremity.* Martin Dunitz/JB Lippincott: London/Philadelphia.

Tupper JW (1989) The metacarpophalangeal arthroplasty, *J Hand Surg* **14A**:371–5.

37
Rehabilitation of metacarpophalangeal joint stiffness

Patrice Morla

Metacarpophalangeal (MP) joints are the link between the more mobile part of the hand and the more stable metacarpals. They are valuable joints, allowing finger orientation for every hand function; MP joint stiffness impairs hand function. Grip strength is difficult if the second and third MP joints have a decreased range of motion. If stiffness affects the fourth and fifth metacarpals, the locking function of the corresponding fingers is lost.

These joints stiffen mostly in extension, and to prevent stiffness immobilization should be performed in the intrinsic plus position, i.e. MP flexion and proximal interphalangeal (PIP) extension.

Main causes of MP stiffness

- *Skin lesions:* sequelae of dorsal skin injuries with adhesions to the extensor tendons (zones 5 and 6). Palmar skin may be involved after complex injuries or after surgical procedures as in Dupuytren's disease.
- *Bone injuries:* metacarpal fractures are less a cause of stiffness than phalangeal fractures. Distal epiphyseal fractures, like the very frequent fracture of the neck of the fifth metacarpal, may be a cause of stiffness. Pluridigital metacarpal fractures after crush injuries are followed by MP stiffness. Proximal fractures of P1 are also a frequent cause.
- *Joint injuries:* from sprain to complete dislocation, capsuloligamentous and volar plate injuries of the MP joint may result in stiffness.
- *Other causes* exist as complex hand injuries, limited amputations and replanted fingers, infections, neurological problems including palsies and spasticity. Neurosympathetic dystrophy is also a frequent cause of hand stiffness with the MP in flexion or extension.

Treatment

During treatment, the therapist is confronted with the need to improve various problems: pain, oedema, range of motion and, finally, function. All these problems are treated simultaneously, but pain will be the guide for the frequency and duration of the rehabilitation sessions. These begin with physiotherapy, bathing the hand in lukewarm water, combined with vibration tools to obtain cooling and limbering up the soft tissues. Massage is the next step. This is the privileged period of the session, allowing the hand therapist to take care of the patient, not only in the physical sense, but also psychologically. It is at this time that the special patient–therapist relationship enables the establishment of a programme of treatment and goals to be reached, taking into account the magnitude of pain and stiffness. From the technical point of view, a global circulatory hand massage is undertaken by scuffing, and by sliding superficial pressure, then deeper in the metacarpal spaces. When scars exist, they should be massaged early, before stitch removal (the manoeuvre of Jacquet–Leroy employs alternate superficial kneading with twisting for this purpose). The M50 device from LPG systems may be used against fibrosis on scars and venous and lymphatic stasis since it allows separation of the different planes by aspiration. Varying the sequences of the M50 allows a painfree and efficient programme to be adapted for each case. Ultrasound waves, used in water for better propagation, are useful for their antalgic and anti-inflammatory properties. The micromassage performed by the ultrasonic waves results in an increased permeability of the cell membranes and a local decrease of the vasopressure combined with a fibrolytic action. It seems more suitable to use frequency modulation (there is less penetration, but a better concentration of the ultrasound waves, reaching more skin elements). To fight oedema, cooling of the hand by ice is used, mainly at the end of the session. At night, an elastic band, not too tightened, improves the results.

Electrotherapy

Two types of electric current are useful: constant unidirectional and variable modulated. Tissues rapidly become accustomed to constant waves, so modulated currents are more efficient: T-E-N-S (antalgic current). Constant unidirectional current (galvanic) prevents the onset of painful sensations by hyperpolarization under a positive electrode, and we use this current to transmit an ionizable substance (ionophoresis). Sodium chloride and potassium iodide are useful for their fibrinolytic action, sodium salicylate for analgesic action and magnesium sulphate or chloride for anti-inflammatory action.

Rehabilitation of the MP joint

Early passive mobilization is the basic technique. True passive mobilization is performed in flexion–extension and unintentional passive mobilization is the axial rotation which is a physiological movement.

At the beginning of the treatment, the tenodesis effect of the wrist on finger flexion is used. MP joint flexion with PIP extension is first performed passively, followed by complete flexion of the fingers with particular emphasis on the MP joints. This is combined with sagittal mobilization of the fingers to obtain a stretching of the capsuloligamentous structures. Passive mobilization of the MP joint, strictly in the axis of this articulation, helps to remodel this joint during the healing period, particularly after an intra-articular fracture. Continuous passive motion may be used after or during the sessions to complement passive work and also to improve hand trophicity. The Kinetec 8091 is relatively easy to fix around the hand, and respects hand physiology (Fig. 1).

Holding the MP joints in a flexed or extended position for any length of time should be performed manually, to allow prompt adjustment to the patient's pain and flexibility. Continuous passive

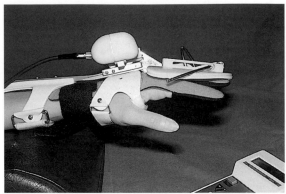

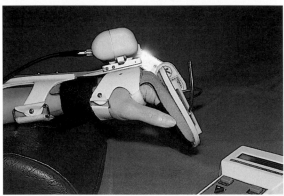

Figure 1

Passive motion using the Kinetec 8091. (a) extension position; (b) flexion position

motion is combined with massage to try to prevent pain, circulatory and retraction problems and to increase the efficiency of the joint.

Dynamic splints complete the techniques of joint rehabilitation; they are used for 10–20 minutes, four times a day, and help to sustain the benefit of manual rehabilitation and the progress of the range of motion (Fig. 2). The traction force is applied on the first phalanx and directed towards the hand axis. For significant stiffness, it is necessary to advance the application of the traction force with an anterior buttress to retain its efficiency. The dynamic force should be applied on the first phalanx to act only on the MP (Fig. 3).

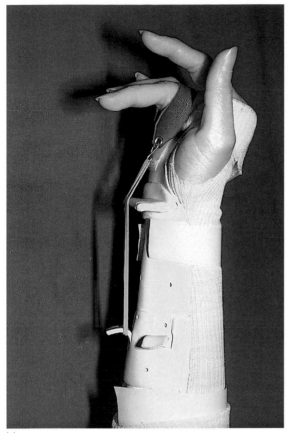

(a)

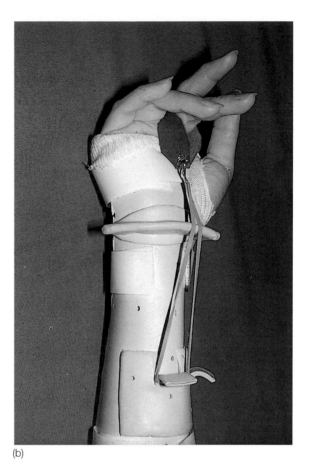

(b)

Figure 2

(a, b) Joint rehabilitation using a dynamic splint

Functional and muscular rehabilitation should increase progressively during all the sessions while pain and joint problems should decrease. The return of action motion may be facilitated by the use of electrostimulation with a fast impulse; an excito-motor quadrangular current is used to produce a period of contraction, a period where the contraction is maintained and a period where the muscle is relaxed. Muscle enhancement is the result of work against resistance and is easy to adapt for these small joints. Ergotherapy can also be added: this would consist of improving digitopalmar grip with large devices allowing active flexion and extension against resistance (or by practising grip of cones, weaving, woodwork, manipulation of rice or of sand in a box. Small diameter grip using complete finger flexion, e.g. using a screwdriver,

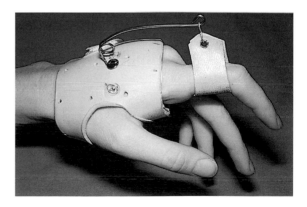

Figure 3

Digitopalmar grip is improved by devices allowing active flexion and extension against resistance

particularly favours the work of the fifth finger. Fingers are also wrapped with 'buddy' splints during sessions.

Conclusion

We have reported on the possible use of rehabilitation, devices and splints to fight MP stiffness. The causes of MP stiffness are so diverse that it is difficult to establish a standard treatment. The therapist must adapt the available techniques to the particular problems of the patient, always keeping in mind that the goal of the treatment is to reinsert the hand into the motor scheme of the upper limb.

38

Extrinsic causes of stiffness of the proximal interphalangeal joint

Constantin Sokolow

Introduction

Curtis (1954) stated that the proximal interphalangeal joint (PIP) joint is the epicentre of surgery of the hand. This joint, which has only a degree of freedom, presents a highly complex anatomical structure at its volar aspect which is even more complex at the dorsal aspect. Its position, in the middle of the digital chain, gives this joint a primary role in positioning the finger in space for either precise, fine or strength manipulation. Any impairment of its mobility will affect the function of the entire hand.

The causes of ankylosis of this joint are numerous: they can be classified as extrinsic, or mixed. The treatment of joint stiffness is usually difficult, lengthy and exacting for the patient. A strict preoperative assessment is mandatory to elaborate a precise therapeutic plan that often requires several chronological steps to maximize the ultimate result.

Anatomical review (Sokolow 1995)

The PIP is a trochlear joint that has only a degree of freedom. It has been compared to a pulley, with the proximal base of P2 gliding on the head of P1 resulting from the action of the flexor and extensor tendons. The head of P1 presents two asymmetric condyles separated by a shallow trochlear groove that has a different orientation for each finger. The latter, combined with the asymmetric condyles, contribute in the convergence of the flexed fingers towards the scaphoid tubercle. On a coronal view, the configuration of the condyles is trapezoidal with a volar base twice the size of the dorsal. On a lateral view, the condylar shape is broader at the anterior

aspect which favours a more complete flexion of the joint. Laterally, both condylar surfaces are in continuity with oblique bone surfaces which broaden the base of P1 and allow the insection of the collateral ligaments. The base of P2 is complementary to the head of P1, but the relationship between the area of contact of P1 and P2 is only 50%. This fact allows a flexion–extension arc of approximately 120°.

The main function of the collateral ligaments is to provide lateral stability to the joint. These ligaments are made of two fascicles:

- *The proper ligament*, is a strong and wide structure with an eccentric insertion to the lateral concave surface of the head of P1. This is a thick triangular band or strand that can be as wide as 35% of the total width of the articulation and of which the orientation is oblique through the lateral base of P2 where it inserts. At the dorsal aspect this insertion continues the attachments of the central slip of the extensor tendon, and at the volar aspect the fibres of the collateral ligaments are braided with the volar plate attachments; this complex forms a very strong insertion node (critical corner). Because of its semicircular attachment to the head of P1 and linear attachments to the base of P2, this ligament always has a stabilizing role whatever the amount of flexion or extension of the joint.
- *The accessory fascicle* is situated proximal to and on the posterior aspect of the main fascicle. Its fibres are more vertically oriented, insert on the lateral aspect of the volar plate and, at its proximal portion, to the origin of the check-reins. There is no attachment to P2.

The volar plate is a thick fibrocartilage located on the volar aspect of the joint which limits its hyperextension. Its insertion takes all the width of the base of P2 and is strong on critical corners and loose at the median aspect. Proximally, the volar plate is arcuate and free, and has two horns that insert on the volar aspect of P1 and intermingle with the distal insertions of the A2 pulley, to form the checkreins described by Bowers (1980). This structure is thick and not extensible. During finger motion, the volar plate glides in one block without festoons. It adheres to the terminal portion of the flexor digitorum superficialis (FDS) and increases its moment of action.

The joint capsule is thin, loose and supple. Its length can double during finger flexion and extension. The capsule has a volar cul-de-sac that is located at the level of the free border of the proximal portion of the volar plate and intermingles with the emergence of the vincula. The dorsal cul-de-sac is situated between the volar aspect of the extensor mechanism and the dorsal aspect of the condyles. Those two culs-de-sac have a cartilaginous type of surface that, when combined with the volar plate, double the length of the gliding surface of the base of P2, allowing constant homogeneous gliding surfaces of contact. The lateral cul-de-sac provides a lining to the deep portion of the collateral ligaments.

The motor elements of the PIP joints are the flexor tendons and the extensor mechanism of which the anatomy is well described. The extensor mechanism trifurcates at the level of the PIP joint; the central slip attaches to the dorsal base of P2 and the two lateral bands continue distally on both sides of the PIP joint at the apex of its widened portion. These structures are united by the transverse retinacular ligament.

The oblique retinacular ligament is a structure that extends from the flexor tendon sheath at the level of the A2 pulley, continues distally towards the PIP joint on the deep aspect of the transverse retinacular ligament where it adheres with the collateral ligaments in front of the plane of flexion of the PIP joint, merges with the lateral slips of the extensor tendons to form the conjoined lateral band and inserts in the dorsal base of the distal phalanx. On cadaver dissection, the oblique retinacular ligament is not always found. When present, it plays a passive tenodesis effect on the distal interphalangeal (DIP) joint. In fact, flexion of the PIP joint automatically extends the DIP joint, and the reserve is also true.

Motion of the joint is, as previously emphasized, primordial; the relative length of the digital skeleton varies during flexion and extension. During flexion,

the length of the anterior aspect of the skeleton decreases while the posterior aspect increases. The difference in length of the skeleton between full extension and flexion is approximately 24 mm (Zancolli 1979). This variation requires an adaptation of all the articular, para-articular and tendinous structures. These structures adjust due to their distension and/or gliding capacities. Any alteration of these capacities will impair the motion of the articulation and result in stiffness.

Definition of ankylosis of the PIP joint resulting from extrinsic causes

Any impairment of the range of motion defines an ankylosis:

- in extension, when the flexion is limited
- in flexion, when the extension is limited.

The useful range of motion of the PIP joint is from 30° to 70°, but this area of motion increases from the second to the fifth finger. Thus, therapeutic guidelines should not be based on these numbers but on the requirements of each patient. In fact, for some patients a greater range of motion than the standard values may be needed depending on patient activity. Other important factors for treatment are the aetiology of the ankylosis and whether there have been any previous surgical attempts to correct the stiffness.

Aetiologies of extrinsic ankylosis of the PIP joint include all extra-articular and para-articular (collateral ligament and volar plate injuries) causes that may provoke joint stiffness. The causes are numerous and their mechanisms often include more than one anatomical structure.

Physiopathology of long fingers stiffness (Green 1993)

Each injury of the hand, whether localized or generalized, induces an oedema which alters articular and para-articular components and consequently decreases joint motion. If this oedema is prolonged, a fixed fibrosis will develop. Moreover, the pain which provokes a decrease of joint motion potentiates the effect of oedema. A decrease of range of motion of the joint impairs lubrication of the cartilage.

Intratissular oedema induces a shortening of the para-articular structures (collateral ligament, joint capsule, volar plate) and intra-articular oedema causes distension of the capsule which brings the joint to a position of maximum content capacity: extension of metacarpophalangeal (MCP) joint and flexion of the interphalangeal (IP) joints. In MCP extension, tension of the flexor tendons is increased and the tension of extensor tendons is decreased, which secondarily puts the IP in a flexed position. When this position is maintained, some modifications of the IP joints occur, affecting cartilaginous and para-articular structures, and most importantly, volar plate and the check-reins. Collateral ligaments and joint capsule are less often involved in joint stiffness in flexion. The check-reins are thin and supple and become hypertrophied and stiff to limit IP extension. This structural alteration may occur due to an injury, but also after prolonged immobilization of the IP in flexion.

Causes of extrinsic stiffness

- Cutaneous by scarring secondary to injury or burn
- congenital: such as camptodactyly
- Dupuytren's disease
- reflex sympathetic dystrophy
- post-traumatic:
  - flexor tendon injury
  - extensor tendon injury: boutonnière deformity, distal to PIP joint
  - extra-articular fractures
- swan neck deformity
- iatrogenic: cast, internal fixation, sepsis.

Cutaneous causes

They are obvious at the time of inspection of the hand and easily confirmed by the history.

Skin contractures

Scar contractures are the sequelae of periarticular contusion injuries over the PIP joint, particularly at the volar aspect where skin and subcutaneous tis-

sue are thick. These contractures are often longitudinally oriented, perpendicular to the flexion creases, and can be acutely painful and neglected by patient or therapists. At the dorsal aspect, the scar can impair the range of motion of the articulation, particularly when there is skin and/or tendinous substance loss. Importantly, there may also be large soft tissue losses of the dorsal or volar aspect of the metacarpals which have healed spontaneously or were grafted and may ultimately impair PIP range of motion.

Burn sequelaes, as in all burned tissue, show an increase of capillary permeability due to liberation of vasoamine substances and accumulation of fluid and interstitial space oedema. Collagen fibres are produced with secondary loss of elasticity of the infiltrated tissues. This oedema is the main cause of the extrinsic deforming force; elasticity of the dorsal skin allows its accumulation between skin and extensor apparatus. The MCP joint adopts a hyperextension position and the strength of the extrinsic extensor mechanism is decreased. Imbalance of forces of flexor and the extensor tendons places the IP joints in a flexed position. For burns of the dorsum of the hand the skin is said to be the only cause of deformity. This may be true in most cases, but the thin skin at the level of the PIP joint can involve the central slip of the extensor tendon with a resulting boutonnière deformity. It also may secondarily involve sepsis of the extensor mechanism. These deformities are mixed.

Burns of the volar aspect of the joint are less common and the resulting deformities are less severe because of the thickness of the subcutaneous tissue. Deformities are essentially due to sclerotic scars. Electrical burns can carbonize subcutaneous tissue and injure flexor tendons. The severity of the injury depends on the causal agent, the duration of contact and the pressure exerted on the severed tissues.

Scar contracture can cause subluxation of the joint, particularly at the dorsal aspect, due to the contracture power of the wound healing process.

Sclerodermia

Sclerodermia is a pathology of unknown aetiology with two evolving phases: first, the oedematous phase is painless, deforms the fingers, decreases the fingers' motion and causes morning stiffness that is usually marked (this is often associated with

Raynaud syndrome). The second phase is characterized by progressive skin fibrosis with thickened and hyperpressured skin. The skin becomes tensed, with disappearance of the creases and limited joint mobility. Typically, the MCP joint is fixed in extension and the PIP joint in flexion. Bones are usually not involved and the main cause of stiffness is the combination of skin and tendinous retraction, particularly of the dorsal aspect of the hand. Characteristically, the skin over the PIP joints is tensed and demonstrates white zones of hyperpressure on top of the condyles of the head of P1. The subsequent risk is exposure of the joint and, eventually, sepsis.

Dupuytren's disease

PIP joint stiffness is a challenge for the surgeon. The fixed flexed deformity of the MCP joint is usually easily corrected even if it is a long-standing flexion deformity. Conversely, a fixed flexed PIP joint deformity is not always easy to correct even if the deformity is recent. This is the main reason why aponevrotomy and aponevrectomy are indicated early when there is secondary involvement of the PIP joint.

The deformity of the PIP joint is due to two factors:

- alteration of the digital fascias structures colonized by myofibroblasts (these fascias are closely related to the skin and the structures of the digital canal)
- retraction of the para- and periarticular structures that have been maintained in a flexed position but are not involved by the pathologic process of the volar and/or digital fascias.

Involvement of the digital fascias

The various digital fascias that have been incriminated in the development of flexum deformity of the PIP joint have been described by Gosset (1986), Thomine (1986), MacFarlane (1986), Masson (Tubiana and Hueston 1986). These are essentially:

- The pretendinous cord which is the principal cause of the PIP flexion deformity. It is the continuation of the pretendinous metacarpal band and inserts distally on the middle phalanx and on the fibrous components of the digital canal. It is usually adherent to the median part of the skin. This cord is not in relation with the neurovascular bundles which run laterally. At its distal end, it is in close relation with the Grayson ligament (prepedicular) and when the deformity is accentuated, those fibres may attract the neurovascular bundles medially.
- The lateral cords are the pathological thickening of the lateral digital sheet described by Thomine (1986). They are continuous with the natatory ligament, and their insertions are mainly at skin level, but may also be on the tendon sheath at the level of the PIP joint via Grayson's ligament. This cord has a moderate influence on the PIP joint because its main insertion is cutaneous.
- The spiral cords are the lateral continuation of the pretendinous cord at the metacarpal level or they may arise at the level of the terminal tendon of an intrinsic muscle (mainly for the fifth finger). In both cases, the cords, distally to the MCP joint, run dorsal to the neurovascular bundle and merge with the lateral digital sheet. Then they cross the neurovascular bundle anteriorly and run parallel to Grayson's ligament and insert on the skeleton and/or the flexor tendon sheath of the middle phalanx. The more severe contractures of the PIP joint are related to the spiral cords which emerge from the insert to the intrinsic muscles, particularly those on the ulnar aspect of the fifth finger.
- The retrovascular cord described by Thomine was distinguished from the ligaments of Cleland. This cord is longitudinally oriented and is closely related to skin posterior to the neurovascular bundle. There is also an insertion on the fibrous tendon sheath. This cord does not cause a flexion deformity of the PIP joint by itself, but, when partially excised, the joint cannot be extended completely. The residual cord may be the cause of recurrence of the retraction of the PIP joint.
- Of particular importance is the pure digital form of Dupuytren's disease that is characterized by an isolated retraction of the PIP joint without involvement of the palm. The involved cords have been described by many authors and detailed further by Strickland (1985). They arise at the level of the periosteum, at the base of P1 or at the insertion of the intrinsic muscles. Their location is different from the spiral cords previously described because they arise posteriorly and dorsal to the neurovascular bundle, continue their course

obliquely, and insert on the tendon sheath anterior of the neurovascular bundle. The bundle is displaced toward the digital axis, but is never enclosed by the cord. Moreover, this form of Dupuytren's disease is found at variable depths laterally.

Secondary flexion deformity

Already stated, flexion deformity of the MCP joint is easily reduced after excision of the pathological fascia, but this is not the case for the PIP joint. This is due to the difference in the anatomy of these two joints. The volar plate is under tension and strongly attached by the check-reins to the neck of P1, the collateral ligaments of the PIP joint are under tension and adherent to the sides of the head of P1 in flexion, and any lengthy adoption of this position creates adhesions. Many other elements participate in the persistence of the deformity, some of which are difficult to correct:

- Cutaneous retraction which may be related to the fascial insertions or to scarring from previous surgeries.
- Retraction of the flexor tendon sheath: mainly in its mobile portion between A2 and A4 pulleys. This is due to infiltration by pathologic tissue and by adhesion caused by the pathologic tissue.
- Retraction of the flexor muscles and/or adhesion to the tendon. Related to the decrease of excursion of the muscle and tendon. The difference can be appreciated by the correction of the flexion deformity while positioning the wrist in flexion. In case of recurrence, the FDS may be adherent to the volar plate.
- Volar plate involvement; thickening of the check-reins which are infiltrated by pathological proliferation.
- Involvement of the oblique retinacular ligament of Landsmeer. Its involvement is debated, but it may exist more commonly on the ulnar side of the fifth finger and may participate to the flexed deformity of the PIP joint.
- Retraction and adhesions of the collateral ligaments; the anterior aspect retracts because it is tensed in flexion.
- Stretching of the extensor mechanism at the dorsum of PIP joint due to a long-lasting flexed position.
- Joint incongruity; a long-standing flexion defor-

mity of the finger may cause adaptive changes of the joint contour with loss of cartilage and of subchondral bone at the area of pressure.

Sequelae of the severed flexor tendons

Repair of injured flexor tendons is one of the most difficult areas of hand surgery. At the beginning of the history of hand surgery, results of primary tendon repair were so poor that Bunnel (1956) described the 'no man's land' area that was the zone 2 of the flexor tendon sheath. It was not recommended to attempt any primary repair because of the almost inescapable failure to restore function. A large exposure and a difficult suturing technique combined with prolonged postoperative immobilization resulted in formation of severe adhesions of the tendon to the surrounding structures and unacceptable results.

Better understanding of the tendon healing process, new techniques of repair and early mobilization by physiotherapists have considerably improved the outcome of this surgery. Nevertheless, some problems still remain, mainly those due to persistent postoperative adhesions that produce flexion deformities of joints such as the PIP, a source of controversies in treatment.

Tendon healing

This is synonymous with adhesion formation because the latter is the mechanism of tendon healing. Adhesions are the vascular support of the extrinsic healing of lacerated tendons. The re-established continuity of severed tendons stimulates scar formation by increasing local vascularization. Vascularization allows the cells to reach the site of tendon repair; this is called extrinsic tendon healing. Other studies have described intrinsic tendon healing which is based on tenocytes and intrinsic vascularization of the tendon. Healing potential comes from the restored synovial digital sheath that helps healing prior to re-establishment of vascular continuity. If the tendon keeps the possibility of mobilization during the healing phase, the increased pressure in the digital sheath potentiates the healing action of the tenocytes and does not produce adhesions. This theory has its application in early mobilization of the tendons and limits the harmful effect of adhesions.

Numerous experimental studies have shown that some factors are responsible for formation of adhesions:

- Contusion has a poor prognosis due to the related devascularization.
- The technique of repair should be as atraumatic as possible, either in the manipulation of the tendon ends or in the selected choice of repair. Any traumatism by an instrument or by striction by the suture material will create local ischaemia which will increase the amount of cells at the repair site and the formation of adhesions.
- The solidity of the repair must be strong enough to allow early mobilization of the repaired tendon without creation of a tendon gap that will cause an increase of tendon length and lessen its efficiency. Numerous suture techniques have been described with experimental advantages that are not all applicable clinically. It is well accepted that an intratendinous suture combined with a running epitendinous suture that regularizes the repair site to give a better strength is the safest technique.
- With lesions of both flexor tendons in zone 2, it is also well accepted that both tendons should be repaired; if the repair site of the FDP is not in direct contact to the bony floor of the digital sheath (by systematic repair of the FDS) less severe adhesions will occur.
- Concomitant fractures at the level of the severed tendons are correlated with bad prognostic factors because the repair tendons and the bone callus create more severe adhesions. Sometimes obligatory immobilization of the injured digital segment increases the risk of adhesions by preventing early mobilization of the repair tendons.
- With time, the physiotherapy protocols have considerably changed. Strict immobilization should be avoided and is reserved for children and for unreliable patients. Immobilization is correlated with an increased risk of residual flexion deformity. The postoperative splint usually keeps the MCP in 70° of flexion and both IP joints in extension. The Kleinert protocol (Kleinert and Kutz 1967) is a potential source of adhesion formation because the passive acting rubber force is distal and the position at rest is flexed. If this information is not understood by the patient, this protocol may expose both PIP and DIP joints to deformation in flexion. Assisted passive mobiliza-

tion or passive mobilization followed by active positioning motion are presently the more common protocols of rehabilitation because they avoid, in theory, the risk of PIP joint flexion deformity (Dap 1992).

Joint stiffness

This is the consequence of two mechanisms:

- Those related to tendon healing; as previously emphasized, adhesion formation at the site of tendon repair will limit the motion primarily of the tendon and secondarily of the joints distal to the repair site. Adhesions will be replaced by fibrous tissues which will produce the adhesion of the tendons to the surrounding structures; this scarring will interfere with vascular and synovial fluid circulation and will contribute to the extension of the adhesions away from the repair site.
- Those related to the joint itself; joint stiffness may result from the limitation of joint motion during the immobilization phase that protects the tendon suture. This ankylosis is more important if the joint has not been mobilized even passively in all its arc of motion. Also, a concomitant injury of the joint and bone may result in primary joint stiffness.

Stiffness in a flexed position is the most common. Adhesions related to tendon healing, postoperative immobilization, selected physiotherapy protocols and associated joint injury may all result in flexion stiffness.

Stiffness in extension is less common. This develops when there is an intratendinous gap at the repair site during the healing process and, in spite of adequate postoperative protocols, the tendinous excursion is insufficient to allow a complete enrolment of the articular chain secondarily. Dorsal and periarticular adhesions due to inadequate motion after extensor tendon and/or dorsal joint injury may occur and provoke joint stiffness in extension.

Swan neck deformity

This deformity is defined by an association of hyperextension of the PIP joint and an hyperflexion of the DIP joint. It represents an example of the interrelation between the digital articulations. The recurvatum of the PIP provokes a combined deformation of DIP joint and the reverse is also true. This dynamic imbalance occurs when the finger is maximally extended and may result eventually in a fixed deformity.

There are many causes of this complex deformity; they are classified by Zancolli (1979) into three groups: the extrinsic causes (recurvatum of the PIP is due to an excessive pull on the extensor tendons), intrinsic causes (the aetiologic factor is an hyperactivity of the intrinsic muscles), and articular causes from injury of the stabilizing structures of the PIP joint (mainly the volar plate). Schematically, the causes are:

• injury and laxity of the volar plate
• spasticity, whatever the cause
• rheumatoid arthritis
• malunion of a fracture of P2 in a recurvatum position
• mallet finger (in association with an hyperlaxity of the volar plate)
• generalized laxity (with a destabilizing injury).

Insertion of the extensor digitorum communi is at the base of P2; hyperextension is prevented by the volar plate placed under tension. In swan neck deformity, a PIP joint hyperextension and dorsal subluxation of the lateral slips of the extensor digitorum communi occurs. Secondarily, there is weakening of the extension power over the DIP joint which cannot be overcome by the action of the FDP and, a flexion deformity of the DIP joint occurs; the volar plate loses its stabilizing role.

The patients may be subdivided in three therapeutic groups:

• those which can completely flex the PIP joint; they only have a dynamic deformity at forced extension
• those with a fixed deformity, and
• those who have a fixed deformity and articular changes.

Iatrogenic stiffness

After injury to the hand by a burn, a crush injury or any other injuries for which immobilization is neces-

sary, it is mandatory to immobilize the hand in a position which will avoid later development of stiffness. The MCP joints must be immobilized in complete flexion and the PIP joint in complete extension; this position is the intrinsic plus position. In this position, the collateral ligaments of the PIP joint are extended and the volar plate is in maximal tension. The volar plates of the MCP and the IP joints react differently to immobilization due to their anatomic differences. The volar plate of the MCP joint composed of multiple criss-crossing fibres is extensible as a crosspiece whereas the ones of the IP joints are not very extensible. The difference in length of the volar plate of the MCP joint between flexion and extension is approximately 30% compared to 10% for the IP joint. Any retraction will rapidly result in a fixed deformity.

Any trauma or surgical intervention will produce an inflammatory reaction inducing collagen formation which in theory, is a stimulus for further adhesion formation. In fact, this newly-formed collagen will be easily lysed by early mobilization. However, if mobilization is started too early, it is possible to increase adhesion formation by creation of haematomas from the injured small vessels, by tendinous mobilization, etc. After some days, this early phase is completed and mobilization may be started without increasing the amount of new fibroblastic cells. It is also important to avoid postoperative or post-traumatic pain because the pain reflex arc will decrease mobility due to the limited contraction of the muscles when pain is generated.

Iatrogenic stiffness occurs essentially because of lack of knowledge of the principles of stiffness development and the wound healing process and especially because of treatment mistakes in the operative and postoperative period.

Reflex sympathetic dystrophy

This pathology, occurring after an injury, is characterized by pain, oedema of variable degree, vasomotor and trophic changes in the upper limb which result in a more or less fixed ankylosis of the joint. The severity of this entity varies. The physiopathology of this condition acts as a dysfunction of the sympathetic system.

The occurrence of this disease is still mysterious and it is important to emphasize that reflex sympathetic dystrophy may happen after any 'aggression'

to the hand – a traumatic injury or a surgical procedure – and that the severity of the symptoms is not
proportional to the 'aggression' that triggered the
syndrome.

There are many clinical presentations of reflex
sympathetic dystrophy:

- a minor form localized to an area of the hand
- a minor form with involvement of the entire hand
- the shoulder–hand syndrome which combines
involvement of the hand and at distance of the
shoulder
- and a rare presentation, the major causalgia with
a more marked pain.

Evolution of reflex sympathetic dystrophy is typically made of several stages:

- The early stage. Its duration is variable and is
characterized by pain that can be severe and will
decrease in the subsequent stages. Oedema is
also a prominent feature; the hand is usually
bluish and sweating is increased. Joint motion is
limited only by pain.
- The second stage. Pain persists with a tendency
toward decreased intensity as well as an oedema
that becomes indurated and fixed. The skin
becomes dry and joint motion decreases because
of thickening of periarticular tissues; atrophy of skin
and subcutaneous tissues occurs. A common radiological finding is demineralization of the bones.
- The chronic phase. This follows the previous
stages by a variable length of time. This stage is
characterized by joint stiffness. The MCP joints
are usually in extension and the IP joints in flexion
with a more severe involvement of the PIP joints.
This stiffness has the same characteristics as that
presenting secondary to burns, but the joints are
painful at any attempt to reduce them in the
proper position, even though flexion of the fingers
is still possible.
    This chronic phase can last a long time (18–24
months) and the risks of sequelae with stiffness
are greater if the diagnosis is delayed, the physiotherapy initiated late, and as this phase persists.
Decrease of pain and restoration of a supple and
dry skin are good prognostic factors.

The psychological makeup of the patient is
important in the prognosis of this pathology which
must be suspected if, during the post-traumatic
period, disproportionate pain or oedema is present.

It is easier to create a Suddeck syndrome than it is
to treat it.

References

Bowers WH (1980) The proximal interphalangeal joint rolar plate. 1. An anatomical and biomechanical study, *J Hand Surg* **5A**:79–88.

Bunnell S (1956) *Surgery of the Hand*, 3rd edn: JB Lippincott: Philadelphia.

Curtis RM (1954) Capsulectomy of the intephalangeal joints of the fingers, *J Bone Joint Surg* **36A**:1219.

Dap F (1992) Les lésions traumatiques récentes des tendons fléchisseurs de la main: évolution des idées et évaluation des résultats. In: *Cahiers d'enseignement de la Société Française de Chirurgie de la Main, no. 4.* Expansion Scientifique Français: Paris: 1–32.

Gosset J (1986) Anatomíe des aponévroses palmo-digitales. In: Tubiana R, Hueston JT (eds). *La maladie de Dupuytren*, 3rd edn. Expansion Scientifique Française: Paris: 30–1.

Green DP (1993) *Operative Hand Surgery.* 3rd edn. Churchill Livingstone: New York.

Kleinert HE, Kutz JE (1967) Primary repair of lacerated flexor tendons in 'no man's land', *J Bone Joint Surg* **49A**:577.

MacFarlane RM (1986) Anatomie de la maladie de Dupruytren. In: Tubiana R, Hueston JT (eds). *La maladie de Dupuytren*, 3rd edn. Expansion Scientifique Française: Paris: 49–63.

Schneider LH, McEntee P (1986) Flexor tendon injuries. Treatment of acute problem, *Hand Clin* **2**:119–131.

Sokolow C (1995) Anatomie et physiologie de l'interphalangi-enne proximale, *Cahiers d'enseignement de la Societé Française de Chirurgie de la Main, no. 7.* Expansion Scientifique Français: Paris: 107–116.

Strickland JW (1985) The isolated digital words in Dupreytren's contractives: anatomy and clinical significance, *J Hand Surg* **10A**:118–24.

Thomine JM (1986) Le fascia digitale: dévelopment et anatomie. In: Tubiana R, Hueston JT (eds). *La maladie de Dupuytren*, 3rd edn. Expansion Scientifique Française: Paris: 11–19.

Tubiana R, Hueston JT (1986) *La maladie de Dupuytren*, 3rd edn. Expansion Scientifique Français: Paris.

Zancolli E (1979) *Structural and Dynamic Bases of Hand Surgery*, 3rd edn. JB Lippincott: Philadelphia.

39

Intrinsic causes of stiffness of the interphalangeal joints

Alberto Lluch

Introduction

Joint stiffness may be secondary to either remodelling of the collagen fibres of the capsule and ligaments or from deposition of new collagen on the surface of the joint capsule. If the proximal interphalangeal (PIP) joint of any finger is immobilized in flexion for a few weeks for the treatment of a proximal phalanx fracture, and the same is done on the opposite finger, we will observe that the uninjured finger will recover full mobility in a much shorter time. Not enough time will have elapsed for collagen remodelling to take place in either joint, which means that the joint stiffness in the injured finger is secondary to collagen fibre deposition over the joint capsule. For this reason the joints should always be immobilized in such a way that their capsular structures are in their most elongated position. As they are not elastic, capsular structures do not retract, and their shortening is secondary to folding or pleating of their collagen fibres. If the capsular structures are immobilized in a shortened position, collagen deposition on their surface will prevent them from regaining sufficient length to permit full joint movement. For this reason, it is very important to know the exact anatomy of the joint to determine the best position for immobilization.

Interphalangeal joint anatomy

The anatomy of both interphalangeal (IP) joints is very similar, with some differences in the proximal attachments of their volar plates and their respective segments of the flexor tendon sheath (Landsmeer 1975). Their major differences are the smaller dimensions and reduced mobility of the distal interphalangeal (DIP) joint. Therefore, in the fol-lowing description, we will only refer to the PIP joint.

The articular surface of the PIP joint has a much larger transverse than antero-posterior diameter, which coupled with the presence of two thick collateral ligaments, gives them great lateral stability. Contrary to the situation at the metacarpophalangeal (MP) joint level, the collateral ligaments of the PIP joint are tight in all positions of joint flexion, and do not play a predominant role in joint stiffness. The dorsal structures (capsule, extensor tendon and skin) are very thin and lax, allowing for both phalanges to flex more than 100°, until the base of the middle phalanx makes contact with the condylar notch of the proximal phalanx. On the contrary, on the palmar aspect there is a thick ligament that prevents joint hyperextension. The distal part of the volar ligament, called the volar plate, is 2–3 mm thick and has a fibrocartilaginous structure, the same as the dorsal plate located just below the insertion of the central slip (Slattery 1990). The presence of chondroitin and keratan sulphate in the dorsal and volar plates is important in resisting compression forces against the condyles of the proximal phalanx (Benjamin et al 1993). These structures provide protection to both the extensor and flexor tendons, whose collagen fibres are strong enough to sustain traction forces. The proximal part of the volar ligament is thinner and more flexible, mainly in its centre. It is reinforced at both sides, inserting into the proximal phalanx, just inside the most distal fibres of the A2 pulley and the proximal part of the cruciform flexor tendon sheath fibres of the C1 pulley. These proximal capsular reinforcements were first described by Gad (1967) and later by Eaton (1971), Kuczynski (1975), Landsmeer (1975) and Bowers et al (1980), and have been named 'check', 'rein' or 'check-rein' ligaments. The accessory collateral ligaments originate at the proximal phalanx and insert distally at the base of the

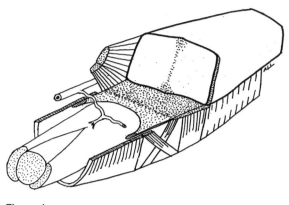

Figure 1

Schematic drawing of the periarticular structures of the proximal interphalangeal (PIP) joint after removing the proximal phalanx. The check-rein ligaments of the volar plate are inserted at the proximal phalanx just inside the most distal fibres of the A2 pulley.

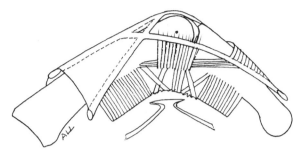

Figure 2

All the structures below the axis of rotation of the proximal interphalangeal (PIP) joint will be remodelled in a shortened position if immobilized long enough: lateral band, transverse retinacular ligament, oblique retinacular ligament, flexor tendon sheath, and volar skin.

middle phalanx, just below the collateral ligament, and at both sides of the volar plate (Fig. 1).

Aetiopathogenesis of IP joint stiffness

Deposition of recently synthesized collagen fibres on the joint capsule

By far the most frequent cause of intrinsic joint stiffness is deposition of recently synthesized collagen fibres on the joint capsule. When the PIP joint flexes, the proximal part of the volar plate and the accessory collateral ligaments fold upon themselves, and, if collagen deposition occurs in the position of joint flexion, extension will be restricted. It is preferable to have fibrosis of the dorsal structures, since they are thinner and more stretchable. This is the main reason why immobilization of the PIP joint in flexion should be avoided. Besides the volar plate and the accessory collateral ligaments, the remainder of structures volar to the axis of rota-

tion of the PIP joint can contribute to joint stiffness: the transverse and oblique retinacular ligaments (Laidsmeer 1944, Shrewsbury and Johnson 1977), Cleland and Grayson ligaments (Milford 1968), the flexor tendon sheath and the volar skin (Fig. 2).

Detailed understanding and knowledge of the flexor tendon sheath anatomy is also important. The annular pulleys A2 and A4 are fixed structures, as they attach to the proximal and middle phalanges, respectively. On the contrary, the C1 and A3 pulleys are attached to the volar capsular ligament, which is a mobile structure. Only the proximal fibres of the C1 pulley attach at the proximal phalanx, confluent with the insertion of the check-rein ligaments, while its distal fibres attach at both sides of the volar plate. Due to this arrangement, when the PIP joint flexes the distal part of the C1 pulley and the entire A3 pulley displace volarly, creating a space at the neck of the proximal phalanx which will be filled by the folding of the proximal part of the volar ligament. During PIP joint flexion, the C1 and C3 pulleys collapse like an accordion, until the A2, A3 and A4 pulleys approximate to one another (Fig. 3). Deposition of collagen on the flexor tendon sheath in this position will also limit PIP joint extension.

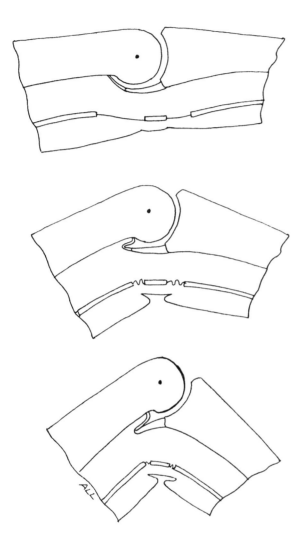

Figure 3

Cross-section of the proximal interphalangeal (PIP) joint and the palmar structures in different degrees of flexion. We can observe the increasing folding of the volar plate, the flexor tendon sheath and the volar skin as the joint progressively flexes.

Remodelling of capsular collagen fibres in a shortened position

This is the main cause of extrinsic joint stiffness, as it requires a much longer period of joint immobilization. Under these circumstances, IP joint stiffness

can occur after long-standing Dupuytren's disease, camptodactyly, claw hand secondary to intrinsic palsy, extensor or flexor tendon rupture, etc.

Causes of intrinsic interphalangeal joint stiffness

The three components of any joint are the capsule, the synovial membrane and the articular cartilage. Alteration of one or more of the above structures can cause intrinsic joint stiffness.

Capsular lesions

Joint stiffness occurs mainly after trauma. If the capsular structures are disrupted by the injury, the fibrosis required for its repair will very likely prevent recovery of full joint mobility, even after short periods of immobilization. The most common capsular injuries are collateral ligament disruption, volar plate detachment and joint dislocation. Unless bone architecture is altered, such as in fracture-dislocations, the joint remains stable even after severe capsular injuries (Kiefhaber et al 1986). This is why joint instabilities are very rare sequelae after joint trauma, while joint stiffness is very common.

As mentioned before, either partial or total *collateral ligament ruptures* are not a cause of joint instability, and for this reason should be immobilized in full extension for only a few days, so as to minimize the inflammatory response to trauma, and avoid joint stiffness. Pure collateral ligament lesions are rare, as they are usually associated with ruptures of the accessory collateral ligament and part of the volar ligament.

Volar plate detachments are secondary to hyperextension injuries of the PIP joint. The volar plate usually detaches from the base of the middle phalanx, and may include a bone fragment of a variable size. Only in the presence of a large bone fragment is immobilization in joint flexion advisable, so as to avoid dorsal subluxation of the middle phalanx. Prolonged immobilization in flexion will lead to a flexion contracture of the joint.

Joint dislocations. The PIP joint can dislocate dorsally or palmarly. In the more common dorsal dislocation, the volar plate and the accessory collateral ligaments have to rupture for the middle phalanx to displace dorsally. Associated rupture of one collateral ligament usually occurs, although the collateral ligaments may be spared from the injury in pure dorsal dislocations. After the joint has been reduced, its lateral stability should be examined, to determine the integrity of one or both collateral ligaments. Joint stability should also be assessed by asking the patient to actively flex and extend the joint after reduction.

Anterior dislocations of the PIP joint are rare, and either a transverse or longitudinal rupture of the extensor mechanism must occur. The central slip of the extensor tendon can rupture from its insertion in the middle phalanx, mainly with detachment of a small bone fragment. If this does not occur, the condyles of the proximal phalanx will protrude dorsally through a longitudinal tear of the interconnecting fibres between the central slip and one of the lateral bands. The displacement of the central slip to one side of the head of the proximal phalanx will cause a moderate rotational deformity of the middle phalanx. Integrity of the extensor mechanism should always be explored after reducing a volar dislocation of the PIP joint.

When the capsule is not disrupted, but is surrounded by a fibroblastic reaction in response to the repair of a nearby structure, it can also become stiff, but it will require a longer period of immobilization. The closer the repair process is to the joint capsule, the greater the chances are for the joint to become stiff. For this reason, the probability of developing a PIP joint stiffness is higher after a fracture of the condyles than of the base of the proximal phalanx.

Synovial tissue diseases

Alterations of the synovial membrane will cause joint stiffness from restriction of mobility secondary to pain, capsular fibrosis, and articular cartilage destruction. The synovial tissue can be altered under different pathological circumstances, mainly in rheumatoid disease. Infections from a great variety of microorganisms are also a frequent cause of joint stiffness and destruction if not treated promptly and adequately. Psoriatic arthritis and other connective tissue diseases such as lupus and scleroderma can also cause joint stiffness. Less frequently, the finger joints can also be affected by

metabolic diseases that will cause crystal deposition in the synovial tissue, such as gouty arthritis (uric acid) and pseudogout (calcium pyrophosphate (Smyth 1972). Arthritis can also be associated with haematologic disorders (leukaemia, lymphomas, myeloma, sickle cell disease, reticulohistiocytosis and haemophilic haemarthrosis). Amyloidosis, sarcoidosis, and ochronosis (alkaptonuria) can also affect the joints, but are very rare in the small joints of the hand (Decker 1972).

Tumours of the synovial tissue, although unusual in the fingers, can also be a cause of joint stiffness and destruction (pigmented villonodular synovitis, synovial chondromatosis and synovial sarcoma) (Decker 1972).

Joint cartilage destruction

Intra-articular fractures will cause joint cartilage destruction, which will be more or less severe according to the degree of comminution and displacement of the osteochondral fragments. In general, fractures of the base of the middle or distal phalanges will have a better prognosis than a fracture of its condyles. In clinical practice, we have observed that the destruction of the concave side of any joint has a better prognosis than an injury to the opposed convex side (elbow, wrist, hip, knee, ankle, etc).

Cartilage destruction can be secondary to any type of joint synovitis, such as those already described. Certain pathologies will cause a more rapid cartilage destruction than others. A bacterial joint infection, for example, will be more destructive than a synovial chondromatosis. Yet even the same pathology, as in rheumatoid arthritis, can manifest itself with a wide spectrum of joint cartilage deterioration.

Ageing of the joint (degenerative arthritis) can be another cause of joint stiffness, mainly of the DIP joints in women, from both articular cartilage destruction and capsular fibrosis.

Finally, we should comment on neuropathic joint disease (Charcot joints) which has the peculiarity of presenting, in some cases, a completely destroyed joint without any signs of joint stiffness. Joint hypermobility and instability, with disproportionately little pain, are characteristic. Neuropathic joint disease can be seen in tabes dorsalis, congenital insensitivity to pain, diabetes, Charcot-Marie–Tooth disease, neuropathy of leprosy, etc. Similar deterioration of joint cartilage has been observed after repeated intra-articular injections of glucocorticoids. It has been suggested that the relief of pain provided by such treatment permits excessive mobility and interferes with normal protective processes, thereby accelerating the progress of the underlying joint disease, usually rheumatoid arthritis or osteoarthritis (Rodnan 1972). This observation leads us to believe that pain is probably the most important factor in the presentation of joint stiffness, as it plays an important role in protecting joint cartilage.

Prevention of interphalangeal joint stiffness

The best treatment for joint stiffness is prevention. Loss of joint motion is most frequently seen after trauma, in which case joint stiffness could be considered iatrogenic. The patient never comes to the emergency room with a joint stiffness, as it is not caused by the initial injury, but rather as a consequence of immobilization. However, immobilization is necessary for the healing of tissues, but it should always be done on the least possible number of joints, for the shortest time, and in the optimal position. It is also very important to avoid oedema and tissue inflammation. The former can be accomplished by limb elevation, and wrapping the finger, with light to moderate pressure, by using an elastic autoadhesive bandage (Coban.3M). Inflammation cannot be totally eliminated as it is a physiological mechanism necessary for tissue repair. Excessive inflammation should be avoided, and can be controlled by careful handling of the tissues and the administration of anti-inflammatory drugs. Fibroblast proliferation is essential for tissue repair, and from the cisternae of their rough endoplasmic reticulum the collagen precursors will be secreted. Once in the extracellular space, tropocollagen aggregation and fibrin formation, responsible for tissue repair, will take place (Peacock and Van Winkle 1976). Unfortunately, collagen fibres will also be laid down on the surface of the joint capsule, which will prevent its unfolding if maintained in a shortened position for a sufficient period of time.

Which is the proper position to immobilize the IP joints?

For many years, immobilization of the IP joints in flexion in what was called the 'functional position' was recommended (Bunnell 1924, Kanavel 1925). The main reason for immobilization in this position was the fact that it was the most functional position if the IP joints became stiff. This circumstance was quite common at that time, prior to the discovery of antibiotics and emphasis on better surgical instrumentation and suture material. Today it is agreed that the IP joints should be immobilized in full extension if stiffness is to be avoided or minimized. This position was called the 'safe position' by James (1970) and the 'protective position' by Beasley (Beasley and Kestern 1969, Lluch 1972). On the other hand, this is not a recommended position for immobilization of a joint expected to become completely stiff or fused. The 'protective position' should only be used for temporary immobilization for the prevention of joint stiffness, and the 'functional position' for permanent immobilization, as in the case of a joint arthrodesis.

References

Beasley RW, Kestern NC (1969) Principles of medical surgical rehabilitation of the hand, *Med Clin North Am* **53**:645.

Benjamin M, Ralphs JR, Shiton M, Irwin M (1993) Capsular tisues of the proximal intephalengeal joint: normal composition and effects of Dupuytren's disease and rheumatoid arthritis, *J Hand Surg* **18B**:371–6.

Bowers WH, Wolf JW, Nehil JL, Bittinger S (1980) The proximal interphalangeal joint volar plate. I. An anatomical and biomechanical study, *J Hand Surg* **5**:79–88.

Bunnell S (1924) Reconstructive surgery of the hand, *Surg Gyn Obst* **39**:259.

Decker JL (1972) Miscellaneous conditions complicating or producing arthritis. In: Hollander JL, McCarty DJ, eds. *Arthritis and Allied Conditions.* Lea & Febiger: Philadelphia: 1283–1390.

Eaton RG (1971) *Joint Injuries of the Hand.* Charles C Thomas: Springfield: 9–17.

Gad P (1967) The anatomy of the volar plate of the capsules of the finger joints, *J Bone Joint Surg* **49**:362–7.

James JIP (1970) The assessment and management of the injured hand, *Hand* **2**:97–105.

Kanavel AB (1925) *Infections of the Hand.* Lea & Febiger: Philadelphia.

Kiefhaber TR, Stern PJ, Grood ES (1986) Lateral stability of the proximal interphalangeal joint, *J Hand Surg* **11A**:661–9.

Kuczynski K (1975) Less-known aspects of the proximal interphalangeal joints of the human hand, *Hand* **7**:31–6.

Landsmeer JMF (1944) The anatomy of the dorsal aponeurosis of the human finger and its functional significance, *Anat Rec* **104**:31–4.

Landsmeer JMF (1975) The proximal interphalangeal joint, *Hand* **7**:30.

Lluch A (1972) Protective position of the hand. Anatomical study, *NY Acad Med Sci,* 8 May 1972.

Milford LW (1968) *Retaining Ligaments of the Digits of the Hand.* WB Saunders: Philadelphia.

Peacock EE, Van Winkle W (1976) *Wound Repair.* WB Saunders: Philadelphia.

Rodnan GP (1972) Neuropathic joint disease (Charcot joints). In: Hollander JL, McCarty DJ, eds. *Arthritis and Allied Conditions.* Lea & Febiger: Philadelphia: 1329–39.

Shrewsbury MM, Johnson RK (1977) A systematic study of the oblique retinacular ligament of the human finger: its structure and function, *J Hand Surg* **2**:194–9.

Slattery PG (1990) The dorsal plate of the proximal interphalangeal joint, *J Hand Surg* **15B**:68–73.

Smyth CJ (1972) Metabolic bone and joint diseases. In: Hollander JL, McCarty DJ, eds. *Arthritis and Allied Conditions.* Lea & Febiger: Philadelphia: 1071–1201.

40

Treatment of stiffness of the proximal interphalangeal joint

Philippe Saffar

Proximal interphalangeal (PIP) joint stiffness is one of the most difficult problems in hand surgery. This joint is in relation:

(a) Dorsally with the complex anatomy of the joint tendon, which is divided in three bands. The central band insert at the base of the middle phalanx in close relationship with the PIP joint. Any injury of the extensor tendon in this area results in malfunction (boutonnière) and then stiffness of the joint

(b) Volarly, there is the flexor tendon chiasma with division of the flexor digitorum sublimis (FDS) through which passes the flexor digitorum profondus (FDP). Part of the vascularization of both tendons is provided by the vincula which emerges from an anastomosis between the two lateral arteries. Injury of the flexor tendons and/or their vincula in this area results in joint stiffness in flexion. The volar plate is an element of stability. Injury of this structure may result in fixed flexed deformity.

Anteroposterior and lateral X-rays are necessary to assess the joint space and the articular contours. Tenolyses and arthrolyses are ineffective if the joint space is narrowed or the cartilage not present. Sequelae of articular fractures should be appreciated. Post-traumatic clinodactyly may be present after extra- or intra-articular fractures.

Tenolysis

Flexor tendon tenolysis

This is a difficult and precise technique.

After flexor tendon injury

In zone 2, where it is most frequently performed, the indication depends on the history:

• type of mechanism: clear-cut section, laceration or crush; isolated or associated injury: open wound, vasculonervous injury, extra- or intra-articular fracture
• type of initial treatment: type of suture, early mobilization, delay since injury, rehabilitation programme.

Tenolysis should never be performed before 4–6 months after injury. The only exception is suspicion of secondary tendon rupture. Preoperative rehabilitation is often useful.

Technique. The best approach is a Brüner oblique approach, which may be modified by previous scars. Exploration should be made first proximally to the suture in a zone where the tendon is normal; proximal traction on the tendon should assess the normal muscle elasticity. Then, we have to deal with tendon status, pulleys, tendon vascularization, joint status and associated injuries.

Tendon status. The suture area should be inspected. It is usually the site of maximum adhesions. The stitches should be removed and the status of the tendon assessed: it is of great importance for the result of tenolysis. The tendon sheath may be adherent to the tendon and after removal of the fibrosis, the underlying tendon may appear normal. If the adhesion zone is less than 2 cm and the tendon has a good aspect, the result will be good. A tendon of bad quality on more than 4 cm, having lost the normal tendon appearance, too thin (danger of rupture) or too thick would imply a bad prognosis and a decision of tendon graft may be evoked. The tendon should be then separated from the bone and from the PIP volar plate, taking care to respect the vincula when this is still present.

Sometimes only one tendon has been sutured, and the other one is retracted and adherent at a level that is often the carpal tunnel. It should be found and proximally resected.

Pulleys. The pulleys should be respected, at least A2 and A4. If adherent to tendons, a special tendon elevator should be introduced between tendon and pulley and going back and forth, separate the two elements and then the tendon from the bone. Normal gliding should be obtained between the two elements and also between the two tendons. It is possible to suppress A1 and perform the tenolysis under the A2 pulley or to suppress the middle part between A1 and A2 and perform the tenolysis under the two pulleys, keeping the retaining action of both pulleys (Fig. 1).

The tendon should not be too thick and should glide easily under the pulley.

Tendon vascularization is assessed by the presence of vincula, existence of lateral artery injuries and, indirectly, by the magnitude of fibrosis that is a feature of bad prognosis.

After a complete tenolysis, the PIP joint may still be non-flexible or fixed in flexion or, rarely, in extension (possibly a problem of associated dorsal injury?) and a decision of PIP arthrolysis should be made.

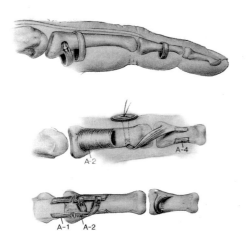

Figure 1

The pulleys.

Associated injuries should be detected preoperatively: previous fractures, neurovascular bundle injury, extensor injury, infection and skin retractions have to be treated at the same time. Artery and nerve exploration is performed on one side or both. If both sides have been injured, this is a bad prognosis.

After fracture

The fracture may have been a diaphyseal fracture or a para-articular fracture. Tenolysis is then easier, the area of adhesion being more limited. However, if it is near the epiphysis, an associated arthrolysis may be necessary.

1   At the level of zone 1, adhesions are mainly with bone and distal intephalangeal (DIP) volar plate. Fibrosis surrounding the tendon is easy to remove but it is difficult and of paramount importance to preserve the A4 pulley to obtain a complete flexion of the DIP. It is also difficult to separate the tendon from the distal part of the volar plate without detaching its insertion from the bone. The PID joint is often fixed in extension and even passive flexion is limited.
2   At the level of zone 4, the tendons are adherent to each other, and this is usually the case in multiple tendon injuries at the palm or the wrist. At this level complex nerve and tendon injuries have often to be repaired, and it may be necessary to resect the FDS tendon to have a good gliding of the FDP tendons.

For the fifth finger, the FDS is often very thin and may be suppressed, but it may be useful to reinforce the FDP after tenolysis with the proximal part of the sublimis, to suture it side by side to the FDP.

For the thumb, tenolysis is easier because there is only one tendon and pulleys are easy to respect. The difficult area is inside the thenar eminence.

Elements of a bad prognosis for flexor tenolysis are:

- bad initial treatment
- extended peritendinous fibrosis
- tendon too thin or too thick
- extended tendon alteration
- absence of pulleys
- bad vascularization
- associated joint stiffness

• long-standing stiffness which may alter the muscle.

Flexor tenolysis is less used than before because tendons are usually well treated now, and a good initial treatment is essential to obtain a good result after tenolysis.

Extensor tendon tenolysis

Stiffness may be the consequence of extensor tendon injuries at the dorsal aspect of the first phalanx (P1), and particularly of the PIP joint. Stiffness in extension may be due to an extensor tendon injury at the dorsum of P1 and at times more proximal, or a P1 or metacarpal fracture. Extensor tenolysis is easy to perform. Adhesions are not only between tendon and bone, but also between skin and tendon. Care should be taken to detach the lateral bands and the interosseous expansions from both sides of P1. Stiffness in flexion is a completely different situation: it is generally a fixed 'boutonnière' deformity and the treatment is not a matter of simple tenolysis. It has to be differentiated from the false boutonnière (McCue et al 1975) that is the consequence of an hyperextension mechanism with detachment of the volar plate and its healing in retraction which results in fixed flexion. The principal difference is that in fixed boutonnière, the patient is unable to flex actively the DIP.

Arthrolysis

This is a challenging procedure. It may be performed alone or combined with tenolysis. The PIP is fixed in flexion in most cases. Causes of PIP joint stiffness are numerous.

Surgeons may be aware that a simple immobilization in flexion of the PIP, even after a distant injury may lead to PIP stiffness in 2 or 3 weeks. The so-called 'position function' in flexion for immobilization of this joint should be totally abandoned and replaced by the 'intrinsic plus' position with PIP in extension.

Other causes are intra- or para-articular fractures and malunions, sprains, volar plate detachment, inflammatory diseases, ischaemic problems and non-sympathetic dystrophy (NSD).

One should avoid every type of manual forced extension on the PIP joint, either during a surgical procedure or during an extra-surgical examination. Adhesions at this level are very strong and will be the last thing to break; sometimes the lateral arteries trapped in the adhesions will break first and result in finger ischaemia. A gentle and progressive extension may sometimes be obtained with an extension splint. However, it can rarely go beyond what is obtained by passive extension of the finger.

1 Volar arthrolysis may be performed by an anterior approach and the 'check-reins' of the joint (Watson et al 1979) should be first resected. This technique is used mainly in association with flexor tenolysis. Distal volar plate detachment has also been advocated.
2 We use an anterolateral approach based on a technique called total anterior tenoarthrolysis that will be described later. The periosteum of the first and second phalanx are in continuity with the volar plate and may be elevated together from the volar aspect of these phalanxes.
   Technique. A lateral approach at the junction of the dorsal and volar skin is performed extending from the middle of the proximal phalanx to the distal part of the second phalanx. This technique is based on a subperiosteal dissection. A direct contact is taken with the lateral aspect of the phalanxes. A periosteal incision is made on the lateral aspect of the first and second phalanx. A subperiosteal elevation of the periosteum is made from the lateral aspect of the phalanx, then from the volar and opposite aspect of the first and second phalanx (Fig. 2). This should be made with care, slowly. The volar plate, which is in continuity with the periosteum, is freed from its attachment to the bone with a scalpel and is then elevated, cutting the accessory ligaments of the PIP joint (Fig. 3). The anterior aspect of the joint is then visible. If this joint is fixed in a flexed position, the anterior part of the lateral ligaments are cut to straighten the finger. This approach is useful when an isolated arthrolysis should be performed.
3 Association of flexor tenolysis and PIP arthrolysis is sometimes necessary. Results have not been rewarding and no more than 20° of increased PIP motion are usually obtained (Mansat et al 1983). In fixed flexed fingers operated on several times and with a good residual flexion, we have

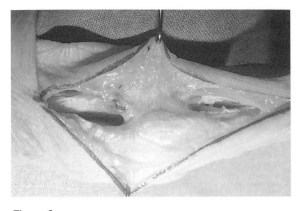

Figure 2

Subperiosteal dissection of P1 and P2.

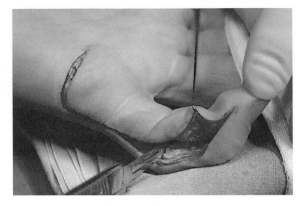

Figure 4

Cutting the proximal interphalangeal (PIP) lateral ligaments to obtain a complete extension.

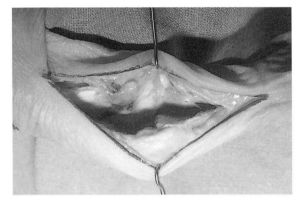

Figure 3

The volar plate is elevated.

4 Dorsal arthrolysis is always combined with extensor tenolysis. It is very difficult to separate the extensor tendon from the joint capsula. This capsula should be divided transversally at its proximal insertion and the lateral ligaments cut from dorsal to palmar until complete flexion is obtained. They may also be detached from their proximal insertion.

Arthrodeses

The approach for PIP arthrodesis may be lateral to avoid cutting flexor or extensor tendons. The joint is easily subluxated, and preparation of the articular surfaces is performed in the same way as for metacarpophalangeal (MP) arthrodesis. Two rounded surfaces are created, one convex and one concave to fit each other with a maximum contact. Fixation is performed in the adapted position of flexion which varies from 20° for the index to 45° for the fifth finger. K-wires, screws or other types of fixation are used.

Arthroplasties
Without prostheses

Arthroplasties have not been frequently reported for the PIP joints. Different techniques have been described.

proposed a procedure called total anterior tenoarthrolysis (TATA) (Saffar and Rengeval 1978). The anterolateral approach and subperiosteal dissection mentioned above is extended to the DIP volar plate and the flexor tendon distal insertion released. PIP lateral ligaments are progressively cut from volar to dorsal until PIP extension is obtained (Fig. 4). Several procedures are associated to keep a good fingertip. This procedure is indicated only when complex finger sequelae of injuries are present.

Carroll and Taber (1954) have reported 30 PIP arthroplasties without interposition and with K-wire distraction by elastic bands through a plaster. The tendons around the joint have not been injured.

Other reported various types of interposition for PIP joints: fascia lata (Payr 1914), fascia and periosteum (Hesse 1922), extensor tendons (Hellum and Vainio 1968), perichondrium (Engvist et al 1975, Skoog and Johansson 1976) and silastic sheet. The use of external fixation without interposition was also reported (Sokolow 1995).

Eaton and Malerich (1980) (Fig. 5a, b) reported a limited PIP arthroplasty by volar plate advancement and transosseous reattachment which is indicated for dorsal PIP subluxation or dislocation associated with a fracture–avulsion of the volar part of the base of the second phalanx.

Modified Tupper arthroplasty

The approach may be volar or dorsal.

The *volar approach* is of the Brüner type. The sheath and the A3 pulley are opened and the flexors tendons and neurovascular bundles are retracted, taking care to preserve the flexor tendon vincula. The volar plate is detached distally from the bony insertion at the base of the second phalanx and from the lateral borders along the joint. A subperiosteal elevation is then performed at the first phalanx since the volar plate is in continuity with the periosteum of the first phalanx (as has been proved with the total anterior tenoarthrolysis). This allows an easy advancement of the volar plate to perform the interposition. Resection of 1 cm of the distal bone of the first phalanx is performed and the bone remodelled in a rounded way. In this process, lateral ligaments are usually detached and are too short to be reattached proximally. There is no resection of the base of the second phalanx, except if realignment of the finger is indicated which cannot be corrected by the distal first phalanx resection. Osteotomy should be calculated and the proximal part of the second phalanx may be resected on a few millimetres. Two stitches are then passed at each lateral part of the distal volar plate. Volar plate advancement and interposition between the two phalanxes is then possible. Each stitch is passed lateral to the lateral bands of the extensor tendon apparatus and through the dorsolateral skin. The two stitches are passed through a button and sutured to each other (Fig. 6).

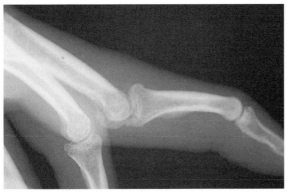
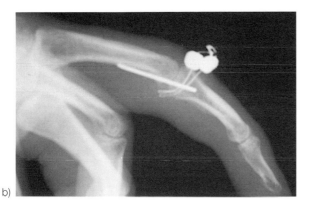
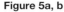

Figure 5a, b

Eaton-Malerich proximal interphalangeal (PIP) arthroplasty.

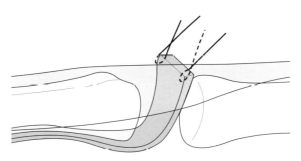

Figure 6

Modified Tupper arthroplasty with interposition of the volar plate.

A *dorsal approach* may be used if there is an associated dorsal procedure to be performed. In this case, subperiosteum elevation should be carefully performed before bone resection and distal volar plate detachment. The stitches are passed, if possible, proximal to the extensor tendon repair.

Prostheses

PIP prostheses provide worse results than MP prostheses. Swanson silastic prostheses are the only ones where large series with a long follow-up have been reported.

Approaches

The PIP joint is surrounded by extensor and flexor tendons and it is very difficult to attain the proper elements of the joint without cutting the extensor tendon dorsally or opening the flexor sheath and the volar plate volarly.

Different approaches have been described.

1 The *posterior approach* has been recommended by several authors:

   • transversal section of the extensor tendon: the section takes place 1 cm proximal to the PIP and the extensor apparatus is elevated distally

   • longitudinal section of the extensor tendon: the tendon is cut in the median axis and the central slip of the extensor tendon detached from its distal insertion

   • elevation of a triangular flap of the extensor tendon (Chamay 1988): a flap distally based at the level of the extensor central slip and including half of both lateral band is elevated and gives access to the joint (Fig. 7).

2 The *anterior approach*

   • cutting the A3 pulley, retracting the flexor tendons and elevating the volar plate.

Different types of prostheses are available:

(a) Implants type spacer: silicone prostheses: Swanson (Iselin and Pradet 1984), Sutter, Niebauer (Niebauer and Landry 1971)

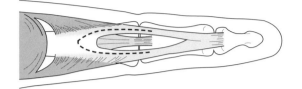

Figure 7

Chamay's dorsal proximal interphalangeal (PIP) approach.

(b) Prostheses: titanium–polyethylene or metal–metal

Technique

The premises are to work on the PIP joint without opening the flexor sheath and without cutting the extensor tendons. Closure of the skin should be made only with the finger in extension to prevent a retraction in flexion of the joint.

Postoperative care

As no tendons have been cut, postoperative active mobilization may be initiated as early as the third day (Fig. 8). This does depend on the type of proce-

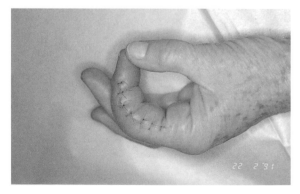

Figure 8

Early postoperative rehabilitation.

dure that has been performed, but is the case for arthrolysis or prosthesis insertion.

This approach should not be used if there is a particular procedure to perform on the extensor tendon apart from extensor tenolysis.

Approaches which cut the extensor tendon do not usually allow early active mobilization. We had to perform secondary extensor tenolysis when using a dorsal approach, even after early passive rehabilitation, and extensor tendon adhesions are frequent.

Whatever the approach used, a procedure on the PIP joint is then possible. Insertion of a prosthesis is made using the ancillary tools to prepare insertion of stems in the shaft.

Common problems to finger joint prostheses

(a) Mechanical complications are common to all types of prostheses: rupture, metal or silicone particles, wear and debris, displacements and dislocations, clinodactyly by displacement of the stems or rupture.

(b) The postoperative course is similar for all types of prostheses. Initially a good range of motion, realignment and pain relief. In the long term the range of motion decreases, deformity and pain recur. This course is partly explained by the 'sinking' of the prosthesis in the diaphysis, even with cemented stems. The joint space decreases and bone abutment leads to joint stiffness (Fig. 9).

(c) Other problems include:
   • the extensor tendons particularly if previously injured
   • skin coverage; if insufficient there may be a postoperative problem
   • periarticular structures which are as important as bone and joints
   • infection.

From the results, it may be said that the more the patient's strength, the more the prosthesis ruptures.

Research is always in progress and the aims are to obtain:

1 low friction between the two components and with the extensor tendons
2 osteoinductive properties around the stems avoiding metal wear and debris

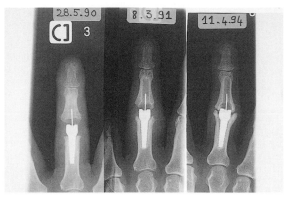

Figure 9

'Sinking' of a proximal interphalangeal (PIP) prosthesis in the diaphyses over the course of 4 years.

3 a better fit of the stem and to prevent the prosthesis sinking in the bone shaft
4 a better load distribution and stress patterns in the bone and surrounding joints.

The PIP joint is a very difficult joint and prevention of stiffness should be borne in mind each time this joint is injured.

References

Carroll RE, Taber TH (1954) Digital arthroplasty of the proximal interphalangeal joint, *J Bone Joint Surg* **36A**:912–20.

Chamay A (1988) A distally based dorsal and triangular flap for direct access to the proximal interphalangeal joint, *Ann Chir Main* **7**:179 83.

Eaton RG, Malerich MM (1980) Volar arthroplasty of the proximal interphalangeal joint: a review of ten years' experience, *J Hand Surg* **5**:260–8.

Engvist O, Johansson SH and Skoog T (1975) Reconstruction of articular cartilage using autologous perichondrial grafts. A preliminary report, *Scand J Plast Reconstr Surg* **9**:203–6.

Hellum C, Vainio K (1968) Arthroplasty of the metacarpophalangeal joints in rheumatoid arthritis with transposition of the interosseous muscles, *Scand J Plast Reconstr Surg* **2**: 139–43.

Hesse E (1922) Beitrage zur Frage der operativen Mobilisierung versteifter Fingergelengke, *Arch Klin Chir* **119**:1–12.

Iselin F, Pradet G (1984) Traitement des lésions enraidissantes des doigts par résection-arthroplastie IPP avec implant de Swanson. In: Tubiana R, ed. *Traité de Chirurgie de la Main*, 2nd edn. Masson: Paris: 937–49.

McCue FC, Honner R, Gieck JH, Andrews J, Hakala M (1975) A pseudo-boutonnière deformity, *Hand* **7**:166–70.

Mansat M, de la Caffinière JY, Delprat J, Bonnevialle P (1983) Post-traumatic stiffness of the fingers and its rehabilitation, *Rev Prat* **33**:429–35.

Niebauer JJ, Landry RM (1971) Dacron–silicone prosthesis for the metacarpophalangeal and intephalangeal joints, *Hand* **3**:55–61.

Payr E (1914) Weitere Erfahrungen über die operative Mobilisierung ankylosieter Gelenke mit Berücksichtigung des späteren Schicksals des Arthroplastik, *Dtsch Z Chir* **129**:341–463.

Saffar P, Rengeval JP (1978) Total anterior tenoarthrolysis. Treatment of fixed flexed deformity, *Ann Chir* **32**:579–82.

Skoog T, Johansson SH (1976) The formation of cartilage from free perichondrial grafts, *Plast Reconstr Surg* **57**:1–6.

Sokolow C (1995) Les nécroses articulaires de l'interphalangienne proximale: traitement par résection-distraction à l'aide du fixateur multicentrique MS3, *Ann Chir Main* **14**:202–6.

Watson HK, Light TR, Johnson TR (1979) Checkrein resection for flexion contracture of the middle joint, *J Hand Surg* **4A**:67–71.

41
Rehabilitation of the proximal interphalangeal joint

Patrice Morla

Proximal interphalangeal (PIP) joint stiffness is one of the most frequent consequences of hand and finger injuries. PIP stiffness may be:

- in extension when flexion is limited
- in flexion when extension is limited
- a combined limitation.

A functional range of motion (ROM) is situated between 25° and 75° and allows all types of prehension if metacarpophalangeal (MP) joints are normal.

Anatomical structures involved in stiffness may be:

- extra-articular:
  - skin: volar or dorsal injuries
  - extensor tendon adhesions
  - volar structures
  - para-articular fractures
- intra-articular:
  - volar plate
  - intra-articular fracture
  - sprains and dislocations
- neurosympathetic dystrophy accounts for 15% of the cases.

Rehabilitation

1 *Skin adhesions and scars* are treated by massage, making the skin slide like a glove on a finger. Ultrasound and cryotherapy treatments are combined with massage treatment. The goals are to make the skin supple so that it glides normally over the subcutaneous planes and to increase blood and lymphatic circulation. An elastic bandage is applied between sessions and especially at night (Coheban) (Fig. 1).

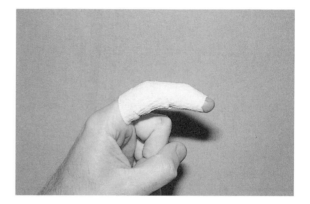

Figure 1

Treatment for skin adhesions and scars using an elastic bandage

2 *Passive motion of the joint*, reaching the maximum amplitude possible, is used against flexor and extensor tendon adhesions. Continuous passive motion maintains the ROM obtained during sessions. *Active motion* follows passive motion exercises in the same amplitude range and is useful for regaining normal tendon gliding. Electrostimulation may help. The use of 'buddy splints' combining active and passive motion is a useful technique which helps to decrease pain (Fig. 2).

3 *Dynamic splints* are indicated for capsuloligamentous stiffness in flexion or in extension. The dynamic splint is made of thermoplastic material. For the dynamic splint *in extension*, a gauntlet is used with a dorsal and volar bar to fix the MP at 45° of flexion and the P1, while a traction

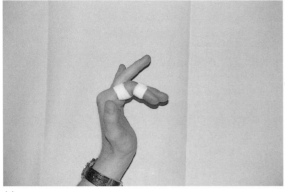

(a)

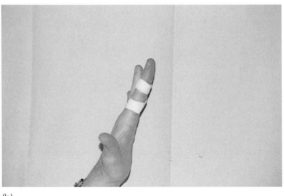

(b)

Figure 2

'Buddy splints' to work (a) the extension and (b) the flexion

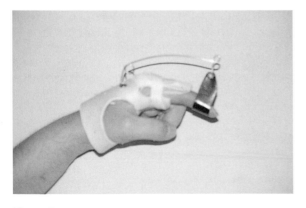

Figure 3

A dynamic splint for stiffness in extension

provided on P2 by a finger cuff attached to a spring wire is applied (Fig. 3). For the dynamic splint *in flexion*, a thermoplastic splint for the wrist and forearm is used. MP joints are maintained in extension by a bar applied on the middle part of P1. Biflex bandages are used for traction, first longitudinally and then transversally to regain complete flexion (Fig. 4). These splints are used sequentially; the duration and intervals for wearing each device depending on pain and oedema. It is important to use the splint sequentially, ie for 20 minutes every 2 hours rather than for longer periods of time.

Finger stiffness is a frequent complication of hand and finger injuries and preventive treatment is essential: after every trauma or surgery, immobilization should be comfortable and painless and not prolonged without a specific reason. The PIP joint should always be immobilized in extension. A fixed flexed deformity is often a significant problem at the PIP joint that is not always cured by surgery.

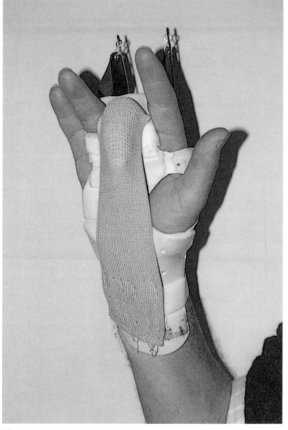

(a)

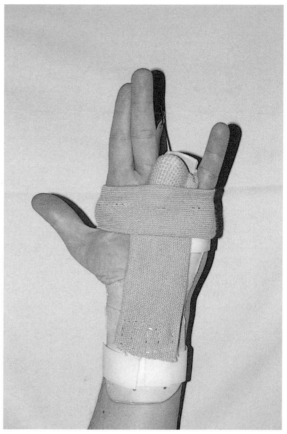

(b)

Figure 4

Biflex bandage (a) longitudinally and (b) transversely for regain of complete flexion

42
Stiffness of the thumb

Antonio Landi, Giuseppe Caserta, Antonio Saracino and Maria Cristina Facchini

Introduction

The definition of joint stiffness remains controversial. According to a new proposal, joint stiffness should be defined as a reduced range of motion in at least one of the three spatial planes. Stiffness may follow trauma or surgical procedures, and may be related to intrinsic or extrinsic causes, or both (Carreri et al 1995). Nonetheless, besides any accepted definition, the functional implications of stiffness of the first ray are almost invariably relevant.

The peculiarity of the thumb is reflected in its different etymology in Greek and Latin cultures. The Latin root for thumb derives from *polleo* ('to be strong'), which denotes its feature of strength; the Greek word is *anti-cheir*, which means 'opposed to the hand' and underscores the importance and functional autonomy of the thumb, based on a dynamic chain of joints, which makes the impact of thumb stiffness particularly severe (Tubiana 1986). The high workload of the thumb in everyday activities and some occupations is compromised if one of the three joint pairs, trapeziometacarpal (TM), metacarpophalangeal (MP), and interphalangeal (IP), has become painful and rigid. Considering the functional anatomy of the above mentioned joints, the TM must be retained as a directional articulation, and the MP (due to its unidirectional configuration and muscle attachments) as a joint of strength. Conversely, the IP plays a double role as the closing phase of the fist contributes to strength, but its integrity remains essential for precision tasks.

These basic considerations should be borne in mind when considering the functional repercussions due to stiffness of the joints of the thumb, in isolation or association. Paradoxically, painful stiffness of one or two joints can be rationally treated by arthrodesis. However, when stiffness of the three joints coexists, even in the absence of pain, normal functioning of the hand is impaired. This is seen with retroposition deformities of the TM and flexion deformity of the MP and IP joints. In contrast, fixation in anteposition of the TM and in neutral position of the MP may not involve a significant loss of function for everyday activities.

The TM joint deserves special consideration; it is a directional joint and should be preserved whenever possible. Stiffness of the TM joint, when the articular surfaces are intact, can be corrected by arthrolysis, which, however, is rarely performed because its surgical steps have not been clearly coded. If the degree of scarring of various tissues surrounding the thumb is severe, in the absence of functional muscles, one must nonetheless resort to arthrodesis of the TM (Tubiana 1986). Suspension arthroplasty and, at times, prostheses designed specifically for the TM joint have been proposed as an alternative to arthrodesis .

The first ray raises the problem of interrelated stiffness, as the more distal joint quite consistently becomes stiff following either an intra- or more often an extra-articular disorder of the proximal joint. When an associated stiffness has evolved, it can be assessed by goniometric evaluation of the individual joints of the first ray (Bostock and Morris 1993, Durham et al 1993) and especially by the simple clinical test of opposition and retroposition introduced by Kapandji in 1986.

As stiffness of the joints of the first ray might lead to severe functional impairment, some general guidelines should be followed when dealing with emergencies having intra-articular fractures or ligamentous injuries of the thumb:

- Internal fixation of intra-articular fractures should be anatomical and reliable so as to allow early mobilization of the affected and neighbouring joints.

- If the joints are not salvageable fusion should be performed in the first instance by a rigid and reliable fixation so as to encourage early passive and active motion.
- Capsular–ligamentous injuries mainly at the MP joints are best treated by intraosseous anchoring (Rehak et al 1994, Buch et al 1995, Carneiro and Kay Wjarnes 1995) as this surgical policy will allow, at least, an immediate mobilization of the neighbouring joints and early motion of the affected ones.
- When dealing with a crush or thermal injury or any other kind of physical trauma to the hand, soft tissues should be strictly monitored. Control of oedema by elevation is imperative, but soft tissue and muscular intracompartmental pressure should also be monitored (Esposito et al 1996) and fasciotomy promptly performed when needed to avoid intrinsic muscles and first web contracture. When consequent severe functional impairment occurs, sophisticated surgical procedures are available, but the original functional independence of the thumb might not be completely restored.

We will now examine the main causes of stiffness of the joints of the first ray separately, and due emphasis will be given to the factors which lead to interrelated stiffness of the entire segment (Landi et al 1995).

Stiffness of the trapeziometacarpal joint

Joint stiffness due to intrinsic causes

The TM, like other joints, is susceptible to joint effusion even in the absence of ligament lesions. This factor *per se* justifies the marked intra-articular synechia that we have observed at surgery when performing arthrolysis (Thomine 1986). Unfortunately, accurate ultrasound studies of this joint in recent trauma are not well coded. On the other hand, capsular–ligamentous lesions of the TM have been studied in detail, both by new radiological observations (Kapandji and Kapandji 1993) and especially by experimental studies (Imaeda et al 1994, Strauch et al 1994). The basic anatomy of the ligaments as described by Pieron (1973) has been confirmed by these authors. What has changed is the stabilizing role attributed to the oblique anterior ligament, dorsoradial ligament, and oblique posterior and intermetacarpal ligaments. Instability in acute dorsal dislocation was once thought to be tied to rupture of the anterior oblique ligament (Eaton and Littler 1973), but it is now assumed that the primary stabilizing structure is confined to the dorsal radial ligament (Imaeda et al 1994, Strauch et al 1994). Loosening of the anterior oblique ligament represents an epiphenomenon in chronic dorsal dislocation, and this might explain the inconsistent results of ligament reconstruction according to the Eaton technique (Eaton and Littler 1973). In our experience, stabilization by the above-mentioned method provided favourable results in four out of five patients; in one case of pure dorsal dislocation it did not resolve the stiffness and chronic dorsal instability.

Another cause of intrinsic stiffness of the TM is represented by articular fractures. When considering only the Bennet fracture, the general concept that true symptoms of post-traumatic arthritis of wrist and hand appear much later than those of the corresponding joints of the lower extremities holds true. In fact, in a medium term study with 10 year follow-up (Timmenga et al 1994), no problems with joint stiffness or significant differences between conservative or surgical treatment for this type of fracture were reported, even if the incidence of arthritis correlates well with the quality of the initial reduction. However, in a series with a mean follow-up of 26 years (Livesley 1990), which referred just to conservative treatment, the outcome deteriorated over time.

In a comparative study between direct osteosynthesis and extrafocal synthesis for fractures of the base of the first metacarpus, the group treated with internal fixation had statistically significant improvement in thumb opposition (Brazier et al 1996), though there were no significant differences from the radiological standpoint with the group treated with osteosynthesis. These recent studies seem to confirm the concept that anatomical reduction of a fracture is the best guarantee for long-standing favourable outcomes.

Intra-articular comminuted fractures at the base of the metacarpus or trapezium justify immediate arthrodesis for particular occupational activities, bearing in mind that the hand cannot be fully flattened in about 45% of treated patients and that handling of small objects may become difficult (Chamay and Piaget-Morerod 1994).

Joint stiffness due to extrinsic causes

The most frequent causes are related to the absence of preventive measures when dealing with paralysis of peripheral nerves, crush injuries and any kind of physical trauma to the hand. Contraction in adduction of the first web can be classified in a way similar to that of burns:

- in first degree contracture, retraction is limited to the skin
- in second degree contracture, this is mainly related to fibrotic retraction of the intrinsic muscles which, however, retain the potential for functional recovery

- in third degree contracture, the first web is 'frozen', and stiffness of the TM joint coexists.

This last occurrence will be discussed under the heading of interrelated stiffness, since there is simultaneous involvement of MP and IP joints (Zancolli 1979).

First degree contracture can be treated by simple skin plasties. In second degree lesions, skin contracture can be dealt with similarly or, if the retraction is confined to the deep structures, by a simple straightforward incision (Fig. 1). Release of the first web follows the sequence: detachment of the first dorsal interosseous muscle from the first metacarpus, Z-lengthening (Fig. 2) or reinsertion of the

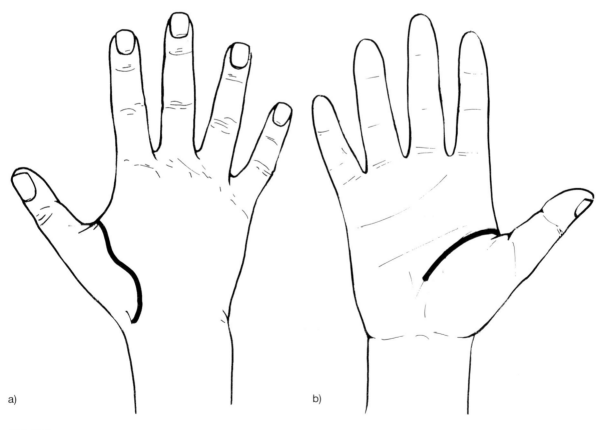

a)   b)

Figure 1

(a) The skin incision adopted when skin plasties are not needed for treatment of a first web contracture. (b) Volar incision used under the same circumstances.

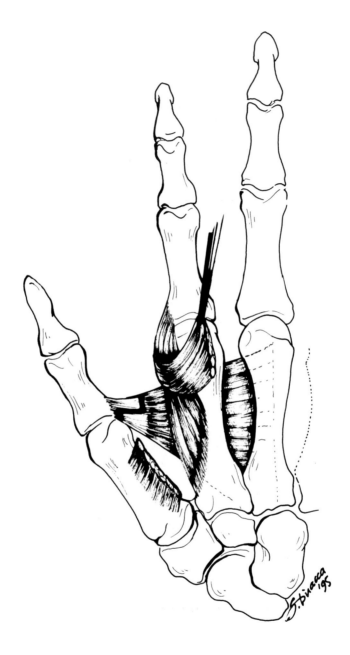

Figure 2

The first dorsal interosseous muscle has been detached from the metacarpus. The mild contracture of the adductor muscle can be dealt with by Z-lengthening of the myotendinous junction.

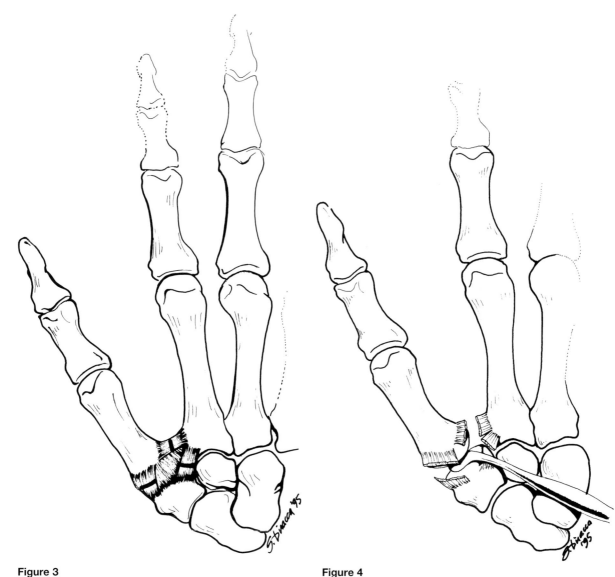

Figure 3

Further opening of the first web may be obtained by release of the first intermetacarpal ligament. The dorsal release of the TM joint is achieved by syndesmotomy of the dorsal-ulnar and dorsal radial ligaments. A complete dorsal capsulotomy should also be added.

Figure 4

The intrinsic stiffness of the TM joint represents the ultimate obstacle to obtaining full passive mobility of the first ray. Joint release is usually performed by a curved rougine. Care is taken not to damage the volar oblique ligament.

adductor muscle at a lower site, detachment of the flexor pollicis brevis. If full range of motion of the first ray is achieved, the procedure is completed. Conversely, if associated stiffness of the TM joint coexists, the following steps are performed in succession: syndesmotomy of the intermetacarpal liga-

ment and dorsal capsulotomy (Fig. 3). Finally, explorative arthrotomy allows removal of all intra-articular adherences (Fig. 4). When cutaneous reconstruction is required at the end of a complete

(Figure 5 follows)

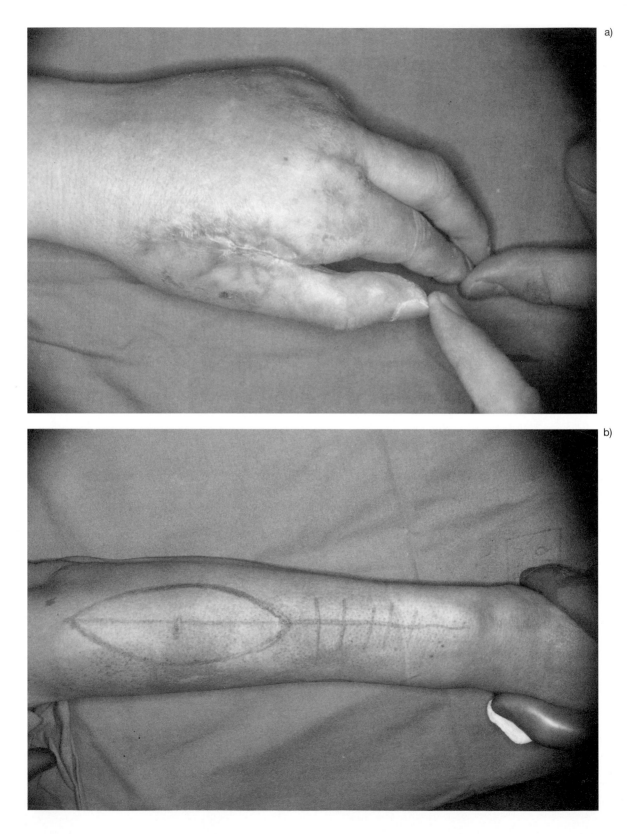

a)

b)

c)

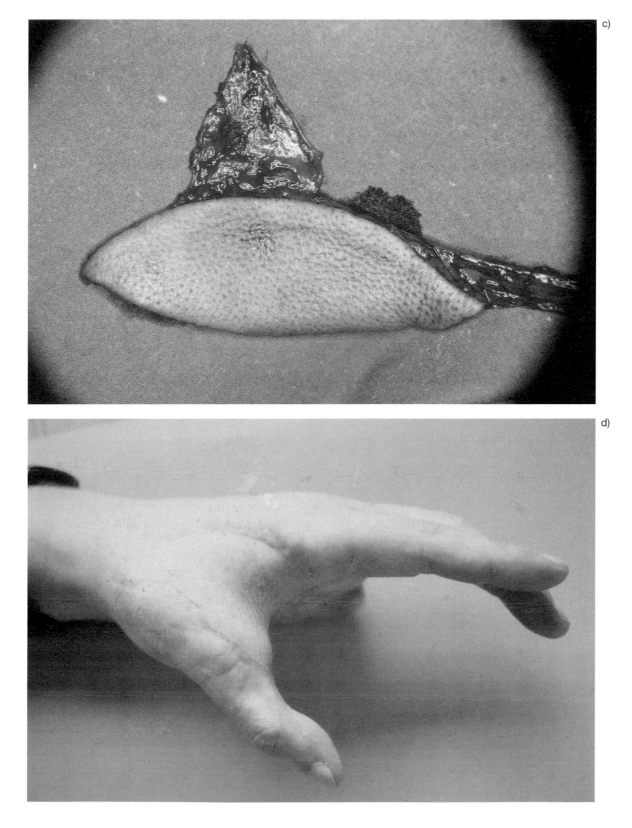

d)

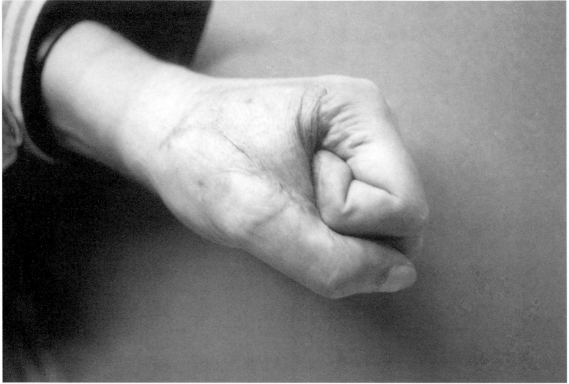

e)

Figure 5 *(contd)*

(a) Sequelae of a fireworks injury to the left hand of a 36-year-old man. The first web is completely 'frozen'. (b) A distally-based posterior interosseous flap is outlined to cover the skin defect that results from the surgical release of the web. (c) The flap has an elliptical shape and a fascial extension is included to cover the ulnar skin defect of the base of the thumb. All surgical steps of muscular, capsular and TM joint release have been performed in this case. (d), (e) Good functional results at 4 years follow-up. Some residual interrelated stiffness is still present at the MP and IP joints.

release of the first web, one must resort to reconstruction techniques that have evolved over the years from local, axial and free flaps (Soragni et al 1985) to the latest preference of regional flaps. An example is the distally based posterior interosseous flap (Fig. 5), which we have used in 70% of reconstructions of the first web (Landi et al 1991). Recently, in two patients where the communicating vessels of the posterior interosseous artery were found to be absent at surgery, the flap was successfully resecured by including a large fascial component nourished by the recurrent branches of the anterior interosseous artery.

Stiffness of the metacarpophalangeal joint of the thumb

Joint stiffness due to intrinsic causes

Painful post-traumatic stiffness, if readily predicted as the consequence of intra-articular fractures or complex trauma such as replantation of the thumb, can be prevented by performing immediate fusion. In dislocations, there is a marked difference in the functional outcomes between conservative and surgical treatment of the dorsal variant. If dislocation is reduced according to the Farabeuf manoeuvre (Sedel 1989) and the joint is stable after reduction, there are usually no sequelae. Instead, if dislocation is irreducible, stiffness of the MP joint often follows surgical reduction. Volar dislocation is much less common than the previous variant and leads to a certain, though not significant, degree of stiffness after both conservative and surgical treatment, even when emergency stabilizing techniques have been used for highly unstable lesions (Kohut et al 1994). Conversely, in lesions of the ulnar collateral ligament, the range of motion of the MP joint does not seem to be compromised after surgery (Bostock and Morris 1993).

In a revision of the case series by one surgeon in our Institution, this finding seems generally confirmed in 10 patients divided into subgroups where fixation of the ligament has been achieved by pull-out sutures (six patients) or Mitek fixation (four patients) (Table 1). Only cases one and four present a significant interrelated stiffness, and they both belong to the pull-out group. It appears that early mobilization as consented by intraosseous anchoring devices will lead to better functional outcomes.

The unfavourable cases belong to group IV or V of the Landi classification (Sacchetti et al 1990), and the stiffness, beyond any considerations on technique, may be related to a simultaneous lesion of the dorsal capsule and adhesions between this and the abductor extensor hood. Lesions of the radial collateral ligament are usually missed and are not treated in emergencies. In the chronic phase, surgery for reinsertion or ligament reconstruction might lead to asymptomatic joint stiffness (Durham et al 1993).

Joint stiffness due to extrinsic causes

The most frequent causes are related to adhesions subsequent to tenorrhaphy of the extensor and flexor tendons. For the flexor apparatus, this area is comprised in zone 2, or 'no man's land', and thus tenolysis becomes necessary in 10–30% of subjects, depending on the surgical and rehabilitative techniques used (Landi et al 1994).

In particular, flexion deformity of the MP as com-

Table 1 Stener lesion

Patient no./ age/ affected hand	Return to work (days)	Follow-up (years)	Flexion deficit MPJ[2]	Extension deficit MPJ[2]	Flexion deficit IPJ	Extension deficit IPJ	Interrelated stiffness MPJ + IPJ	Surgical procedure	Final judgment
1) right*38	–	1.3	−23°	−10°	−35°	−10°	78°	Pull-out	Good
2) right*48	40	6.5	+15°	−5°	+5°	+5°	20°	Pull-out	Very good
3) left*34	75	5.6	0°	0°	0°	0°	–	Pull-out	Very good
4) left*28	180	3.2	−20°	−40°	−5°	−10°	75°	Pull-out	Good
5) right*34	40	4	+15°	−12°	−10°	0°	17°	Pull-out	Very good
6) left*36	–	3.4	−20°	0°	−15°	0°	35°	Pull-out	Very good
7) right*17	60	1	0°	0°	−5°	0°	5°	Mitek	Very good
8) left*48	45	4 months	−10°	0°	0°	−25°	35°	Mitek	Good
9) right*39	21	3 months	0°	−30°	−20°	−5°	55°	Mitek	Good
10) right*46	120	2.4	+5°	−10°	−20°	+5°	20°	Mitek	Very good

[1]The deficit is related to the unaffected site
[2]MPJ = metacarpopharyngeal joint; IPJ = interphalangeal joint
*Dominant hand

plications of hand or thumb replantations often represents the sum of ischaemic retractions of the short flexor and adductor muscles and adhesions of the flexor apparatus.

Lastly, two particular aspects emerge concerning the complications of treatment of trigger finger. We have observed in adult patients with long-standing lesions that persistent pain after surgical release was related to a localized reflex sympathetic dystrophy (RSD) affecting the MP joint. The diagnosis has been confirmed by X-rays and resolved when causal treatment was undertaken.

In children, a boutonnière type deformity might be observed in very late follow-up, and it is probably connected to excessive release of the pulley system (Castaldi et al 1991, Zissimos 1994).

Stiffness of the interphalangeal joint of the thumb

In most cases, stiffness follows an apparently simple sprain of the joint which has, in effect, caused an often missed lateral dislocation. When the lesion becomes symptomatic, the dislocation cannot usually be reduced and arthrodesis is envisaged. The same reasoning holds for joint fractures, which follow the same fate, and may benefit from reconstructive treatment with possible preservation of joint function only when one surface is involved. Under these circumstances osteochondral transplant may allow recovery of a useful range of motion. With increasing frequency, within complex lesions of the thumb (injuries from fireworks, amputations, burns, etc.), we observe a flexion deformity of the distal phalanx even in the presence of an intact joint. In these cases, in addition to the procedure for skin reconstruction by local or regional flaps, volar plate release needs to be carried out, and lengthening of the flexor pollicis longus might also be needed. The overall correction following these sequential surgical steps will be maintained by nocturnal splinting holding the joint in neutral position for a minimum of 2 months.

Interrelated stiffness of the thumb

Rarely this is due to a simultaneous traumatic involvement of two joints of the same ray. In sports traumas, one may find a Stener lesion associated with some kind of injury located at TM joint (Sacchetti et al 1990). Conversely, interrelated stiffness is more frequently found in long-standing Stener lesions, where volar subluxation of the first phalanx occurs and is associated with contracture of the abductor and adductor extensor hoods, therefore limiting flexion of the distal phalanx. We have seen these deformities developing in manual workers and becoming painful over time. Treatment may consist of fusion of the MP joint and release of the dorsal hood with the aim of improving flexion of the distal phalanx.

Frequently, interconnected stiffness of the thumb is due to extrinsic causes. Recognition of the origin of the deformity and its correction may also resolve distal joint deformities, but this is not the rule.

In post-ischaemic contracture of the first web, the surgical approach to flexion deformities of the MP joint and extension deformity of the IP joint includes, as surgical steps beyond skin release, resection of the extensor hoods to improve flexion of the IP joint.

In spasticity, which might broadly be considered an extrinsic type of stiffness of the upper limb, a relatively common fracture is represented by the association of retropulsion with dislocation of the TM joint and flexion deformity of the IP joint. At the TM joint we recommend fusion in a functional position, but tenotomy of the tendons of the first dorsal compartment must be added to prevent the risk of a delayed consolidation of fusion due to the underlying muscle spasticity. Likewise, flexion deformity of the thumb should be managed by myotendinous lengthening and adductor release.

These are some of the most frequent examples of interrelated stiffness of the first ray which, however, are rarely seen by the specialist. Incredibly, most isolated and interrelated thumb stiffness is still due to the surgeon's complete lack of knowledge of the available rehabilitation options. This knowledge cannot therefore be transmitted to the rehabilitation team, which is especially important when they are dealing with patients who need to be convinced that they do not have to delegate their functional recovery for reintegration into work and social life to others.

Acknowledgements

The authors acknowledge their gratitude to Dr John M Pradelli for assisting in the English revision.

References

Bostok S, Morris MA (1993) The range of motion of the MP joint of the thumb following operative repair of the ulnar collateral ligament, *J Hand Surg* **18B**:710–11.

Brazier J, Moughabghab M, Migaud H, Fontaine C, Elia A, Tillie B (1996) Les fractures articulaires de la base du premier métacarpien, *Ann Chir Main* **15**:91–8.

Buch BD, Innis P, McClinton A, Kotani Y (1995) The Mitek mini G2 suture anchor: biomechanical analysis of use in the hand, *J Hand Surg* **20A**:877–81.

Carneiro RS, Kay Wjarnes RN (1995) PA-C: The use of bone anchors in hand surgery. In: *6th Congress of the International Federation of Societies for Surgery of the Hand, Helsinki, Finland*, 3–7 July 1995.

Carreri G, Di Leo P, Santucci A, Barbarella R (1995) Le rigidità articolari post-traumatiche e post-chirurgiche: definizione, classificazione, eziopatogenesi. *Giornale Ital Ortop Traumatol* **XXI**(suppl):13–16.

Castaldi G, Amelio E, Testoni R, Cugola L (1991) Il dito a scatto nel bambino, *Riv Ita Chir Mano* **28**:247–50.

Chamay A, Piaget-Morerod F (1994) Arthrodesis of the trapeziometacarpal joint, *J Hand Surg* **19B**:489–97.

Durham JW, Suheil Khuri, Myung Hyo Kim (1993) Acute and late radial collateral ligament injuries of the thumb metacarpophalangeal joint, *J Hand Surg* **18A**:232–7.

Eaton RG, Littler JW (1973) Ligament reconstruction for the painful thumb carpometacarpal joint, *J Bone Joint Surg* **55A**:1665–6.

Esposito M, Caserta G, Saracino A, Barca F, Landi A (1996) La misurazione della pressione intracompartimentale nella sindrome compartimentale acuta. In: Gagg A, ed. *Progressi in Medicina e Chirurgia del Piede: Le Sindromi Compartimentali Acute Della Gamba e Del Piede, Vol. 5.* Bologna: 55–62.

Imaeda T, Glen Niebur, Kai-Nan An, Cooney III WP (1994) Kinematics of the trapeziometacarpal joint after sectioning of ligaments, *J Orth Res* **12**:205–10.

Kapandji A (1986) Cotation clinique de l'opposition et de la contre-opposition du pouce, *Ann Chir Main* **5**:67–73.

Kapandji II TG, Kapandji AI (1993) Nouvelles données radiologiques sur la trapézometacarpienne, *Ann Chir Main* **12**:263–4.

Kohut M, Droz C, Della Santa (1994) La dislocation palmaire de la metacarpo-phalangienne du pouce, *Ann Chir Main* **13**:50–5.

Landi A, Luchetti R, Soragni O, De Santis G, Sacchetti GL (1991) The distally based posterior interosseus island flap for the coverage of skin loss of the hand, *Ann Plast Surg* **27**:257–536.

Landi A, Cavana R, Caserta G, Esposito M, De Luca S, Stacca R (1994) Il punto sulla tenolisi dei tendini flessori nella zona 2, *Giornale Ital Ortop Traumatol* **20**:347–58.

Landi A, Caserta G, Saracino A, Facchini MC (1995) Le rigidità del primo raggio, *Giornale Ital Ortop Traumatol* **XXI**(suppl):205–10.

Livesley PJ (1990) The conservative management of Bennett's fracture-dislocation: a 26-year follow-up, *J Hand Surg* **15B**:291–4.

Pieron AP (1973) The mechanism of the first metacarpal joint, *Acta Orthop Scand* **148**(suppl):7–104.

Rehak DC, Sotereanos DG, Bowman MV, Herndon JH, Pittsburgh PA (1994) The Mitek bone anchor: application to the hand, wrist and elbow, *J Hand Surg* **19A**:853–60.

Sacchetti GL, De Luca S, Alfarano M, De Santis G, Landi A (1990) La lesione intraarticolare del legamento collaterale ulnare del pollice, *Atti SERTOT* **XXXII**:59–64.

Sedel L (1989) Luxations de l'articulation métacarpophalangienne du pouce et des doigts. In: Tubiana R, ed. *Traitè de Chirurgie de la Main.* Vol. 2. Masson: Paris: 790–6

Soragni O, Luchetti R, Landi A (1985) Il lembo libero della prima commissura del piede nella ricostruzione del primo spazio della mano, *Riv Chir Mano* **22**:403–6.

Strauch RJ, Behrman MJ, Rosenwasser MP (1994) Acute dislocation of the carpo-metacarpal joint of the thumb: anatomic and cadaver study, *J Hand Surg* **19A**:93–8.

Timmenga EJF, Blokhuis TJ, Maas M, Raaijmakers ELFB (1994) Long-term evaluation of Bennett's fracture, *J Hand Surg* **19B**:373–7.

Thomine JM (1986) Raideurs de l'articulation trapèzometacarpienne et retractions posttraumatiques de la commissure du pouce. In: Tubiana R, ed. *Traitè de Chirurgie de la Main.* Vol 2. Masson: Paris: 958–65

Tubiana R (1986) *Traitè de Chirurgie de la Main.* Masson: Paris:

Zancolli E (1979) *Structural and Dynamic Bases of Hand Surgery.* Lippincott: Philadelphia.

Zissimos AG, Szabo RM, Yinger KE, Sharkey NA (1994) Biomechanics of the thumb flexor pulley system, *J Hand Surg* **19A**:475–9.

43
Stiffness of the base of the thumb

Giorgio A Brunelli and Giovanni R Brunelli

Stiffness of the basal joint of the thumb is a severe impairment as thumb mobility is essential to hand function. Stiffness may be partial or complete, painful or not, and more or less disabling according to the spatial position of the stiff metacarpal. Causes of stiffness may be articular or extra-articular (Curtis 1984, Saffar 1990).

Articular lesions may be arthritic, traumatic, infectious or congenital. An incomplete ankylosis may be very painful, but a complete one may be very disabling if it is fixed in a bad position (i.e. adduction). In contrast stiffness in mild abduction–opposition may be fairly well tolerated and is even searched for (arthrodesis) in painful arthritis for young labourers doing heavy work.

Extra-articular causes depend on skin, intrinsic muscle, fascia and extrinsic tendon retractions or scar substitution following open lesions, infections, ischaemias, long-lasting immobilization and any kind of swelling. Stiffness due to soft tissue retraction is often more disabling than that due to joint lesions. In fact, as aforementioned, stiffness of the carpometacarpal (CM) joint in a good position is often painless and well tolerated.

This is not the place to describe the anatomy and the infinite anatomical variations of the trapeziometacarpal (TM) joint and musculo-tendineous units. Nevertheless, we want to recall that the 1st intermetacarpal space has a variable geometry and can be completely annulled, being responsible (with its plasticity) for the most specialized movement of the hand: the opposition. Morphological and functional abnormalities of the 1st space may be due to retraction or complete scar substitution of the soft tissues contained in it. The 1st metacarpal is retracted in adduction and supination with flexion in the metacarpophalangeal joint (MPJ) depending on the muscle retraction, whereas in the fixed adduction of the first metacarpal due to articular alter-ations of the trapeziometacarpal joint, the MPJ is generally in hypertension (for compensation).

Aetiology

Causes of soft tissue (*extra-articular*) stiffness are traumatic or non-traumatic lesions of skin, muscles and fascias (Chanson and Michon 1979, Apoil et al 1982, Masquelet 1992). Traumatic agents may be mechanical, thermal or chemical (Rousso 1975). Non-traumatic lesions are infections, Dupuytren's disease, connectivitis (sclerodermia), arthrogryposis, spastic palsies (with the typical thumb-in-palm), ischaemia (Volkmann, Finocchietto syndromes) and oedema. Also a prolonged incorrect immobilization may lead to skin, muscle, fascia and ligament retractions which are often iatrogenic. Furthermore, we must consider congenital malformation (syndactyly of the 1st and 2nd ray, muscular anomalies or agenesis) (Rushforth 1949). Very seldom stiffness in abduction–supination occurs due to scar retraction of the laterovolar skin or of the adductor pollicis brevis (APB) muscle.

Articular lesions producing stiffness of the base of the thumb (Forestier 1937, Kuhlmann 1987, Brunelli et al 1988, Ebelin 1993, Kadiyala et al 1996) are: sequelae of intra-articular fractures, rhizarthrosis at the last stage, some types of arthritis and pyogenic osteoarthritis (occasionally due to intra-articular injections). Stiffness is more disabling (and painful) when arthritis involves not only the trapeziometacarpal joint but also the scapho-trapezio (and trapeziotrapezoid) joint (panarthritis or peritrapezium arthritis).

Even a total ankylosis given by an arthrodesis may prove uncomfortable or disabling for the patient, or it can give, after years, painful scaphotrapezial arthritis and require surgery. In general, the rhizarthrosis at stage 3+ and 4 gives stiffness in adduction, which is the disabling position, and requires progressive hyperextension of the MP joint. Adduction becomes progressively irreducible introducing the Z deformity of the thumb. Surgery may involve the soft tissues (often including TM capsulotomy) or TM joint (seldom requiring soft tissue release).

Soft tissue surgery

Treatment of 1st web retractions must consider: 1, release of the 1st metacarpal; 2, repair (motor reanimation and skin coverage) (Masquelet 1992).

Release

This must involve the skin, the superficial and deep palmar and the deep dorsal aponeurosis, the muscles and often the trapeziometacarpal capsule which is generally secondarily retracted. From the onset the approach must take into consideration the type of final skin repair (Z plasty, local rotational flap or free or pedicled flap).

After skin and deep dorsal fascia opening, two conditions may occur: 1, the muscular tissue looks normal; 2, no muscles are left and only a scar block is present.

In the first case, the 1st interosseous insertion on the 1st metacarpal is detached. The underlying deep volar fascia is cut longitudinally taking care to spare the radial artery. If the abduction–opposition of the 1st metacarpal is not yet possible, the transverse bundle of the adductor pollicis is detached from the 2nd and 3rd metacarpals. If necessary the deep part of the short thumb flexor is also cut. A tenolysis of the extrinsic muscles or their lengthening at the musculotendineous junction may even be necessary.

In the second case removal of the scar may be done only up to complete mobilization of the 1st metacarpal. Immobilization in forced antepulsion (abduction–opposition) must follow for 4 weeks.

Repair

This must consider skin coverage and sensory–motor reanimation. Various procedures may be used in isolation or combined:

(a) Z-plasty or derived-plasty (VYZZ) is useful for web retraction with intact or fairly good skin.
(b) Local rotational flap from the dorsal aspect of the base of the index finger or from the dorsal aspect of the thumb.
(c) Sometimes the index finger may be sacrificed and all its dorsal skin used to reconstruct the skin of the web. It gives sensory coverage and allows deepening of the web.
(d) Distant flap (mainly the McGregor groin flap): currently seldom used due to its thickness. The 'cross-arm'-plasty may supply very good skin from the anterior aspect, but this flap is also seldom used due to the inconvenience of arm immobilization for 4 weeks.
(e) Pedicled flaps: Chinese flap: seldom used today due to the sacrifice of the radial artery.
(f) Dorsal interosseous flap: the most used nowadays (Scheker et al 1988).
(g) Free flaps: lateral arm flap and in some cases dorsalis pedis flap with the skin of the 1st web of the foot.

The use of free flaps requires more skill and implies a percentage of failures. It is generally used in units with extensive microsurgical experience. The dorsalis pedis free flap also fulfils the sensory reconstruction goal.

Motor reconstruction of adduction and abduction–opposition is obtained in a second stage by classical tendon transfer techniques.

Articular surgery

Surgery for articular stiffness includes:

1 Resection of the trapezium (partial or total) (Magnusson et al 1985) Burton and Pellegrini 1986, Brunelli et al 1989, Schernberg 1990, Brunelli and Brunelli 1991, Kleinmann and Eckenrode 1991, Nylen et al 1993, Young and Nemecek 1994,
2 Interpositional resection arthroplasty (Eaton et al 1985)
3 Silicon rubber spacer arthroplasty (Swanson et al 1981)
4 Cardan silicone replacement (Kapandji 1990)
5 Partial replacement (plastic or metallic)
6 Total replacements (de la Caffinière 1984, Chaise et al 1994, Mele 1996)

Different types: metal to metal
                metal to plastic
                constrained or not

7 Osteotomies to improve the position of the stiff 1st metacarpal when arthroplasty cannot be done (Molitor et al 1991)
8 Arthrodesis when TM stiffness is incomplete and painful in young labourers doing heavy work (Kwarnes and Reikeras 1985)

Trapezometacarpal surgery may be done through various approaches, mainly:

1 dorsal approach in between the abductor pollicis longus (APL) and extensor pollicis longus (EPL) when surgery involves the extensor carpi radialis longus (ECRL) tendon
2 the lateral approach above the APL (in between APL and extensor pollicis brevis, EPB)
3 volar approach (curved incision) on the base of thenar eminence (includes the proximal detachment of thenar muscles from their insertion)
4 anterior approach (Le Viet et al 1996) along the ulnar aspect of flexor carpi radialis (FCR) tendon (includes the severance of the volar carpal transverse ligament and follows the FCR tendon up to its insertion on the base of the 2nd metacarpal)

All these incisions are often modified by the different authors by means of bayonet-like course in order to reach the different tendons.

Resection of the trapezium was first done by Gervis (1949). Good results were presented. Subsequently, various authors suggested varied techniques of total or partial trapeziectomy with or without interposition of autologous soft tissue (tendon, fascia lata, fat tissue) or alloplastic materials such as Goretex (Young and Nemecek 1994).

A simple resection of the trapezium gives instability of the thumb with recession of the 1st metacarpal which often becomes painful due to the impingement of its base with the scaphoid. To avoid this impingement, either interpositional arthroplasty or stabilization using tendon slips (by different techniques) or both simultaneously are used (Brunelli et al 1989, Nylen et al 1993). The interpositional material is often tendon, the so-called 'anchovy' procedure. The tendon is rolled up like an 'anchovy' or a ball and interposed between the 1st metacarpal and the scaphoid. The fascia lata has also been used to provide a sufficient amount of fibrous tissue to be interposed.

Whatever the technique of interposition and stabilization it is important to spare the capsule when removing the trapezium. The capsule may be cut longitudinally or by means of an H-shaped incision in order to allow the capsule to be closed at the end of the operation. Trapeziectomy either in 'monobloc' or piecemeal must spare both the capsule and the tendon of the deep FCR. When removing the trapezium special care must be taken to remove all its medial osteophytes to avoid residual dislocation and painful impingement. Also, any osteophytes of the base of the metacarpal must be removed.

Simple interposition arthroplasty with a tendon anchovy has proved unable to prevent the recession of the metacarpal. Revision surgery has shown that the interposed soft tissue often disappeared with painful impingement. Therefore 'stabilization' of the base of the metacarpal or its 'suspension' by means of a tendon passed through the bones in various ways are done by most surgeons either in isolation or in combination with interposition. Stabilization may be achieved by techniques originally conceived for stabilizing the base of the thumb (without removal of the trapezium) or by techniques which were especially introduced for resection–interposition with tendon stabilization.

These techniques are:

(a) Epping's technique (Saffar 1990) is the simplest. A slip of FCR (left inserted distally to the base of the 2nd metacarpal) is passed through the base of the 1st metacarpal (Fig. 1a).
(b) Eaton and Littler's technique (Eaton et al 1985). A slip of the FCR tendon is passed through a tunnel pierced in the volar–dorsal direction in the base of the 1st metacarpal: the tendon slip is passed under the APL, then under and around the remaining FCR and eventually sutured to the fibrous tissues of the radial aspect of the capsule (Fig. 1b).
(c) Lanz (Saffar 1990) uses a very similar technique. The only variant consists in the final suture of the tendon slip around the APL (Fig. 1c).
(d) Kleinmann (Kleinmann and Eckenrode 1991) uses a slip of the FCR which is passed several times in and out, around the APL and FCR (without any perforation of the base of the metacarpal) (Fig. 1d).
(e) Magnusson et al (1985) again use a slip of the FCR first passed under the carpal transverse ligament then through a tunnel pierced in the base of the first metacarpal in the radioulnar

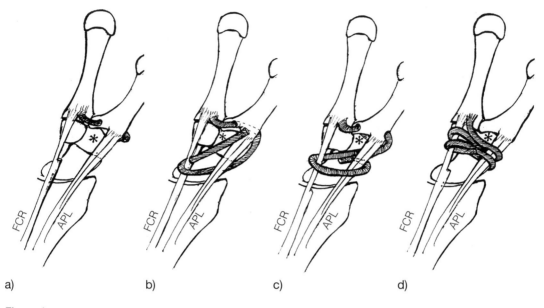

a)   b)   c)   d)

Figure 1

a   Epping's technique
b   Eaton and Littler's technique
c   Lanz's technique
d   Kleinmann's technique

direction, then under the slip itself at the base of the 2nd metacarpal and sutured on itself at the base of the 1st metacarpal (Fig. 2a).

(f) Burton and Pellegrini (1986) use a slip of FCR after removal of the trapezium and the base of the 1st metacarpal. The slip is introduced from the resection surface and goes out to the radial aspect of the base of the metacarpal. It is then rolled up like a ball and put as a spacer in the cavity left by the trapeziectomy. The authors add the proximal transfer of the EPB (Fig. 2b). Nylen et al (1993) modified Burton and Pellegrini's technique in various ways without resecting the base of the 1st metacarpal. Nigst (and then Shernberg 1990) use a very similar technique which does not resect the base of the metacarpal but passes the slip throughout a transverse tunnel. Other authors use a free ten-

don graft: the palmaris longus acting as an 'anchovy'.

(g) Jones (Saffar 1990) passes the graft in a tunnel at the base of the metacarpal and sutures it to itself after passing it around the FCR (Fig. 2c).

(h) Chaise et al (1994) use practically the same technique of stabilization, but they add more interpositional material (Fig. 2d).

All the above-mentioned techniques use a volar approach in order to reach the FCR tendon.

(i) In contrast Thompson (Saffar 1990) (Fig. 3a) uses a dorsal approach and takes the tendon of the APL, a slip of which is passed first through the base of the 1st metacarpal from which it goes out dorsally and then through the base of the 2nd metacarpal, to reach and transfix the ECRL.

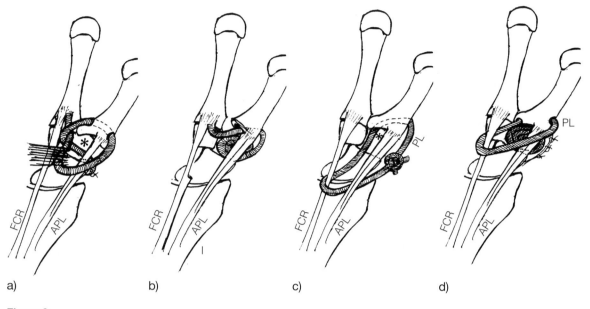

a)   b)   c)   d)

Figure 2

a   Magnusson's technique
b   The technique of Burton and Pellegrini
c   Jones's technique
d   The technique of Chaise et al

(j) Martini (Saffar 1990) uses a dorsal approach and uses a slip of the ECRL for stabilization.

All these methods have in my opinion some drawbacks:

• a certain difficulty in performing the operation
• the construction of neoligaments different from the anatomic ones
• a high ratio of failure or of fair results (declared by the authors themselves)
• some postoperative stiffness common to all of them.

With the goal of reconstructing the most important anatomic ligament (the interosseous or beak ligament) while preserving the normal range of movements by means of a simple and easy opera-

tion, we have studied and perfected a surgical protocol which uses one of the various tendons of the so-called APL for stabilization and another one for interposition (leaving at least one tendon for abduction to avoid postoperative adduction of the thumb) (Fig. 3b).

Our technique (Brunelli et al 1988 and 1989) is as follows: radial approach along the APL tendon, 7 cm long. The sensory branches of the radial nerve are recognized and protected. There is much anatomical variability of the tendons. Very seldom only one big tendon of the APL muscle is found. In a recent anatomical research on 100 hands we found one tendon in only two cases and 24 different patterns of insertion of several tendons (up to seven).

Insertions are multiple: 100% on the base of the 1st metacarpal (one, two or three tendons), 72% on

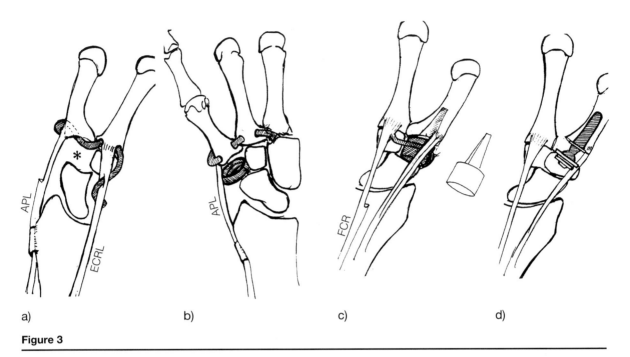

a)   b)   c)   d)

Figure 3

a   Thompson's technique
b   The Brunelli technique
c   Swanson's implants
d   De la Caffinière's prosthesis

the trapezium (one or two tendons), 60% on one of the thenar muscles (more frequently the APB but also the opponens muscle) (Brunelli and Brunelli 1991). We found that when the insertion on the trapezium is present it is rare to have arthritis occurring, while when it is not present the frequency of arthritis at a certain age is very high. In fact, the absence of this *normal* insertion produces a harmful shearing effect on the TM joint.

Two of these tendons are cut 7 cm proximal to this distal insertion. As mentioned above, one abductor tendon must be spared to avoid the possibility of a very disabling adduction of the 1st metacarpal. The cut tendons are pulled distally out of the 1st dorsal compartment of the wrist (sparing the pulley). One is severed at its distal insertion and will serve as an 'anchovy', the other one is pulled distally and will be used for stabilization. As we said

before, the trapezium bone is removed piecemeal leaving all the capsule in place.

The selected tendon (or slip of tendon) is gently pulled distally and 5–6 mm of cortical bone of the base of the metacarpal are freed by scalpel to allow the passage of the drill. The distal insertion must be spared.

A tunnel of 3 mm diameter is pierced throughout the base of the 1st metacarpal parallel to its articular surface in the direction of the base of the 2nd metacarpal where the beak ligament attaches. The base of the 2nd metacarpal is also pierced. The drill exits at the dorsal aspect of the base of the metacarpal. A second small incision of the skin is done at this point. The drill must have a button-hole on its point. A nylon thread is passed through the button-hole and withdrawn to the entrance point of the drill serving to pull the tendon, taken by a slip

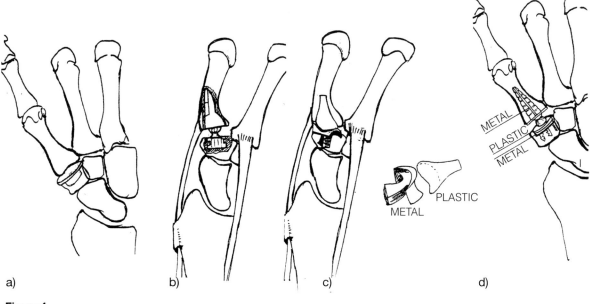

a)   b)   c)   d)

Figure 4

a   Ashworth's discs
b   The Mayo prosthesis
c   Linscheid's prosthesis
d   The prosthesis of Bedeschi and Mele

knot, throughout the two tunnels.

The stump of the tendon is pulled while keeping the first metacarpal in abduction–opposition and sutured to the fibrous tissues of the base of the 2nd metacarpal (capsule and even the distal insertion of ECRL). The other tendon, which had been selected for 'anchovy', is moulded by two crossed injection needles with various sutures to maintain the shape, and is put in the empty space left by trapezium removal. To keep the 'anchovy' in place, one stitch is made to take the FCR tendon into the depths with more stitches applied to the capsule. A K-wire is passed transversally through the shafts of the 1st and 2nd metacarpal in opposition–abduction for 30 days.

Partial implants

These have been almost completely abandoned due to the great number of failures. We can list only the plastic discs (Ashworth et al 1977) (Fig. 4a). The plugs consist of a convex plastic disc with a stem to be implanted in the base of the metacarpal and the metallic implants.

Total implants (replacements)

• Silicone rubber implants (spacers): first described by Swanson in 1972 (Fig. 3c).
  This is a thick plug of silicon rubber which must take all the space left free by trapeziectomy and is fixed into the base of the 1st metacarpal by a

stem after removal of the articular cartilage. The approach is dorsal and the capsule reconstruction is meticulous with reinforcement by a slip of FCR. Similar implants made of titanium have been suggested. Nye and Eaton (Saffar 1990) suggested a silicone implant with a tunnel to allow associated ligamentoplasties. The silicone implant was also prepared with Dacron coating to allow integration with the scar.

- Soft cardan silicone implant of Kapandji (1990).

It has two degrees of freedom and two stems: one to be introduced into the resected base of the 1st metacarpal and the other in the trapezium which must be partially removed.

Total replacement

De la Caffinière (1984) (metal to plastic retaining, total replacement) (Fig. 3d). The metacarpal component is made of chromo-cobalt alloy and has a 5.5 mm diameter head which is joined to a 10 mm diameter polyethylene cup to be cemented into the trapezium. The original design has been modified during the years. The idea is good and the manufacture very precise. Nevertheless the small dimensions of the trapezium and its structure and mineral stock alterations often allow loosening. Also the stem often becomes loose with reabsorption of the metacarpal shaft.

The Guepar total replacement (Alnot) (Saffar 1990) is very similar to de la Caffinière's. The two components however cannot be separated and must be cemented at the same time. The stem has some circular furrows. Also the Guepar prosthesis has the same drawbacks as de la Caffinière one.

Another cemented prosthesis has been used at the Mayo Clinic (Saffar 1990) (Fig. 4b).

Ledoux (Saffar 1990) has used an uncemented prosthesis with a self-locking metacarpal component and a trapezial component containing a polyethylene cup and having six tongues which automatically diverge when inserting the cup, thus obtaining a pretty good anchorage.

Beckenbaugh et al (in press) have recently presented a plastic to metal cemented prosthesis with anatomical reconstruction of the joint shape (Fig. 4c).

Bedeschi and Mele have proposed a tripodal prosthesis (Mele 1996) which get its anchorage in the trapezium by means of three feet (Fig. 4d).

There may be local or general individual reasons which exclude the trapeziectomy and interpositional arthroplasty. In these cases the surgeon may perform either a surgical fusion in abduction–opposition which eliminates scarce but painful residual movements, or an osteotomy (Molitor et al 1991) at the base of the metacarpal which opens the 1st space, restituting the grip and grasp capacity.

Associated surgical procedures

When a long-lasting adduction has caused MP hyperextension (more than 40%) a volar capsuloplasty must be done by suturing the volar plate to the bone with temporary fixation in moderate flexion by means of a K-wire. If the interphalangeal (IP) joint of the thumb is hyperflexed (in a Z deformity) this joint must be fixed in very slight flexion (8–10°). If the hyperextension is less than 40° a simple transfixion of the MP joint in flexion may be done with the goal to obtain MP joint stiffness in moderate flexion. Flexion should be maintained for 4–8 weeks according to the severity of the hyperextension.

When the soft tissues of the 1st metacarpal space are retracted as a result of long-lasting stiffness of the TM joint in adduction, disinsertion of the adductor pollicis or of the 1st interosseous from the 3rd and 2nd metacarpal have to be done. This disinsertion has to be preferred to distal tenotomies. Disinserted muscles may spontaneously get reinsertion on the aponeurosis with faster recovery of the muscular function.

Critical consideration comparing the various surgical procedures (Connolly and Roth 1993)

We have already mentioned the drawbacks of simple trapeziectomy. Trapeziectomy associated with interposition and ligamentoplasty allows restitution of mobility and almost complete absence of pain to the thumb with slight differences depending on the different techniques.

For many of these techniques the drawbacks are the constant diminution of strength and the slowness in getting the result. Sympathetic reflex dystrophy seems to be more frequent when a volar approach through the carpal tunnel is used. Furthermore, at long-term control there is generally a severe diminution of the space between the base of the 1st metacarpal and the trapezium with a relapse of pain and even of Z deformity.

The Swanson (or other silicone) implants can supply very good results provided that the surgery has been meticulous and correct in reconstructing the capsule and reinforcing it by means of a slip of FCR. At long-term control anyway the implant shows wear especially of the medial–proximal part with instability and subluxation. Furthermore, the tiny debris produce the so-called siliconitis – a proliferation of invasive granulation tissue which invade the surrounding bones and provokes pseudocysts and partial destruction of the bone.

Total replacements have the advantage of providing quick results with total painless recovery of the normal range of movements, but there are some difficult technical details, and a sound trapezium bone is required. Mobilization or fragmentation of the trapezium is frequent, as well as fractures or dislocation of the implant.

Overall, at present the most suitable operation seems to be resection arthroplasty provided that the stabilization is effective in avoiding proximal recession of the 1st metacarpal.

References

Apoil A, Karren C, Augerau B, Papin P (1982) Pathogénie du syndrome de Volkmann de la 1ère commissure de la main, *Ann Chir Main* **3**:210–13.

Ashworth R, Blatt G, Chuinard RG, Stark HM (1977) Silicon rubber interposition arthroplasty of the carpometacarpal joint of the thumb, *J Hand Surgery* **2A**:345–57.

Beckenbaugh RD Cooney WP, Linscheid RL (in press) Metacarpophalangeal surface replacement prosthesis: a randomised, prospective clinical trial.

Brunelli GA, Brunelli GR (1991) El musculo abductor del carpo, *Rev Espanola Cirug Mano* **18**:47–53.

Brunelli GA, Monini L, Brunelli F (1988) Stabilizzazione della trapeziometacarpale nella rizartrosi, *G It Ort e Traum* **14**:371–6.

Brunelli GA, Monini L, Brunelli F (1989) Stabilization of the trapeziometacarpal joint, *J Hand Surg* **14B**:209–12.

Burton RI, Pellegrini VD (1986) Surgical management of basal joint arthritis of the thumb. Part II. Ligament reconstruction with tendon interposition arthroplasty, *J Hand Surg* **11A**:324–32.

Chaise F, Friol JP, Gaisne E, Bellemere P (1994) Les arthroplasties de stabilization interposition dans les lesions arthrosiques péri-trapéziennes, *Ann Chir Main* **13**:153–61.

Chanson L, Michon J (1979) Corrections plastiques des retractions de la commissure du pouce, *Ann Chir* **33**:689–95.

Connolly WB, Roth S (1993) Revision procedures for complications of surgery of osteoarthritis of the carpometacarpal joint of the thumb, *J Hand Surg* **18B**:533–9.

Curtis RM (1984) Management of the stiff hand. In: Hunter J, Schneider L, Mackin E and Callahan A, eds. *Rehabilitation of the Hand.* Mosby: St. Louis: 209–10.

De la Caffinière JY (1984) Prothèse totale trapézo-métacarpienne. In: Tubiana R, ed. *Traité de Chirurgie de la Main.* Masson: Paris: 505–11.

Eaton RG, Glickel SZ, Littler JW (1985) Tendon interposition arthroplasty for degenerative arthritis of the trapezio-metacarpal joint of the thumb, *J Hand Surg* **10A**:645–54.

Ebelin M (1993) La rhizarthrose. In: *Cahier D'enseignement de la Société Française de Chirurgie de la Main,* Vol. 5. Expansion Scientifique: Paris: 113–27.

Forestier J (1937) L'osteoarthrite sèche trapézo-métacarpienne. Rhizarthrose du pouce, *Presse Med* **45**:315–17.

Gervis WH (1949) Excision of the trapezium for osteoarthritis of the trapezio-metacarpal joint, *J Bone Jt Surg* **31B**:537–9.

Kadiyala RK, Gelbermann RH, Kwon B (1996) Basal joint arthrosis. Radiographic assessment of the trapezial space before and after ligament reconstruction and tendon interposition arthroplasty, *J Hand Surg* **21B**:177–81.

Kapandji AI (1990) La prosthèse "cardan" sample de l'articulation trapeso-métacarpienne. In: Saffar P, ed. *La Rhizarthrose.* Expansion Scientifique: Paris: 154–60.

Kleinmann WB, Eckenrode JE (1991) Tendon suspension sling arthroplasty for thumb trapeziometacarpal arthritis, *J Hand Surg* **16A**:983–91.

Kuhlmann JN (1987) Le poignet et la colonne du pouce. Thesis, Faculté de Medecine, Pitie Salpetrière, Paris.

Kwarnes L, Reikeras O (1985) Osteoarthritis of the carpometacarpal joint of the thumb: an analysis of operative procedures, *J Hand Surg* **10B**:117–20.

Le Viet DT, Kerboull L, Lantieri LA, Colbius DE (1996) Stabilized resection arthroplasty by an anterior approach in trapezio-metacarpal arthritis: results and surgical technique, *J Hand Surg* **21A**:194–201.

Magnusson A, Bertheussen K, Weilby A (1985) Ligament reconstruction of the thumb carpo-metacarpal joint using a modified Eaton–Littler technique, *J Hand Surg* **10B**:115–16.

Masquelet AC (1992) La première commissure de la main. Anatomie et principes de reconstruction. In: *Cahiers d'ein-segnement de la Société Française de Chirurgie de la Main*, Vol. 4. Expansion Scientifique: Paris: 33–48.

Mele R (1996) La protesi tripodal e la sua evoluzione. *Abstract, Convegno Sulla Rizartrosi, Milano, 1996.*

Molitor PJ, Emery RJH, Meggit BF (1991) First metacarpal osteotomy for carpometacarpal osteoarthritis, *J Hand Surg* **16B**:424–8.

Nylen S, Johnson A, Rosenquist AM (1993) Trapeziectomy and ligament reconstruction for osteoarthritis of the base of the thumb, *J Hand Surg* **18B**:616–19.

Rousso M (1975) Brulures dorsales graves de la main. Reconstruction de la commissure. Technique à cinq lambeaux, *Ann Chir* **29**:475–9.

Rushforth AF (1949) A congenital abnormality of the trapezium and first metacarpal bone, *J Bone Jt Surg* **31B**:543–6.

Saffar P (1990) *La rhizarthrose*. Expansion Scientifique Française: Paris.

Scheker LR, Lister GD, Wolff TN (1988) The lateral arm free flaps in releasing severe contracture of the 1st web space, *J Hand Surg* **13B**:146–50.

Schernberg F (1990) Les techniques de trapézectomie totals, *Ann Chir Main* **9**:172–5.

Swanson AB (1972) Flexible implant arthroplasty for arthritic finger joints: rationale, technique and results of treatment, *J Bone Joint Surg* **53A**:435–55.

Swanson AB, De Goot Swanson G, Watermen JJ (1981) Trapezium implant arthroplasty, *J Hand Surg* **6**:125–41.

Young VL, Nemecek JR (1994) The interpositional material: Goretex roll. In: Kasdan ML, Amadio PC and Bowers WH, eds. *Technical Tips for Hand Surgery*. Hanley & Bezfus: Philadelphia: 53.

44
Rehabilitation of the stiff thumb

Jacques Otthiers

Introduction

The essential function of the thumb is to place itself in front of the other fingers and so enable pretensile activity. This opposition is the only motion indispensable for efficient thumb action. If a significant loss of mobility in the metacarpophalangeal (MCP) and interphalangeal (IP) joints is generally well accepted (even normal hands may show differences at these levels), maximum mobility in the trapezometacarpal (TMC) joints is necessary for good use of the thumb column.

The aim of the rehabilitation team is to keep or to recover a painless and movable TMC and a good muscular strength so the thumb has its maximum potential.

We will try to define the guidelines for recovery for the most important injuries (rheumatoid and traumatological) which result in a stiff thumb. The splinting of the thumb column will be described in the second part of this chapter.

The rheumatoid thumb

Osteoarthritis of the base of the thumb

At the onset of the evolution of this disease, treatment is essentially prevention of joint deformities and joint economy. Therefore small static splints are used: thermoplastic gloves which stabilize the thumb column in the most functional position.

After surgery (trapezectomy, arthroplasty, etc.) and immobilization, during which the same thermoplastic glove is maintained, all usual rehabilitation techniques are used to recover mobility, strength

and function with special attention to proprioceptors. Technical aids in everyday life help the patient to recover independence.

Rheumatoid arthritis

We will often be confronted with a 'Z' deformation of the thumb column. A lever orthosis is used for correction of the axis of the first metacarpal bone and re-equilibration of the thumb.

Traumatic injuries

'The best treatment of a stiff limb is . . . not to let it become stiff . . .'

Fractures

The first part of the treatment – reduction and retention of the fracture – must be done as soon as possible to allow the earliest mobilization of all the limb parts that can be mobilized.

After retention, normal re-education, alternated with dynamic splints (if needed), will recover mobility.

Joint injuries

Strains of the MCP joints are very frequent. When surgery is not needed for suture of the wounded ligament (Stainer injury, for example), a combined treatment of antalgy and early mobilization may begin as soon as possible and will normally not lead to any loss of mobility.

Tendon injuries

After flexor tendon ruptures, we prefer an early mobilization technique following Kleinert. During the splinting period, passive thumb flexion will be achieved by gentle and careful passive mobilization in a protected position.

After the splinting period, massage of the scars and aspiration techniques should be perfomed to keep flexor and extensor tendons free of adherences.

Complications: adherences, tenolyses, arthrolyses

After tenolyses, mobilization must be introduced very early in the treatment, reinforced by electrical stimulation. This stimulation of the adherence has been successfully combined with an aspiration technique. Continual passive motion may be a good complement in this treatment. Arthrolysis, especially for the MCP joint, will become an essential part of the treatment.

Splintage

Because of its configuration and its essential function of opposition, the thumb presents very particular problems for the conception and the preparation of orthoses. The decentralized position of the thumb with respect to the axis of the hand, the distance to the stablest parts of the hand skeleton, the relative deficiency of its length that impose the use of very short levers, and, finally, the great mobility of the base of the thumb column make the technical realization of suitable splints very complex.

When considering the numerous thumb pathologies that can be found, it is preferable initially to define each splint, to describe and to class it by its various actions and to find the best application for each type of splint in dealing with particular thumb pathologies.

Definition

A splint is a device which can be adjusted and fixed to a limb to modify its anatomical and physiological properties. Splints can be used:

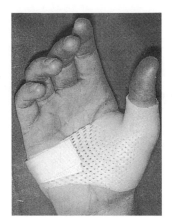

Figure 1

Total immobilization of the thumb

- to prohibit or to limit mobility
- to assist mobility.

Splints which prohibit or limit mobility

Whole immobilization

In our example (Fig. 1), the thumb column is fixed by a thermoplastic glove to the stablest parts of the hand skeleton (second and third metacarpals and second carpal range). The thumb segments may be fixed as needed for treatment of the particular lesion. This kind of splint is used for:

- phalanx fracture
- strain of the MCP joint between mobilization and antalgic treatment
- osteoarthritis of the base of the thumb.

The whole immobilization splint can also be used with a posture effect to prevent or to correct some deformations.

A 'Z' deformation of the thumb in a patient with rheumatoid arthritis is corrected by a posture splint (Figs 2 and 3).

Incomplete immobilization

Either axis or amplitude motion can be limited.

In axis limitation the splint permits motion in one plane. The joint is protected from unwanted devia-

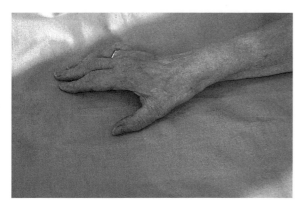

Figure 2

'Z' deformation of the thumb

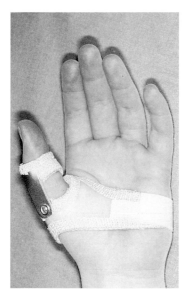

Figure 4

Axis limitation: extension of MCP

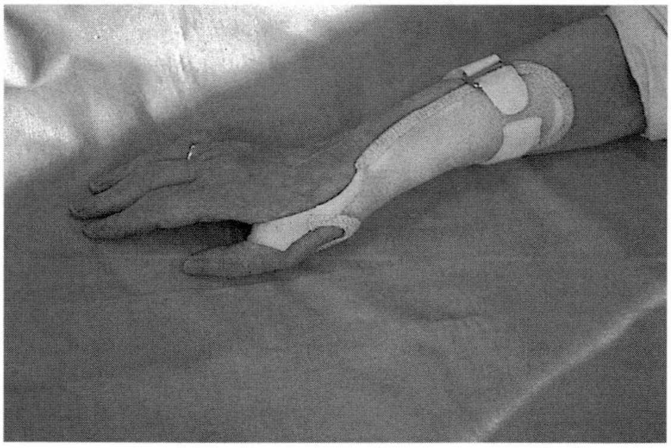

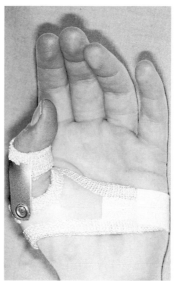

Figure 3

A posture splint for 'Z' deformation of the thumb

Figure 5

Axis limitation: flexion of MCP

tion and ligamentous traction. These splints, articulated in the axis of the MCP joint, permit exercises in flexion and extension of the thumb without traction on the wounded MCP ulnar ligament (skier strain) (Figs 4 and 5).

In amplitude limitation the splint will put the wrist and the thumb in a position that will protect the tendon suture during active extension, and the elastic achieves return to flexion (Figs 6 and 7). This would be used after a Kleinert surgical procedure for repair and rehabilitation of a severed flexor tendon.

Splints which assist mobilization

These splints will assist the rehabilitation of joint amplitude deficiencies. It is very important to remember when using such dynamic splints that both traction power and duration must be adjusted to suit the injury.

Flexion splints

For recovering the flexion amplitude of the thumb (MCP and IP) we use an elastic strap and two pieces of hook and loop fastener fixed to a glove

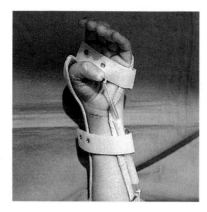

Figure 6

Amplitude limitation: Kleinert technique (passive flexion)

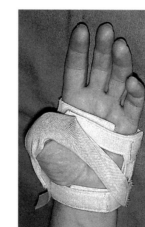

Figure 7

Amplitude limitation: Kleinert technique (extension)

made of thermoplastic or cotton and straps (Fig. 8). This splint can be used for recovering thumb flexion, in traumatology, after MCP strain, tendon adherences, and so on.

Extension splints

The classical 'Levame orthosis' can be adapted for the particular conformation of the thumb (Fig. 9). Capener splints can also be easily adapted for the thumb and will have the same applications. We prefer to use them for traumatological problems, tendon adherences or sequelae after strains (Fig. 10).

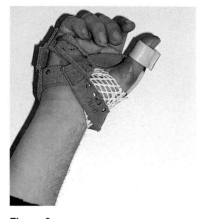

Figure 8

Dynamic flexion splint

Figure 9

Dynamic extension splint (Levame orthosis)

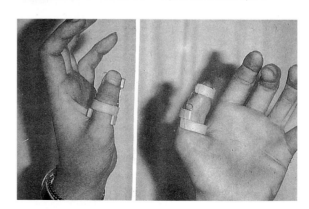

Figure 10

Dynamic extension splint (Capener splint)

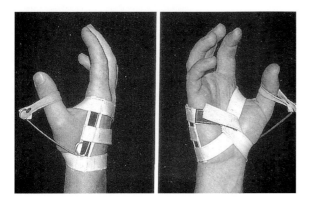

Figure 11

Dynamic abduction splint

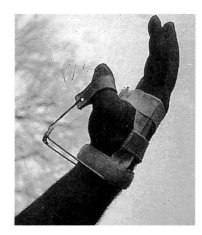

Figure 12

Dynamic antepulsion splint

Antepulsion and abduction

With little gallows fixed on the same glove as used for the flexion splints, and oriented to the side of the traction, we can achieve a good opening of the first commissure in both rheumatoid and traumatological pathologies (Figs 11 and 12).

Conclusion

Each therapist will have to choose from these technical possibilities, – using their knowledge of the materials and their technical expertise – the best solution for the patient that completes surgical treatment and rehabilitation.

Part V
Interrelated stiffness

45

Clinical and neurophysiological aspects of the spastic upper limb

Rudolf Schoenhuber and Francesco Teatini

Many patients with neurological diseases affecting the motor system are first seen by an orthopaedic or hand surgeon; the classical example is that of patients with Duchenne muscular dystrophy. Motor neurone disease (amyotrophic lateral sclerosis) is also often erroneously considered to be cervical radiculopathy or cubital syndrome. An increasing number of patients suffering from diseases affecting the central nervous system (CNS), such as Parkinson's disease or focal dystonia (writer's cramp) are seen at our movement disorders clinic after referral by hand surgeons. This is because the patient understands the words stiffness, cramps, palsy etc. to mean that the arm or hand cannot be moved at will. The physician has to interpret the patient's complaints in terms of disability. The distinction between subjective symptoms and objective signs is very important, as is the distinction between positive (due to increased activity within the CNS or the nerve), and negative (due decreased activity) (Table 1). Within this framework the inability to move the hand properly can be due to either excessive involuntary activity arising within the CNS or reduced activity due to pain or to non-neurological reasons such as arthritis or a ruptured tendon. This distinction is the first step to uncover the underlying pathology. Optimal outcomes can only be expected if treatment of motor symptoms, such as paresis or spasticity, is rational, i.e. based on a systematic approach correctly addressing the underlying pathology.

All movement, whether reflex or voluntary, normal or abnormal, is the result of global neural activity derived from many sources acting upon the primary motor neurones (the final common pathway) with their peripheral nerves, neuromuscular junctions and muscle fibres. Motor dysfunction may result from involvement of muscle, neuromuscular junction, peripheral nerve or CNS. Damage to almost any portion of the CNS can disturb motor performance. Most striking disturbances are seen when the motor pathway (pyramidal and extrapyramidal,

Table 1 Neurological signs and symptoms

	Motor	Sensory	Vegetative
Negative signs	Loss of strength, muscle atrophy	Sensory loss	Anhidrosis, vasodilatation, trophic skin changes
Negative symptoms	Subjective loss of strength	Sensory loss	None
Positive signs	Cramps, dystonia, fasciculations	None	Hyperhidrosis, vasoconstriction
Positive symptoms	Cramps	Pain, paraesthesias	Pain

Table 2 Clinical differences between peripheral and central motor lesions

	Lower motor neurone syndrome	Upper motor neurone syndrome
Lesion	Peripheral	Central
Force	Reduced	Reduced
Dexterity	Reduced	Reduced
Trophism	Reduced	Less reduced
Tonus	Reduced	Increased
Reflexes	Reduced	Increased
Associated sensory loss pattern	Absent or radicular/plexus/nerve pattern	Absent or cortical/radicular pattern

lower motor neurones in the brainstem and the spinal cord, and also the cerebellum) is damaged. Two major syndromes can easily be differentiated: the upper and lower motor neurone syndrome (Table 2).

Important characteristics differentiating central and peripheral lesions are reflexes and muscle tone (the resistance of a muscle to passive movement). At least six reasons for increased limb resistance to movement or stiffness can be differentiated from clinical and neurophysiological points of view:

- increased resistance to stretching because of viscoelastical changes of the muscle; passive stiffness with retractions and very important contractures prevails
- irregular myotactical activity (static phase) due to either an inconstant and insufficient presynaptical Ia inhibition or a sudden fall of the antidromic inhibition of Renshaw cells
- increased automatic flexor and extensor activity following exteroceptive stimuli (model of spinal type spasticity)
- increased and prolonged myotactical activity in the static phase for hyperexcitability of alpha and reticular neurones, and low threshold to the sensory afferents (model of cerebral type spasticity)
- decerebration model, with mostly phasic hyperactivity, prevalence of extensor tonus, hyperreflexia and no electrical activity at rest (dynamic gamma type spasticity)
- increased muscular activity secondary to states of anxiety (model of the behaviour hypertonus following cortical excitement).

The most frequent and most clinically relevant reason for stiffness is the alteration of the muscle tone known as spastic hypertonus (Burke 1988, Meinck et al 1985, Brown 1994, Rothwell 1994, Young 1994). Spastic hypertonus can and must be differentiated clinically and neurophysiologically from other reasons for stiffness such as rigidity and dystonia. Passive, static or intrinsic stiffness depends on the viscosity and elasticity of the muscles and tendons. Necrosis or fibrosis of muscle tissue, as seen in Volkmann's disease, also belong to this category. Hand surgeons do not need assistance from neurologists to deal with these cases. Some basic knowledge of neurology and clinical neurophysiology may be helpful in cases of active or dynamic stiffness (Delwaide 1985b), i.e. the force with which the muscle opposes changes to its length, and which is due to a pathological hyperactivation of physiological reflexes mediated by proprioceptive afferents from muscle spindles (Ia fibres) and from tendons (Ib fibres).

In this chapter we will try to explain how different motor complaints can be differentiated clinically and how methods available in clinical neurophysiology laboratories can be of some use.

Clinical evaluation

Patients seldom complain of increased or decreased tone but generally refer to the associated disorder of motility. In rigidity and spasticity, spontaneous complaints usually refer to the dragging of a limb or to slowness of movement. Occasionally, a patient will speak of stiffness, heaviness, weakness or even 'numbness' when referring to increased tone in an extremity. Either rigidity or spasticity may lead to pain, especially in the axial and girdle muscles. Hypotonia is usually ignored by patients.

From a clinical point of view, spasticity is one of the components of the upper motor neurone syndrome, characterized by a series of negative signs and symptoms such as loss of strength and dexterity, and of positive signs such as hypertonus and increased deep tendon reflexes, flexor spasms, abnormal exteroceptive responses (Babinski sign), loss of cutaneous (abdominal and cremasteric) reflexes (Table 2). These elements do not always exist simultaneously in the same patient, and any of them could predominate. Spasticity itself is the speed-dependent increase of muscular resistance to passive movement.

In everyday practice muscle tone, strength and dexterity are evaluated clinically. A standardized clinical examination, possibly with some accepted scoring system, is useful, particularly in view of follow-up examinations (Table 3).

Muscle tone is difficult to quantify. Adequate evaluation of muscle tone is a matter of personal experience requiring that the patient be as relaxed as possible. Spasticity, rigidity and dystonia have to be differentiated when assessing a patient with upper extremity stiffness (Table 4). In hypertonus, particularly spasticity, the extremities at rest tend to assume a fixed posture of overextension or, more often, of increased flexion. The examiner moves each extremity through its full range of motion at each joint. Normally a mild even resistance to movement is noted through the entire range. Following lesions of the pyramidal system spasticity develops. Spasticity is a speed-dependent sudden increase of resistance (clasp knife phenomenon), and is more prominent in arm, hand and finger flexors than extensors. Diseases of the extrapyramidal system may lead to an increased muscle tone which affects both extensors and flexors alike and is not speed dependent. The typical rigidity of

Table 3 Clinical scoring systems for spasticity, spasms and reflexes

Score	Ashworth scale	Spasm scale	Stretch reflex scale
0	No increase in muscle tone	No spasms	Missing reflexes
1	Slight increase, manifested by minimal resistance when the affected part is moved in flexion or in extension	Spasms only by strong cutaneous or motor stimulation	Reduced
2	More marked increase, but affected part is however moved in flexion	Rare or easily evoked spasms	Normal
3	Considerable increase, passive movement difficult	<10 spontaneous spasms/hour	Brisk
4	Affected part rigid in flexion or extension	>10 spontaneous spasms/hour	Clonus

Table 4 Differential diagnosis of spasticity, rigidity and dystonia

	Spasticity	Rigidity	Dystonia
Strength reduced	Yes	No	No
Associated pain	Sometimes	Sometimes	Sometimes
Flexors more affected	Yes	No	Sometimes
Speed dependent	Yes	No	No
Task related	No	No	Yes

parkinsonism is the resistance of the resting limb to passive flexion and extension, while dystonic coactivation of both extensors and flexors arises most often when a patient is involved in a particular task, such as writing or playing the piano or strings. Such patients suffering from writer's cramp (Marsden 1990) or other occupational dystonias are increasingly seen by hand surgeons.

Tonus can also be indirectly assessed by passively displacing the arm upwards, and then allowing it to fall down and swing freely. A regular pendular movement results that slowly dampens, like a pendulum (Boçzko and Mumenthaler 1958). This pendulousness may be increased or decreased in range and duration. One should observe the number of oscillations, their regularity, the pattern described by the movement, and compare the two arms. Tonus can also be tested by moving the patient's shoulders back and forth through an arc with the trunk as a pivot point. One shoulder is pulled forward as the other is pushed backward and vice versa. The resultant to-and-fro swinging of the upper extremities due to centrifugal forces is observed by the examiner. For the same purpose the examiner places his hands on the patient's hips and briskly flips the patient's arm away from the body. The speed, range, regularity and pattern of movement may be seen, heard and felt by the examiner as the arms swing away from the body and return. Patients with spasticity and rigidity will have less arm swing on the affected side, while patients with dystonia show either no difference at all between arms or the affected limb will swing more due to hypotonus.

In patients with neurological reasons for increased muscle stiffness, a careful and complete neurological examination is mandatory. Routinely discussing these cases with a neurologist would probably be in the best interests of both the patient and the hand surgeon.

Neurophysiological methods

Every surgeon interested in the treatment of peripheral nerve lesions, and particularly every hand surgeon, knows the objective and quantitative advantages of neurosphysiological methods compared to clinical evaluation. Precise stimulation of specific nerves and recording from nerves or, more frequently, muscles allows a good topographical localization with an extremely fine time discrimination (in the millisecond range). Several neurophysiological methods have been proposed in recent decades to assess muscle tone. We will describe in more detail a few methods that are more commonly used. Tests proposed for the neurophysiological evaluation of the motor system go back to the methods of electromyography (EMG) and reflex recording (Burke 1988, Knutsson 1985, Brown 1994, Meinck et al 1993, Rothwell 1994, Young 1994). There are three main groups of neurophysiological tests: those assessing globally the whole muscle (kinesiological and surface EMG methods); those assessing the behaviour of single motor units (needle EMG); and the response of global muscle activity or single unit to experimentally applied stimuli (reflex studies).

The electrical activation of muscle fibres can be globally assessed with a simple EMG recording during the active and passive execution of movements at one or more joints, and at different speeds. Surface electrical activity is recorded from at least one agonist and one antagonist muscle recording on a slow time base (Hallet et al 1975). If possible acceleration and the angular shift should also be recorded simultaneously. With a setup as simple as a two-channel EMG machine, the extension and timing of voluntary movement and the presence of co-contraction can be easily recorded. Speed dependence can be assessed by asking the patient to make fast alternating movements. Those patients in whom a motor deficit is suspected, but a contemporary activation of muscles to the opposite action (paralysis by subtraction) is found, can also be diagnosed using this technique.

The availability of several channels allows simultaneous recording from several muscles. Dynamic multichannel EMG is now available in many clinical neurophysiology laboratories and is the easiest and most effective electrophysiological method for evaluating spasticity. The examination of patterns of muscular activation during voluntary movement is called electromyographic kinesiology (EK) or polyelectromyography (polyEMG). It can be used to study the mechanism involved in the production of abnormal movements. For example, in a spastic patient unable to fully extend the elbow there could be either a limited ability to generate voluntary activation of the triceps, an inappropriate overactivity (either tonic contraction or transient co-contraction) of a particular elbow flexor or combination of elbow flexors, or even fixed contracture of an elbow flexor.

These problems are usually addressed in research laboratories where instead of recording biological potentials from the muscles only by means of surface EMG, more sophisticated methods which record body movement are also available (Knutsson 1983 and 1985, Meinck et al 1993, Young 1994). The description of body movement itself without regard to the underlying forces is called kinematics. Kinematic variables include linear and angular displacement, velocity and acceleration of body segments. Modern systems employ digital computers to obtain image data to derive the space–time trajectories of the motion under study. This can then be used to compute joint angle kinematic variables using standard trigonometric techniques. Several methods have been proposed over recent decades as sources of biomechanical data. They can be classified into kinematic and kinetic methods. The latter consider direct measurement of force by strain gauges, dynamometers or force platforms. The former deal with the measurement of motion either by electrogoniometers and accelerometers or cinematographic, and more recently, videographic or optoelectronic spotting devices. Kinetic or kinematic methods are often used in combination with surface EMG recording to study the problem of controlling hand position in space (i.e. co-ordination of shoulder–elbow mechanism), hand grasp and release functions (i.e. wrist and extrinsic finger flexors and extensor) and fine pinch using the thumb with activation of intrinsic hand muscles (e.g. lateral pinch). The design of the examination, the selection of motor tasks and the selection of muscles to be studied will generally depend upon the specific question to be addressed in the examination with respect to disordered motor control or limb deformity.

Using needle electrodes, electrical activity in spastic muscle is normal and no spontaneous activity or motor unit (MU) potentials can be recorded at rest. There are, however, modifications in the recruitment pattern of MUs during maximal effort: the number of voluntarily activated MUs and the variability of the discharge frequency of MUs are both reduced (Andreassen and Rosenfalk 1978, Rosenfalk and Andreassen 1980, Young and Shahani 1980). Generally, in muscles of healthy subjects, a long interval between the potentials is followed by a short one and vice versa. This correlation is known as serial negative correlation and can be visualized graphically by an interval histogram. In spastic muscles this negative correlation disappears. Longer intervals between potentials tend to follow on from other long intervals, short intervals follow other short intervals. This positive correlation is more evident and constant in patients in whom spasticity is related to supraspinal lesions than in patients with spinal lesions.

The muscle response to mechanical stretch, to electrically induced stretch or to stimulation of sensory fibres can be recorded electromyographically to examine the function of the myotactic reflex arc. The advantage of neurophysiological reflex testing is the high time resolution, the possibility of fine tuning the stimuli and of easily quantifying the response in terms of simple numerical parameters such as latency, amplitude and duration.

The neurophysiological equivalent of the deep

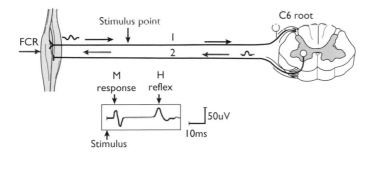

Figure 1

Direct electrical stimulation of an afferent nerve fibre to elicit the H reflex. FCR, flexor carpi radialis

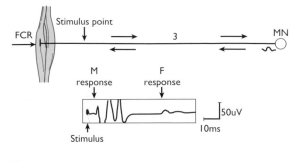

Figure 2

Disappearance of the H reflex following increased stimulus intensity. The F wave is a result of the antidromic stimulation of the motor fibres. FCR, flexor carpi radialis; MN, motor neurone

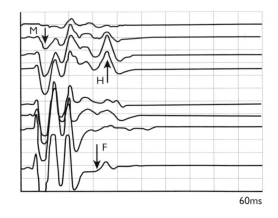

Figure 3

Recording from forearm flexors following stimulation of the median nerve at the elbow. With increasing stimulus intensity, the H reflex (H) appears first, then the M response (M). With further increase of intensity the H reflex is replaced by the F wave (F)

tendon reflex (also called T reflex or Tendon reflex) can be recorded in response to mechanical percussion of a tendon (using a modified reflex hammer which electrically triggers the acquisition of the EMG signal) using surface electrodes on the examined muscle.

The H reflex is more often used in clinical routines (Angel and Hoffmann 1963). Direct electrical stimulation of afferent fibres of nerve trunks, bypassing neuromuscular spindles, elicits a reflex response analogous to that evoked physiologically by stretching the tendon. A stimulus of low intensity is sufficient to excite the high diameter and low threshold Ia fibres to evoke the H reflex. This intensity is too low to evoke the direct motor M response. However, increasing stimulus intensity evokes the direct M response at a lower latency. Further increasing stimulus intensity causes the H reflex to disappear (Figs 1, 2 and 3). The ratio between the two maximal responses one can evoke, H [max]/M [max], is an important index of the excitability of the motoneuronal pool (Delwaide 1985a, Delwaide 1985b, Rothwell 1994).

With double pulse stimulation a second H reflex cannot be elicited between 10 and 100 ms after the appearance of the first response. There is another period lasting several seconds during which the excitability of the reflex is also abnormal. The amplitude of the reflex response gradually increases up to the interstimulus intervals of 200–300 ms (Fig. 3). This facilitation is followed by a later depression period of the reflex, after which the amplitude of the response returns gradually to normal values.

In patients affected by spasticity, flaccid paralysis or parkinsonian rigidity this H reflex recovery cycle is usually altered (Diamantopoulos and Olsen 1967, Olsen and Diamantopoulos 1967, Delwaide 1985b). It must also be said that the H reflex recording is subject to many technical limitations and is particularly sensitive to peripheral factors such as incomplete relaxation in anxious patients, tremor in Parkinson's disease or clonus in spastic patients. The clinical usefulness of the H reflex in the analysis of spasticity is therefore still uncertain.

Another way to examine muscle spindles is the TVR, the tonic vibration reflex. A vibratory stimulation, at frequencies from 100 to 150 Hz, applied directly onto the muscle or tendon causes a subcontinuous muscle contraction by activation of primary terminations of muscle spindles through Ia afferents ending both monosynaptically or via excitatory interneurons onto spinal alpha motor neurones. The EMG recording will show a recruitment pattern following the application of the vibration stimulus. The TVR is notably reduced under the level of a section of the bone marrow and in patients with cerebellar lesions (Hagbarth and Eklund 1968).

In most clinical neurophysiology laboratories F wave recording is now a routine investigation. The F wave is obtained by antidromic stimulation of the motor fibres which evoke a late response after the direct motor M response (Figs 1 and 2). With the same recording setting of the H reflex, further increasing stimulus intensity to maximum following the supramaximal M wave, gives a much smaller F wave. This F wave has a variable morphology and latency due to antidromic excitation of motor fibres, some of them firing back orthodromically. The probability of each single F wave firing back depends on the excitability of its motor neurone. In spasticity, F waves are more easily evoked and of higher amplitude (Schiller and Stalberg 1978, Eisen and Odusote 1979, Fischer 1996, Leis 1996). Drugs effective in spasticity have been evaluated recently using the F wave.

All these methods have been proven to be of limited practical value because of the technical problems (long duration of the examination, methodological complexity) and the limited diagnostic reliability of the results, given the ample range of inter- and intraindividual variability seen in normal control groups of healthy subjects. Their major use is still limited to research issues, particularly the evaluation of drug treatment for spasticity and rigidity. However, their use for assessing the outcome of surgical or rehabilitative intervention, will probably increase in the near future.

References

Andreassen S, Rosenfalk A (1978) Impaired regulation of the firing pattern of single motor units, *Muscle Nerve* **1**:416–8.

Angel RW, Hoffmann WW (1963) The H reflex in normal spastic and rigid subjects, *Arch Neurol* **8**:591–6.

Boçzko M, Mumenthaler M (1958) Modified pendulousness test to assess tonus of thigh muscles in spasticity, *Neurology* **8**:846–51.

Brown P (1994) Pathophysiology of spasticity, *J Neurol Neurosurg Psychiatr* **57**:773–7.

Burke D (1988) Spasticity as an adaptation to pyramidal tract injury, *Adv Neurology* **47**:401–23.

Delwaide PJ (1985a) Electrophysiological analysis of the mode of action of muscle relaxant in spasticity, *Ann Neurol* **17**:90–5.

Delwaide PJ (1985b) Electrophysiological testing of spastic patients: its potential usefulness and limitations. In: Delwaide PJ, Young RR, eds. *Clinical Neurophysiology in Spasticity*. Elsevier: Amsterdam:185–201.

Diamantopoulos E, Olsen PZ (1967) Excitability of motor neurones in spinal shock in man, *J Neurol Neurosurg Psychiat* **30**:327–31.

Eisen A, Odusote K (1979) Amplitude of the F wave: a potential means of documenting spasticity, *Neurology* **29**:1306–9.

Fischer MA (1996) Are H reflex and F responses equally sensitive to changes in motoneuronal excitability? *Muscle Nerve* **19**:1345–6.

Hagbarth KE, Eklund G (1968) The effects of muscle vibration in spasticity, rigidity and cerebellar disorders, *J Neurol Neurosurg Psychiat* **31**:207–13.

Hallet M, Shahani BT, Young RR (1975) EMG analysis of stereotyped voluntary movements in man, *J Neurol Neurosurg Psychiat* **38**:1154–62.

Knutsson E (1983) Analysis of gait and isokinetic movements for evaluation of antispastic drugs or physical therapies. In: Desmedt JE, ed. *Motor Control Mechanism in Health and Disease*. Raven Press: New York: 1013–34.

Knutsson E (1985) Quantification of spasticity. In: Struppler A, Weindl A eds. *Electromyography and Evoked Potentials*. Springer: Berlin: 85–91.

Leis AA, Stetkarova I, Beric A, Stokic D (1996) The relative sensitivity of F wave and H reflex to changes in motoneuronal excitability, *Muscle Nerve* **19**:1342–4.

Marsden CD, Sheehy MP (1990) Writer's cramp, *Trends Neurosci* **13**:148–53.

Meinck HM, Benecke R, Conrad B (1985) Spasticity and the flexor reflex. In: Delwaide PJ, Young RR, eds. *Clinical Neurophysiology in Spasticity*. Elsevier: Amsterdam: 41–54.

Olsen PZ, Diamantopoulos E (1967) Excitability of spinal motor neurones in normal subjects and patients with spasticity, Parkinsonian rigidity and cerebellar hypotonia, *J Neurol Neurosurg Psychiat* **30**:325–31.

Rosenfalk A, Andreassen S (1980) Impaired regulation of face and firing pattern of single motor units in patients with spasticity, *J Neurol Neurosurg Psychiat* **43**:907–16.

Rothwell J (1994) *Control of Human Voluntary Movement*, 2nd edn. Chapman and Hall: London.

Schiller HH, Stalberg E (1978) F responses studied with single fibre EMG in normal subjects and spastic patients, *J Neurol Neurosurg Psychiat* **41**:45–53.

Young RR (1994) Spasticity: a review, *Neurology* **44**(suppl):S12–20.

Young RR, Shahani BT (1980) A clinical neurophysiological analysis of single motor unit discharge patterns in spasticity. In: Feldman RG, Young RR, Koella W, eds. *Spasticity: Disordered Motor Control*. Year Book: Chicago: 205–18.

46

Hyponeurotization in spastic palsy

Giorgio A Brunelli and Giovanni R Brunelli

Spastic palsies are still a challenge to the surgeon. In fact traditional surgery often fails despite repeated operations.

Traditional surgery to diminish spasticity and secondary deformities includes various techniques: tendon lengthening, tendon transfers, tenodesis, bone fusions, deafferentation and others (Braun et al 1970, Braun et al 1973, Lusskin et al 1968). Hyponeurotization can be considered a more target-related operation.

It was conceived at the beginning of this century by Stoffel (1913). First he tried to diminish the innervation of the spastic muscles by cutting (at the elbow) some of the motor fascicles inside the median nerve (Stoffel, 1st technique). As denervation was poorly 'selective', he later divided the muscular branches to the single muscles (Stoffel, 2nd technique).

At that time this operation gave inconsistent and unpredictable results probably due to the poor conditions for surgery. Rapid surgery with small incisions was necessary because of primitive anaesthesia and the lack of antibiotics, of sophisticated electrical apparatus and of the data we have available today.

Microsurgery has allowed us to review these concepts with improvement to both technique and results (Brunelli and Brunelli 1983). Two new concepts have been introduced. First the approach has to be large enough to allow a check to be made on all the motor branches going to spastic muscles. Secondly, the adoption phenomenon has to be taken into account because denervation obtained by operation will be consistently reduced by the 'adoption' of some denervated muscular fibrocells by axon sprouts branching from the spared nerve fibres at both the Ranvier nodes and the motor end plates.

This phenomenon demands a denervation larger than might be expected. Very careful, repeated physical examination with repeated muscular testing has to be done. Prior to surgery it must be decided which motor branches of which nerves are to be denervated (usually median, but often ulnar and musculocutaneous). This is fundamental for determining with a good approximation which muscles have to be denervated and to what extent, although this is always difficult to foresee exactly.

Young patients present with different features at different times according to their current physiological attitude, tiredness, fear of the doctor and temperature, so that only by averaging the results of repeated examination can a good surgical decision be drawn.

Also, adoption phenomenon vary according to various factors: age, health, individuals' type of muscles and type of nerve resection.

A second operation has to be planned 6 months later which patients and parents must be informed about. A second operation may include further denervation and supplementary tenotomies if the adoption phenomenon was very effective or, conversely, reconstructive procedures if the first denervation was too great.

Indications include any degree of spasticity (with different extents of denervation) in collaborating patients or in babies with collaborating parents. Patients with athetosis, severe brain impairment or with low IQ will be excluded as well as uncooperative ones.

The approach varies according to the number and site of the muscles to be denervated. It can be done on the anterior aspect of the arm for denervation of biceps and brachialis anterior muscle or the volar aspect of the forearm and the hand to denervate the flexor muscles as well as the pronators (pronator teres and pronator quadratus).

In the hand it may be necessary to denervate some intrinsic muscles, namely the adductor pollicis which often has to be removed due to the possibility of its re-innervation after simple denervation.

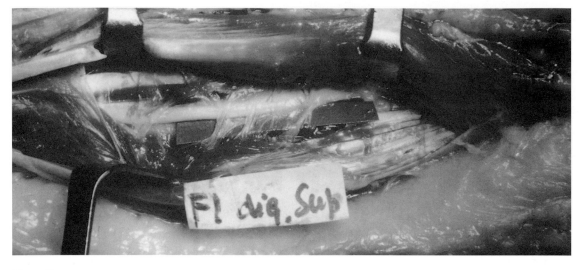

Figure 1

Photograph of four branches going to the flexor digitorum superficialis. When several branches are present, hyponeurotization is easy to perform.

The median nerve is found at the elbow after having divided the lacertus fibrous.

The pronator teres belly is retracted to inspect its muscular branches. According to the severity of spasticity and to the foreseen capacity of re-innervation (adoption phenomenon), one-half, two-thirds or three-quarters of the fascicles going to the muscle are severed (and removed for about 1 cm to avoid spontaneous repair) (Fig. 1).

Denervation is done under the operating microscope and with the help of repeated electrical stimulation. If there are three motor branches to a muscle it is easy to denervate one- or two-thirds, but if there is only one motor branch, epineurotomy is necessary to separate the fascicles, recognize them, and cut and remove the desired number of fascicles.

The pronator teres is retracted while the flexor carpi radialis is pulled down medially allowing visualization and denervation of the motor branches to the flexor carpi radialis itself and to the flexor digitorum superficialis. The latter is then retracted laterally allowing denervation of the flexor digitorum profundus and flexor pollicis longus. In the lower part of the forearm the nerve to the pronator quadratus is found and hyponeurotized or resected in its entirety.

If necessary, in rare cases, the nerve to the abductor pollicis brevis and the opponens muscles are also partially divided and removed. Occasionally it may be necessary to do selective denervation of the extrinsic as well as of the intrinsic muscles innervated by the ulnar nerve.

The extrinsic muscles are approached through the same incision as for the median nerve. The flexor carpi ulnaris and the medial bellies of the flexor digitorum profundus are selectively hyponeurotized with the above-mentioned technique.

As regards the intrinsic muscles innervated by the ulnar nerve, the adductor pollicis is the one which gives the most important problem.

In the past we first did denervation in Guyon's canal and later removal of the muscular branches under the muscle. Practice taught us that denervation can lead to failure because adoption phenomenon takes place not only from the fibres of its own nerve, but also from surrounding muscles. Therefore for many years I have been removing the muscle. Adductor pollicis myoectomy evidently gives rise to a Froment's sign but, in my opinion, this is the only surgery able to solve 'thumb-in-palm' spasticity (Fig. 2). This is the main operating protocol, but in some cases in which retraction is also present (in addition to spasticity), tendon lengthening or even tenotomies are added (especially of flexor carpi radialis and flexor carpi ulnaris muscles). After surgery a hypercorrecting splint must be worn for 45 days.

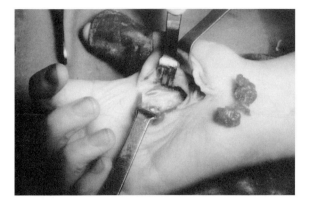

Figure 2

The adductor pollicis denervation is generally unsuccessful therefore complete myoectomy of the muscle is performed even though it leads to a Froment's sign.

Generally the adoption phenomenon takes place within 45–60 days restoring some muscular tone to the muscles which, after denervation, were more or less flaccid. This phenomenon generally ends in 3–4 months.

Sometimes the result is good with the first operation. More often a second operation is necessary to further denervate some muscles in which the adoption phenomenon was too effective, in rare cases to supply some strength to muscles which have been denervated too much, and in some cases to correct residual deformities (e.g. swan neck deformity). With the second operation a good result, satisfying to both patient and surgeon, is generally obtained. In only two out of 56 cases was a third operation performed.

In general results (Fig. 3) are better in young patients with perinatal spasticity of the upper limb. Less good results are obtained in the lower limb or in adults with acquired hemiplegia.

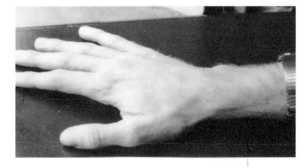

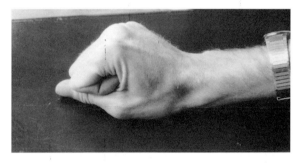

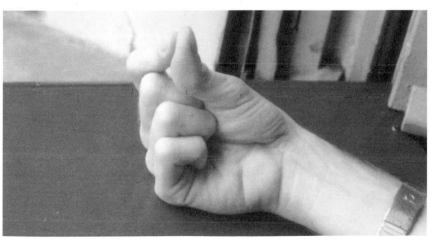

Figure 3

Long-term (15 years) result of hyponeurotization for a middle–severe case. The patient graduated as a medical doctor and is in regular practice.

Established muscular retractions (which can be evaluated under anaesthesia) as well as bony deformities are other conditions which can indicate tendon and bone surgery.

We have done 53 upper limb hyponeurotization in 26 years: 40 cases required a second operation at 6 months; two cases needed a third operation.

A great improvement has been obtained in all cases; the final function being inversely proportional to the severity of the preoperative conditions. Only one female was not satisfied because she wanted a perfect result after a hemiplegia depending on the removal of a brain tumour.

A classification of results is impossible as they depend on the severity of spasticity, the number of muscles involved, added retraction, etc. In cases with moderate spasticity an almost perfect result can be reached. One of our patients became a doctor, another a priest and many have entered upon manual work without handicap.

In conclusion, hyponeurotization must be considered as one of the most effective operations for improving the quality of life of spastic patients.

References

Braun RM, Mooney V, Nickel VL (1970) Flexor origin release for the pronation-flexion deformity of the forearm and hand in the stroke patient. An evaluation of the early results in 18 patients, *J Bone Joint Surg* **52A**:907.

Braun RM, Hoffer MM, Mooney V, McKeever J, Roper B (1973) Phenol nerve block in the treatment of acquired spastic hemiplegia in the upper limb, *J Bone Joint Surg* **55A**:580.

Brunelli G, Brunelli F (1983) Selective microsurgical denervation in spastic paralyses, *Ann Chir Main 2* **3**:277–80.

Lusskin T, Nemunaitis J, Winer J, Grynbaun B (1968) Corrective surgery in adult hemiplegia, *Arch Phys Med* **49**:437.

Stoffel A (1913) Treatment of spastic contractures, *Am J Orthop Surg* **10**:611.

47
Spasticity after prolonged coma

Antonio Landi, Giuseppe Caserta, Lidia Buscaroli, Marco Esposito and Antonio Saracino

Introduction

Severe head injury is the leading cause of death under the age of 45 years in the Western world (Kraus and McArthur 1996). For 15- to 60-year-olds, rates in males are about twice those in females with peak incidence in the 15- to 30-year age group. Case-fatality ratios vary in different countries and according to selection criteria. For head-injured patients admitted to neurosurgical departments, it is about 15%. It ranges between 33% and 50% for those in coma (Kraus and McArthur 1996).

A significant proportion of survivors are left with considerable and prolonged disability. In USA (Kraus 1987) there are two patients per 100 000 individuals with severe disability and 4/100 000 with moderate disability.

The most important and disabling sequela of head injury is cognitive impairment, which can affect the domains of memory, perception, language, attention, abstract reasoning and executive functions.

Motor impairments are also a frequent complaint after severe head injury. Decorticate posture typically shows spastic flexion involving arms, hands and fingers (see Chapter 49), whereas extension of the metacarpophalangeal (MP) joints is very uncommon and recorded when lesions also involve the thalamus.

Because of the complexity and difference on the neuromotor and mental outcomes following prolonged coma, each patient is a case on its own with social aspects proving predominant. The role of surgical rehabilitation is strictly limited to selected cases belonging to functional groups which are likely to have a favourable outcome.

Despite its limited role, surgery can contribute, in unexpected ways, to improve the functional prognosis, restoring the original functional dignity to the upper limb.

General considerations

Coma is unconsciousness from which the patient cannot be awakened. Although reflex movements may be evoked, speech and purposeful eye and limb movements are absent. Unconsciousness derives from a dysfunction of the reticular activating system or from diffuse bilateral hemisphere dysfunction (Marini and Wheeler 1989).

Only four basic pathophysiological mechanisms can cause coma (Plum and Posner 1982):

1 supratentorial mass lesion
2 subtentorial lesion
3 metabolic and diffuse cerebral disorders (including concussion)
4 psychiatric disorders.

A lesion involving exclusively one hemisphere does not produce coma unless it secondarily effects the functions of the contralateral one. Bilateral hemispheric lesions should be suspected in any comatose patients with a history of trauma or headache (Strittmatter 1992). Clinical factors affecting the final outcome in patients with bilateral hemispheric lesions are the depth, progression and duration of coma (Marini and Wheeler 1989, Bosch Blancafort et al 1995, Sorbi et al 1995, Childs and Mercer 1996).

Neurorehabilitation in prolonged coma

After prolonged coma 1.5% of survivors present neurological sequelae of the hemiplegic kind due to focal damage of the central nervous system (CNS), and only 0.4% have true neurological decerebration syndromes associated with disorders of consciousness included in the broad heading of vegetative (or apallic) coma. In the first group where, after awakening from a prolonged coma a hemiplegic syndrome is recorded, the clinical picture matches pathologies typical of the post-ictal syndrome and must be treated by rehabilitation and functional surgery peculiar to this neuromotor disorder.

Much more complex are the therapeutic problems that one must face for the second group, where a clinical picture of decerebration appears, without regaining consciousness. In fact, in apallic comas the rigidity affects the entire soma, although generally the motor deficit will be prevalent on one side.

This pattern of spasticity worsens because of musculotendineous contractures, articular ankyloses and paraosteopathies, in addition to a global disorder of the neurovegetative trophic regulation which is not present in focal syndromes. The contracture typical of long-lasting apallic coma also reveals primordial motor schemas. The spastic palsy, poorly controlled with medical therapy, causes substantial morphological derangements of the musculoarticular structures, which hinder the patient's rehabilitation programme in the rare case of recovery from unconsciousness.

Difficulties in rehabilitation are worsened by the presence of multisystemic, pyramidal, extrapyramidal and cerebellar disorders, associated with swallowing, phonation, ocular-motor, and sensitive-sensorial disorders.

Usually after an apallic state, awakening proceeds slowly with a difficult contact with the surrounding world, a slow reorganization of the personality, and a more or less severe distress of superior functioning. Therefore this post-apallic patient is not capable of actively participating in the rehabilitation programme.

Splints, constant passive motion (CPM) devices, and a great variety of instruments can help patients to stand and walk, and start the rehabilitation procedure. This programme can proceed independently from the actual active participation in the initial phase, and this passive treatment will remain the only possible chance for maintaining the patient's physical integrity. It is possible to aim for a better posture of the patients, but verbal expressiveness and the capacity for gesticulation linked to the upper limb are mainly cortical functions and may thus improve only by co-operation from the patient.

Hence, if prolongation of deep coma represents an unfavourable prognostic factor *quoad vitam*, the prolongation of an apallic coma is an unfavourable prognostic factor *quoad valetudinem*.

At the end of the rehabilitative programme, only 37% of apallic patients will be able to express themselves satisfactorily. In a similar percentage of cases patients appear to interact with the environment but have clear limitations reacting to it.

This makes the treatment to prolonged coma a difficult and an unrewarding task. Difficult because within the complexity of the problems raised by these patients it is necessary to outline priorities, times and methods. Unthankful because from the beginning one already knows that the results that can at best be achieved only after years, will be a far cry from normality.

Very often the exiguity of the resources remaining is the reason for the patient's deep gratitude for outcomes that would otherwise be considered modest in different scenarios.

Assessment of the final outcome after severe brain damage

Persisting disability after brain damage usually combines both structural and physical handicaps.

The mental component is often the most important in contributing to overall social disability (Jennet and Bond 1975, Bryan 1977). It has been stated that most patients who have recovered after prolonged coma have developed little in the way of severe mental symptoms, and most will be able to return to productive work and not remain a burden on their family or society. This reflects the tendency to optimize about the outcome, understandable in those who have worked hard to save the patient's life in the acute stage.

Therefore the need to attempt to realistically classify the nature of disability in survivors of brain damage is an absolute necessity. Some patients are euphoric and make little of their disability, and personality change is the most frequent permanent symptom.

Spasticity and dysphasia may improve for years. However, neuropsychological follow-up indicates that function recovery is most likely to occur within 12 months, whereas in stroke patients this takes 2 months (Waters et al 1990).

Patients who are submitted for surgical evaluation are usually assessed in a multidisciplinary team environment (Schoenhuber et al 1990). The Glasgow assessment scale remains a useful evaluation instrument for the surgeon, as these patients usually belong to the most favourable groups (3, 4, 5) of this scale. In group 3 the patients are conscious but severely disabled. In group 4 they are disabled but independent, as they can travel by public transport and can work in a sheltered environment. In group 4, good recovery implies resumption of normal life even though there may be minor neurological and physiological deficits. A more detailed scale related to specific tasks in spastic patients has been proposed by Lindon (1963). We will expand on this scale later in the chapter as this is the classification we have adopted.

Clinical examination

For surgeons who commonly deal with children affected by cerebral palsy or adults with stroke, survivors after a prolonged coma present very peculiar aspects.

The two hemispheres are normally differently affected by diffuse axonal damage. On one hand, a clinical picture of frank paralysis can be observed. While, on the other, a spastic hemiparesis with predominant myostatic contracture can usually be appreciated. The two sites will therefore carry different prognostic outcomes.

As a general rule, the post-comatose patients will be referred to the upper limb surgeon soon after the best possible independence has been achieved through rehabilitation. The need to handle assisting ambulatory devices is often the 'motivation' for consulting an orthopaedic surgeon with specific experience with 'neurologically impaired' upper limbs. The peculiar clinical features in the sequelae of prolonged coma are the following:

- The compromised general medical status, communication and learning ability, ambulatory capacities and social skills of the patient (Braun 1982).
- Presence of para-articular ossifications mainly located at the elbow joint.
- A great variety of clinical pictures and severity of neurological damage which vary considerably from a posture of bilateral abduction and retropulsion of the shoulder, and flexion deformity

of the forearm with a closed fist (see Chapter 49), to a limited focal dystonia usually localized at the forearm of one limb.
- Any painful condition (untreated skeletal injuries, subacromial conflict, etc.), should be identified and treated as they will interfere with the rehabilitation programme and might trigger a reflex sympathetic dystrophy (RSD).
- Motor power is obviously assessed but it cannot be graded in the same way as in brachial plexus or peripheral nerve lesions. It is generally sufficient to perceive that adequate power is present in the spastic muscles.
- Motor spasticity is usually assessed by means of the Ashworth rating scale (Grazko et al 1995, Reiter et al 1996, Schoenhuber et al 1997; see also Chapter 45).

The muscle tone will be rated from 0 (no increase in tone) to 4 (complete rigidity in flexion or in extension). The surgeon often has to deal with group 3 patients, where the considerable increase in tone renders passive movements difficult.

Grazko et al (1995) have added a spasm frequency scale, with no spasm being present in group 0 and more than 10 spasms per week being recorded in group 4. Spasticity and rigidity are strictly related to the nature and duration of coma.

Spasticity and rigidity examination remain the most difficult part of the overall assessment. Several examinations need to be performed to limit the adverse effects of emotional stimuli linked to the first assessment.

The frequency of spasms in the post-comatose patients can be kept under control by pharmacological agents such as baclofen, but rigidity is scarcely influenced. Furthermore, differential diagnosis between rigidity and joint stiffness is often difficult, but if passive range of motion is not influenced by different positions of the neighbouring joints, joint stiffness should be presumed.

Further investigations and guidelines for treatment

X-rays will reveal if stiffness is also linked to extra-articular factors such as para-articular ossifications, which are in most cases concentrated at elbow level and more rarely at the shoulder and proximal interphalangeal (PIP) joints. This will obviously influence the surgical treatment, but quite often an intra-articular type of contracture is associated with extra-articular factors. Therefore, a formal joint release needs to be added if functional recovery of the limb is aimed for.

When spasticity affects both upper limbs, surgical rehabilitation is performed first in the less impaired one to release the myostatic contracture. Once a functional result is achieved, surgery can be considered for the other limb to improve cosmesis and personal hygiene. Sometimes extensive release of a completely paralysed limb can yield functional improvements, as an open hand can better handle different kinds of walking aids.

When only one limb is affected and spasticity is equally distributed over the entire limb, the shoulder and elbow should be treated first, and spasticity at the wrist and fingers second.

In general, we envisage that simple tenotomies should be carried out for spasticity at the shoulder.

At the elbow, lengthening procedures of the biceps and brachialis muscles are often associated with release of the medial and lateral epicondyle muscles. When para-articular ossifications are present they should be removed if they interfere with joint excursion.

If stiffness is of the intrinsic type, a formal joint release should be added.

Muscle sliding is preferred when dealing with functional muscles, otherwise a combination of tenotomies of the flexor carpi radials (FCR), palmaris longus (PL) and flexor carpi ulnaris (FCU) are associated to the superficialis to profundus (STP) procedure (Braun 1982). In both circumstances, the motor function of antagonist muscles (forearm, wrist and finger extension muscles) can be improved when activity of spastic muscles is reduced to some extent (Landi et al 1990, Priori et al 1995, Reiter et al 1996).

If spasticity of the intrinsic muscle is present, muscle release of the thenar or adductor and remaining muscles is initially performed.

Frequently, due to adaptation phenomenon, adduction contracture of the first web tends to recur, especially when hyponeurotization or neurectomy of the deep branch of the ulnar nerve have previously been carried out (see Chapter 46). In those circumstances, and whenever focal dystonia is the only clinical manifestation, local injection of botulinum toxin is indicated (Jankovic and Schwartz 1993), Reiter et al 1996, Priori et al 1995, Dunne et al 1995).

We dislike the extensive use of this method as, due to the considerable size of the proximal muscles, a dose exceeding the consented 400 units would be required. Furthermore, the cost, need for repeated injections, development of immunity (Dunne et al 1995), occurrence of pain and the possibility of remote weakness (Sheenan et al 1995), specifically at the upper limb, should be taken into account.

Functional assessment before and after surgery

Motor impairment causes various disabilities, listed in the International Classification of Disability and Handicap (ICIDH), such as personal care disabilities (personal hygiene, dressing), locomotor disabilities (deambulation, confining, lifting), dexterity disabilities (daily activities, manual activity, foot control), and situational disabilities (dependence and endurance) (Reiter et al 1996).

For simplicity we have adopted the functional classification introduced by Lindon in 1963, where patients are grouped in six classes as reported in Table 1.

Table 1 Classes of functional assessment

1 Essentially normal hand with no loss of functional efficiency in speed, dexterity, flexibility or power. No limitation in job capabilities. Capable of working in open competition.

2 Mild functional limitation with slight decrease in co-ordination and fine controlled movements. Able to perform all activities, but slower compared with Grade 1. Good power grip.

3 Reduced co-ordination and dexterity with slower reactions resulting in lower standards of hand efficiency and competence in fine work. Adequate controlled grip that can be used for gross motion. Hand can be used for feeding; can occasionally write and button clothes, but poorly.

4 Can function individually for coarse grasping, but control, co-ordination, power and dexterity are more limited than Grade 3. No useful thumb–finger apposition or function present. Works as a helping hand when unilateral.

5 Marked limitation of use with little or no individual function. Can be used for some support to a less involved or unaffected hand. No individual effectiveness, and if bilateral the patient requires constant care and supervision.

6 Functionally useless hand, due to deformity, spasticity, or lack of co-ordination, singly or in combination. No effective grasp or release.

Anaesthesiological guidelines

It is important to make a preoperative evaluation of the patient, who is generally in fair general condition, but often bears the consequences of prolonged tracheal intubation, tracheotomy for mechanical ventilation, and septic respiratory and urinary complications. These patients are also under pharmacological therapy that may interfere with anaesthetic procedures; they show a reduced muscular trophism and distal oedemas that sometimes make it hard to find a valid venous access. This happens because the superficial venous system has already been exploited over many years of treatment, and prolonged vasoconstriction that is provoked even for modest stimuli due to alterations of the autonomic nervous system.

Our experience with anaesthesia for surgical procedures of the upper limb, especially on patients with coma outcomes, has led us to improve the conventional peripheral anaesthesiological techniques. These improvements allow peripheral block which can be associated with sedation without the need to resort to general anaesthesia and tracheal intubation.

The use of electrostimulation (TENS) undoubtedly simplifies execution of brachial plexus block.

The visual examination of muscular fascicular contractions allows identification of the different nervous structures and a selective block with consistent reduction of local anaesthetic dosage and corresponding side effects (Greenblatt and Denson 1981, Pither et al 1985, Tassi et al 1993). The neurovegetative liability in patients with outcomes of deep coma, which often have cardiovascular impairment with severe hypotension, must in fact be carefully considered.

Axillary block is recommended in forearm and distal arm surgical procedures as well.

Interscalenic block ensures a complete anaesthesia of the superior branches of the brachial plexus, but sometimes an incomplete anaesthesia of the distal ones (ulnar, brachial, cutaneous-medialis of the arm and forearm (Kulenkamff and Persky 1983)). Therefore, we recommend its use for surgery of the shoulder and elbow.

Personal experience, surgical techniques, results and conclusions

Our experience is based on 21 surgically treated cases where spasticity of the upper limb was the result of prolonged coma (Table 2). Of these cases, 17 were revised by an independent assessment team with a follow-up of more than 1 year (Table 2).

One of the features of this group of patients was their young age (minimum 11 years, maximum 51 years, average 26.6 years).

In only two cases (cases 17 and 19) surgery was performed at the shoulder level. In four cases spasticity of the elbow was the only relevant feature, and surgery was confined to this area. In two cases elbow release was followed by an extensive muscle sliding procedure of the forearm muscles.

In four cases spasticity and myostatic contracture was so severe that a distal tenotomy or lengthening at the myotendinous junctions of the wrist flexors was also needed after the extensive flexor muscle sliding procedure (FMS).

In case 6 (Table 2), there was a functional gain of four classes according to the Lindon scale. In two cases improvement was of three classes, while in most cases this was of two classes. Only two cases were unmodified among patients followed for more than 1 year.

Therefore, according to our experience the following procedures might be indicated for postcomatose patients:

At the shoulder: surgical release is recommended (Fig. 1) when spastic contracture causes severe pain or prevents axillary hygiene (Waters et al 1990).

Six muscles are responsible for adduction and internal rotation contractures of the shoulder: the pectoralis major, subscapularis, coracobrachialis, latissimus dorsi, teres major and the anterior belly of the deltoid.

Surgery is performed through a deltopectoral incision. The pectoralis major and subscapularis are released in addition to the teres major and latissimus dorsi if they were tight preoperatively (Fig. 1). The most frequent combination of release in our practice, at least in stroke patients, regarded the pectoralis major, subscapularis and anterior deltoid muscles.

The rehabilitation programme has to be initiated immediately postoperatively.

At the elbow: spasticity is usually confined to the

Table 2

Patient	Aetiology	Duration of coma	Final Neurological diagnosis	Preoperative Lindon class	Surgical procedures	Follow-up (years)	Postoperative Lindon class	Improvements	Residual problems
1 24 years Male	Head trauma following RTA	3 M	Spastic hemiplegia on the right side	6	B,ZL BR release FSP Neurectomy deep branch UN	5	4	Improved autonomy with tripod	–
2 25 years Male	Head trauma following precipitation injury	8 M	Bihemispheric spastic tetraparesis	6	Elbow arthrolysis and triceps release	1.5	5	Improved ADL	–
3 16 years Male	Deep silvian spontaneous haematoma	not reported	Spastic hemiparesis on the right side	6	FSP BR to EPL Add R	9	4	Better personal hygiene Can drive a car	–
4 22 years Male	Head trauma following RTA	40 D	Left spastic hand	5	TNT FCR FS long fingers TNT of EIP, APL to EPL	1.3	5	Improved wrist function	Need for stabilization of PIPJ TNT 2nd finger to be repeated
5 27 years Male	Head trauma following RTA	9 M	Spasticity of upper limb on the left side	-MEMR 6	MEMR STP, IMR, + ADD R TNT FPL on the left side	1.4	5/6	Improved personal hygiene and ADL	Further release for recurrence IMC
6 21 years Male	Head trauma following RTA	21 D	Spastic tetraparesis	6	MEMR and TNT FCU, FCR, FS and MTL FP on the right side	1.1	2	Complete independence in ADL	–
7 20 years Male	Head trauma following RTA	Deep coma 40 D vigilant coma 8 M	Spastic hemiplegia on the left side	1 5	MEMR on left side	3	2	Ties shoes and buttons sleeves etc.	–
8 22 years Male	Head trauma following RTA	Deep coma 1 M vigilant coma 16 D	Spasticity and stiffness right elbow	3	Arthrolysis of the elbow joint BR, release and ZL of B on right side	2.5	1	Complete independence in ADL	–
9 37 years Male	Head trauma following RTA	8 M	Spastic tetraparesis	3	TNT FCU and LSS. 2nd and 3rd finger on right side IMR 3rd finger	4.5	2	Significant improvement in ADL	Recurrence swan neck of 3rd finger
10 19 years Female	Head trauma following RTA	5 M	Outcomes of apallic syndrome	6	LEMR + MEMR and MTL of FPL	2.5	6	No real improvements in ADL	–
11 51 years Male	Hemiplegia probably due to left carotic stenosis (ictus)		Spastic hemiplegia on the left side	6	FSP, MTL of FPL Neurectomy of motor branch of UN - fusion TMJ TNT APL, FPL, ADD R	1.5	5	Improvements in ADL	Suggested procedures: 1) Release of the apo-nevrotic septum of the radial extensors 2) Transfer of ECRL to EPL

12 22 years Male	Head trauma following RTA	Vigilant apallic coma 2 M	Right spastic hemiplegia of upper limb on the right side	3	MEMR IMR and TNT FCR and PL	1,1	2	GI	–
13 28 years Male	Head trauma following RTA	3 D	Tetraparesis with spastic elbow on the right side	6	LEMR LNG of B, arthrolysis of elbow joint	1,1	4	Independent in dressing and grooming	–
14 17 years Male	Head trauma following RTA	4 M	Spasticity on the right side in tetraplegia	5	TNT FCU and MEMR on the right side	2,8	2	Significant improvement in ADL	–
15 33 years Male	Head trauma following RTA	Apallic coma 8 M	Spastic hemiparesis on the right side and spastic hemiplegia on the left side	6 L 5 R	Arthrolysis of the elbow and FSP on the right side Fusion of PIPJ 2nd, 3rd and 4th, + STP 3rd, 4th and 5th finger on the left	4,3	3 on the right	Improved walking with device Resumed original job as attorney	–
16 39 years Female	Head trauma following RTA	3 D	Contracture flexion of 4th and 5th finger of right hand in patient with infantile psycosis	6	Fusion PIPJ and MTL of flexors 4th and 5th finger	1	4	Improvement in ADL She can now sweep with broom	–
17 32 years Male	Head trauma following RTA	not reported	Spasticity of the left upper limb	6	TNT PM and 2/3 of anterior deltoid M, MEMR, TNT FCR, PL and FCU	1	4	Improvement in ADL	–
18 29 years Male	Head trauma following RTA	4 M	Spasticity of the right upper limb	NR	MEMR, TNT FP and FS, FCR and FPL	11 M	NC	NC	NC
19 37 years Female	Head trauma following RTA	3 M	Spastic tetraplegia	6	PM and B release, MEMR on left side	10 M	NC	NC	NC
20 18 years Male	Head trauma following RTA	2 M	Focal dystonia of left upper limb	3	Botulinum toxin	5 M	NC	NC	NC
21 11 years Male	Head trauma following RTA	Deep coma 5 M	Spastic hemiplegia on the left side	6	MEMR partial TNT FPL and FS of 3rd and 4th fingers	6 M	NC	NC	NC

Anatomical structures
APL: abductor pollicis longus
B: biceps
BR: brachioradialis
EIP: extensor indicis proprius
ECRL: extensor carpi radialis longus
EPL: extensor pollicis longus
FCR: flexor carpi radialis
FCU: flexor carpi ulnaris
FP: flexor profundus
FPL: flexor pollicis longus
FS: flexor superficialis
PIPJ: proximal interphalangeal joint
PL: palmaris longus
PM: pectoralis major
TMJ: trapezium metacarpal joint
UN: ulnar nerve

Procedures
ADD R: adductor release
FSP: flexor sliding procedure
IMR: intrinsic muscle release
LEMR: lateral epicondylar muscle release
LNG: lengthening
LSS: lasso technique
MEMR: medial epycondylar muscle release
MTL: myotendineous lengthening
STP: superficialis to profundus release
TNT: tenotomy
TT: tendon transfer
ZL: zed lengthening

Overall assessments
ADL: activities of daily life
D: days
GI: general improvement
IMC: intrinsic muscle contracture
M: months
NC: not controlled
NR: not reported
RTA: road traffic accident

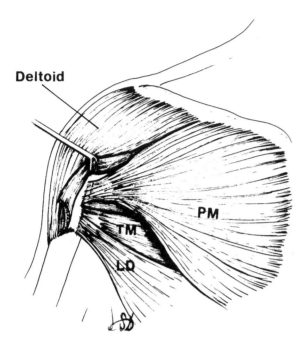

Figure 1

Muscle release of the spastic shoulder is accomplished step by step. Release of the pectoralis major (PM) is sufficient in most cases. Release of the anterior group of the deltoid muscle (DM) sometimes needs to be added. In subsequent order the subscapularis tendon (not reported in the figure) might be divided followed by the release of latissimus dorsi (LD) and teres major (TM).

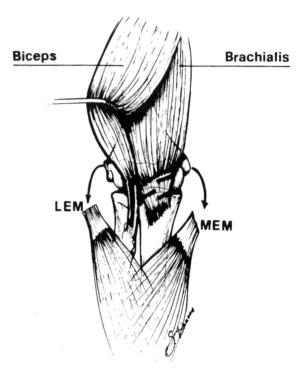

Figure 2

Surgical treatment of the spastic elbow is usually accomplished by Z-lengthening of the biceps. The brachialis might be released through multiple incisions at the myotendineous junction. Very often release of the medial epicondylar muscles (MEM) is required and, on a case by case basis, detachment of the brachioradialis (not represented in the figure) and lateral epicondylar muscles (LEM) might be necessary.

flexors. Very rarely spasticity of the triceps is associated, and this will lead to rigidity of this joint.

Different muscles might contribute to flexion deformity; therefore, each single case will require a personal type of release (Braun 1982).

In some patients it is possible to release an elbow contracture by lengthening the biceps tendon and by simple partial myotomy of the brachialis across the anterior antecubital space. In other cases, the contracture is so severe as to require lengthening of the biceps, myotomy of the brachialis, release of the brachioradialis and of the medial and lateral epicondylar muscles (Fig. 2).

If para-articular ossifications need to be removed, an anterior approach is adequate if they are located anteriorly. When ossifications are present on the posterior aspect, a double approach is selected (Kiaergard-Andersen et al 1993). When flexion/contracture of the elbow is due mainly to overactivity of the brachioradialis muscle, the posterolateral approach is ideal (Tsuge and Mizuseki 1994) as it allows detachment of this muscle, anterior capsulotomy, and consents a simultaneous joint release whenever required. Under these circumstances tenotomy of the biceps is often associated.

Release of the spastic elbow has constantly produced a considerable improvement of the upright posture of the entire body.

When detachment of the medial and lateral epicondylar muscles is performed, spasticity at the wrist level often resolves or improves significantly. Correction of a flexion deformity at the elbow is maintained by a dorsal slab in extension for 3 weeks. If arthrolysis has been associated, passive flexion exercises are performed on a daily basis.

At the forearm and wrist: flexor muscle sliding represents our technique of choice in the post-comatose patients (Fig. 3), as strength is preserved as compared with other techniques such as non-invasive (botulinum toxin), surgical (such as hyponeurotization; see Chapter 46) or chemical (such as denervation; Waters et al 1990, Braun 1982).

Residual spasticity at the wrist, which is present after an extensive muscle sliding procedure, may be corrected by functional lengthening of the wrist flexors at the myotendineous junction (Fig. 3). An arm–forearm thumb spica cast is applied continuously for 3 weeks. A formal rehabilitation programme is initiated soon afterwards. When dealing with a non-functional type of contracture surgery is still indicated, and we usually utilize the STP procedure.

At the hand, a long-standing contracture might have led to a marked flexion deformity of PIP joint, whereas contracture of the forearm muscles might not be very relevant. Fusion of the PIP joint (case 15 and 16, Table 2) in a functional position is then indicated. Contracture of the deep distal extensors might lead to retropulsion of the thumb. Besides the PIP joint, the only case when a joint fusion is considered is at the level of the teres major, but it should be associated with tenotomy of the long abductor to avoid delayed union caused by the underlying hyperactivity of this muscle (case 11, Table 2).

The intrinsic type of contracture has not frequently been observed in post-comatose patients. Tenotomy or muscle release of the adductor muscle or botulinum toxin injections are the procedures we usually select.

The place for tendon transfer in post-comatose patients is very limited. We stick to the rule that muscles that are active both during grasp and release are not suitable for transfer procedures. Basically, FCR or FCU have been used for wrist extension, when spontaneous recovery of the original wrist extension muscles has not occurred after flexor release, and brachioradialis to extensor pollicis longus (McCue et al 1970) have been used in

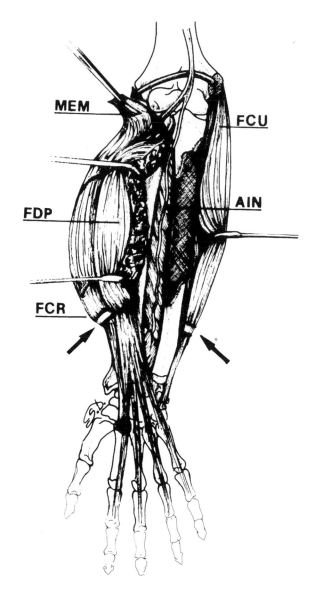

Figure 3

The flexor sliding procedure (FSP) begins with release of the medial epicondylar muscles (MEM) including the epitrochlear head of flexor carpi ulnaris (FCU). The olecranon head of FCU is left in place and further lengthening is achieved, when required, by release at its myotendineous junction (lighter arrow). Detachment of the flexor muscle bulk is accomplished in the proximal–distal direction by detaching it from the ulna and interosseous membrane. Preservation of the anterior interosseous nerve (AIN) and artery is imperative. If further release becomes necessary it can be achieved by tenotomy of palmaris longus and flexor carpi radialis (FCR) at its myotendineous junction (darker arrow).

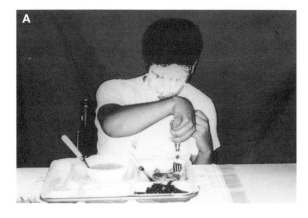

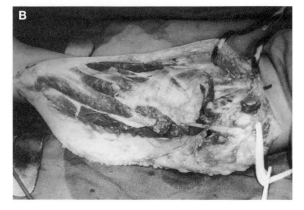

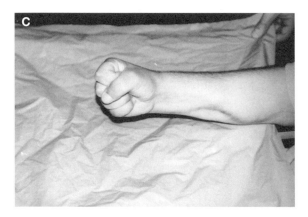

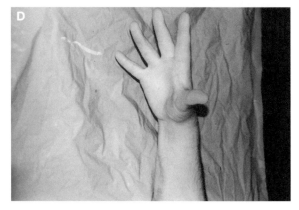

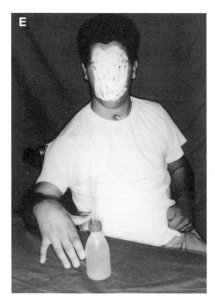

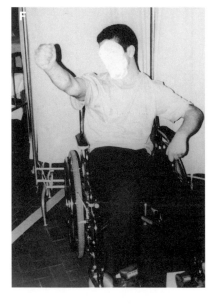

Figure 4

General improvement 15-year-old male (14 in Table 2). (A) Prolonged coma lasting 3.5 months following head injury. The dominant (R) upper limb was mainly affected, with obvious problems in daily life activity. (B) A muscle sliding procedure associated with tenotomy of the flexor carpi ulnaris (FCU) was performed. (C)(D)(E) At nearly 3 years follow-up the patient has achieved complete independence, moving from class 5 to class 2 of the Lindon rating scale. (F) Distal release has indirectly positively influenced elbow function and the overall posture.

addition to surgical treatment of the thumb in palm deformity to facilitate displacement of the thumb from the palm.

In conclusion, we have been positively impressed by the functional outcomes related to surgical treatment of spasticity, rigidity and stiffness in post-comatose patients (Fig. 4).

The factors behind this success have to be related to the fact that myostatic contracture, at least at one site when dealing with a bilateral involvement, depends on the shortening of the supporting connective structures which gives the misleading impression of severe spasticity or rigidity. The functional results that can be obtained in a motivated patient appear to be at least comparable to the surgical outcomes usually achieved in the cerebral palsy and the stroke group of patients (Zancolli et at 1983, Zancolli 1979).

Acknowledgements

The authors acknowledge Professor R Schoenhuber for providing an independent assessment of the operated cases, Professor P Nichelli for assisting in the revision of the neurological concepts, Dr E Bertellini for her contribution to the anaesthesiological guidelines and Dr J Pradelli reviewing the English translation.

References

Bosch Blancafort J, Olesti MM, Poch Puig JM, Rubio Garcia E, Nougués Bara P, Iglesias Berenguer J (1995) Predictive value of brain-stem auditory evoked potentials in children with post-traumatic coma produced by diffuse brain injury, *Child's Nerv Syst* **11**:400–5.

Braun RM (1982) Part II: Stroke rehabilitation. In: Green D, ed. *Operative Hand Surgery*, Vol. 1. Churchill Livingstone: New York: 195–211.

Bryan RS (1977) The Moberg deltoid triceps replacement and key pinch operations in quadriplegia: preliminary experiences, *Hand* **9**:207–14.

Childs NL, Mercer WN (1996) Brief report: late improvement in consciousness after post-traumatic vegetative state, *N Engl J Med* **334**:24–5.

Dunne JW, Heye N, Dunne SL (1995) Treatment of chronic limb spasticity with botulinum toxin A, *J Neurol, Neurosurg Psy* **58**:232–5.

Grazko MA, Polo KB, Jabbari G (1995) Botulinum toxin A for spasticity, muscle spasms, and rigidity, *Neurology* **45**:712–17.

Greenblatt GM, Denson JS (1981) Needle nerve simulator-locator, *Anesth Analg* **41**:599–602.

Jankovic J, Schwartz KS (1993) Use of botulinum toxin in the treatment of hand dystonia, *J Hand Surg* **18A**:883–7.

Jennet B, Bond M (1975) Assessment of outcome after severe brain damage – a practical scale, *Lancet* **i**:480–4.

Kiaergard-Andersen P, Nafei A, Teichert G, Kristensen O, Schmidt SA, Keller J, Lucht U, (1993) Indomethacin for prevention of heterotopic ossification, *Acta Orthop Scand* **64**:639–42.

Kraus JF, McArthur DL (1996) Epidemiology aspects of brain injury. In: Riggs JE, ed. *Neurologic Clinic, Neuro-epidemiology*, Vol. 14. Saunders: Philadelphia: 435–50.

Kraus JF (1987) The epidemiology of brain injuries: the utility of data from population-based studies of brain injured persons. In: *Intern Head Injury Institute. Medical Legal-Rehabilitation*. Emmanuel College, Cambridge, England. Aug. 1st–8th, 1–31.

Kulenkamff D, Persky MA (1983) Brachial plexus anaesthesia: its indications, technic and dangers, *Ann Surg* **87**:883–91.

Landi A, Cavana R, Caserta G, Esposito M, Saracino A (1990) Emiplegia spastica: aspetti epidemiologici ed indicazioni al trattamento chirurgico. In: Lardi A, ed. Atti Hesperia Agg. 'Corso Italiano permanente di Ortesi e Riabilitazione dell' Arto Superiore Vol. 4. 7–9 December 1990. L'arto superiore nelle lesioni nervose centrali.15–26.

Lindon RL (1963) The pultibec system for the Medical Assessment of Handicapped Children, *Dev Med Child Neurol* **5**:125–45.

Marini JJ, Wheeler AP (1989) Coma, seizures and brain death. In: *Critical Care Medicine, The Essentials*. Williams & Wilkins: Baltimore: 237–40.

McCue F, Honner R, Chapman WC (1970) Transfer of the brachioradialis for hands deformed by cerebral palsy, *J Bone Joint Surg* **52A**:171–80.

Pither CE, Raj PP, Ford DJ (1985) The use of peripheral nerve stimulators for regional anaesthesia. A review of experimental characteristics, technique and clinical application, *Regional Anesth* **10**:49–58.

Plum F, Posner JB (1982) *The Diagnosis of Stupor and Coma*. FA Davis: Philadelphia.

Priori A, Berardelli A, Mercuri B, Manfredi M (1995) Physiological effects produced by botulinum toxin treatment of upper limb dystonia, *Brain* **118**:801–7.

Reiter F, Danni M, Ceravolo MG, Provinciali L (1996) Disability changes after treatment of upper limb spasticity with botulinum toxin, *J Neuro Rehab* **10**:47–52.

Schoenhuber R, Gentilini M, Bortolotti P (1990) Il controllo neurologico nell'arto superiore. In: Landi A, ed. Atti Hesperia Agg. 'Corso Italiano permanente di Ortesi e Riabilitazione dell'Arto Superiore – 4th meeting 7–9 December 1990. L'arto superiore nelle lesioni nervose centrali.' pp. 1–8.

Schoenhuber R, Prugger M, Capone L (1997) Valore prognostico delle scale di valutazione funzionale nel traumatizzato cranico, *Fondazione Clinica del Lavoro* Vol. 1. In press.

Sheenan GL, Murray NMF, Marsden CD (1995) Pain and remote weakness in limbs injected with botulinum toxin A for writer's cramp, *Lancet* **346**:154–6.

Sorbi S, Nacmias B, Piacentini S, Repice A, Latorraca S, Forleo P, Amaducci L (1995) ApoE as a prognostic factor for post-traumatic coma, *Nature Med* **1**:852.

Strittmatter WJ (1992) Altered mental status and coma. In: Civetta JM, Taylor RW, Kirby RR, eds. *Critical Care*. JB Lippincott: Philadelphia: 1467–75.

Tassi A, Bertellini E, Grama G (1993) Blocco del plesso brachiale con elettroneurostimolatore. *Atti Convegno 'Modena 93', Anestesia e Rianimazione Terapia Intensiva*: 209–11.

Tsuge K, Mizuseki T (1994) Debridement arthroplasty for advanced primary osteoarthritis of the elbow, *J Bone Joint Surg* **76B**:641–6.

Waters RL, Wilson DJ, Savinelli Hecker R (1990) Rehabilitation of the upper extremity after stroke. Hemiplegia and tetraplegia; In: Hunter JM, ed. *Rehabilitation of the Hand: Surgery and Therapy*. CV Mosby: St. Louis: 953–63.

Zancolli EA, Goldner LJ, Swanson AB (1983) Surgery of the spastic hand in cerebral palsy: Report of the Committee on Spastic Hand Evaluation. *J Hand Surg* **8A**:766–72.

Zancolli E (1979) Structural and dynamic basis of hand surgery, 2nd edn. JB Lippincott: Philadelphia: 263–83.

48
Surgical rehabilitation of the spastic upper limb

Eduardo A Zancolli

The spastic upper limb in patients with cerebral palsy presents one of the most complex problems in reconstructive hand surgery. This is due to the pathology of the central nervous system and the severity of motor imbalance and sensory impairment of the hand. In spite of these difficulties, upper extremity surgery has become an excellent aid in the management of the spastic hand when properly indicated and performed (Goldner 1955 and 1975, Swanson 1968, Zancolli 1968 and 1975). Careful examination, testing and evaluation by the surgeon and the occupational therapist are of major importance in the selection of patients for surgical reconstruction.

Most poor surgical results are due to incorrect indications and poor selection and execution of surgical procedures. Our principal aim is to examine the surgical indications related to the general and local conditions and to explain the surgical techniques we prefer based on the clinical characteristics of upper limb pathology in elbow, forearm, wrist fingers and thumb. Our experience is based on a series of 113 upper limb spastic cases operated on over 33 years. The final results to 47 patients evaluated from a selected group of 91 patients. Of these cases, 84% had operations in the Rehabilitation Center of Buenos Aires (Argentina).

Preoperative evaluation and general surgical indications

The principal parameters studied when selecting cases suited to surgery are:

- aetiology
- general neurological condition
- type of neuromuscular disorder
- extent of limb involvement
- age
- hand sensory impairment
- upper limb deformities (pronator–flexor spastic contracture; elbow, forearm, wrist, thumb and finger)
- classification of hand deformity (voluntary grasp and release patterns of the hand, wrist and fingers).

Aetiology

Cerebral palsy may be defined as an impairment of muscle function due to brain damage. The lesion of the intercranial central nervous system may have its origin in pre-, peri- or postnatal periods. In our experience perinatal brain damage is the most suited to peripheral surgery when the patient is a young hemiplegic.

Perinatal injuries have two main causes: trauma and anoxia during the time of birth. *Prenatal* cerebral palsy may be produced by congenital defects (rubella or other virus disease during the first 3 months of pregnancy) or erythroblastosis fetalis. These defects may produce ataxia or athetosis. *Postnatal lesions* may be caused by infectious encephalitis (most frequent), meningitis, convulsions in a very young child (intercranial haemorrhage) or injury. Blumel et al (1960) found the most frequent lesions were due to trauma at birth (13%), anoxia (24%), prematurity (32%), congenital defects (11%) and postnatal damage (7%).

General neurological defects

Severe neurological defects are usually not found in typical infantile spastic hemiplegia which is the condition most suited to reconstructive surgery of the upper limb. Surgery should be contraindicated when defects in speech, vision and hearing are manifest. These cases are generally associated with tetraplegia, extrapyramidal neuromuscular disorders, convulsions, manifest behavioural disorders, distractibility and learning disability.

Mild alterations of the mental condition are not a surgical contraindication. Surgery is contraindicated when spasticity is markedly increased by emotional stimuli. In this last condition it is very difficult to obtain a reasonable result even if the hand deformity is mild.

The patient must be capable of understanding the surgical goals and be sufficiently motivated to collaborate during postoperative re-education.

Type of neuromuscular disorder

Patients with neuromuscular disorders can be put into one of three groups: *spastic* or *pyramidal*, *extrapyramidal* and *mixed*. Most cases are pyramidal and mixed (60%). It is very important to study the principal clinical characteristics of each type of neuromuscular disorder when selecting candidates for reconstructive surgery.

Pyramidal type

In this type of neuromuscular disorder the classical deformity is characterized by a combination of spastic (pronator–flexor) and paretic or flaccid paralytic (extensor–supinator) muscles. Here we shall study in particular the principal characteristics of the spastic muscle.

(a) *Spastic muscles* through their hypertonicity produce the *typical flexor–pronator deformity of the upper limb*. The most common posture is one of elbow, wrist and finger flexion with forearm pronation and the thumb in adduction or flexion–adduction. These deformities depend on the spasticity of the extrinsic muscles of the forearm and hand and particularly of the flexor–pronator muscular mass. Occasionally, spasticity produces some internal rotation contracture of the shoulder. Flaccid paralysis or paresis affects the supinator–extensor muscles.

(b) It is typical of spastic muscle that its *hypertonic-*

ity increases progressively as the muscle is gradually stretched passively.

(c) *Spasticity is posturally and emotionally induced.* It is rather constant except during sleep or under anaesthesia.

(d) *Synchronous activity or co-contraction* (Samilson and Morris 1964) is a typical characteristic of the spastic muscle. Its clinical manifestation is represented by an abnormal reaction of the spastic muscles during rest or when the muscles are acting as antagonists. Antagonist muscles remain electrically active on both flexion and extension of the involved part of the limb. A typical finding is the persistent activity of the flexor muscles of the wrist when complete finger and wrist extension are attempted, especially at the level of the flexor carpi ulnaris (FCU). Synchronous activity alters the normal grasping and release patterns of the hand.

Co-contraction can be a favourable situation in some tendinous reconstructive procedures (Swanson 1968). Thus co-contraction favours active extension of the wrist after the transfer of a spastic FCU tendon to the extensors of the wrist. Under this condition, the co-contraction of the FCU produces wrist extension due to its synchronous activity (Green's procedure; Green 1942).

(e) *Overactive stretch reflex* is one of the most useful manifestations in the diagnosis of spasticity. It is produced by failure of the normal muscle lengthening reaction on elongation by sudden passive stretching. Owing to the hyperactive stretch reflex, *the spastic muscle contracts at the same point in the arc of motion each time a passive elongation manoeuvre is produced.* Stretch reflex should be investigated for each muscle or group of muscles.

Spasticity and overactive reflexes can be decreased by certain surgical procedures such as lengthening of distal tendons or release of proximal muscle insertions.

Surgical reconstruction of the upper limb through soft tissue procedures, such as tenotomy and tendon transfer, are basically indicated in cases with pure spasticity, and also in spastic patients where mild athetosis is combined with spasticity (mixed group).

(f) *Myostatic contracture* represents a secondary muscular fibrosis after a long-standing flexion contracture. This fibrosis is frequently seen in the flexor muscles of the wrist and digits. It is evaluated with the patient under general anaesthesia or peripheral nerve blocking. This muscular retraction is not a contraindication to surgical reconstruction of the hand. Myostatic contracture is frequently observed during or after adolescence, particularly in permanent and severe contractures. It can be reduced preoperatively by physical methods of stretching with cast or braces. During surgery it is corrected by tenotomy preserving muscular continuity.

Extrapyramidal type

The extrapyramidal type of neuromuscular disorder can be represented by *athetosis*, *ataxia*, *tremor* or *rigidity*. The most frequent extrapyramidal disorder is *athetosis* (25%) which is characterized by:

- abnormal, involuntary and poorly co-ordinated movements with varying degrees of tension (Fig. 1); the deformity decreases at rest and disappears during sleep, but it is accentuated by efforts to move or by any emotional or environmental stimulus; typically the patient may show different finger deformities in the same hand; abnormal hand movements usually reduce if the patient is distracted
- delayed postural development
- hypotonus in infancy, which may change with growth to increased tonus in stress situations
- decreased reflexes in infancy, which may become hyperactive later
- no tendency to muscular contracture
- absence of Hoffman reflex
- frequently preserved sensibility of the hand.

Tremor is represented by involuntary movements that follow a regular rhythmic pattern in which flexor and extensor muscles contract alternately.

Ataxia is characterized by disturbed balance and equilibrium, lack of muscle co-ordination, and hypotonia.

Rigidity is demonstrated by resistance to movement through the hand's entire range, and no exaggerated stretch reflex: both contracting muscles and their antagonists are affected. There is a tendency for diminished motion rather than abnormal motion.

Soft tissue procedures carried out in the pure athetoid patient are absolutely contraindicated since they may produce a new undesirable opposing deformity that may be totally uncontrollable by the patient. In this situation a transference of the initial distorted position to other muscle groups is produced. Soft tissue procedures are also contraindicated in other extrapyramidal muscular disorders such as chorea, ataxia, tremor and rigidity. In athetosis may be exclusively indicated surgical procedures over bones (osteotomies) or joints (fusion).

Soft tissue procedures are absolutely contraindicated in a young child with extrapyramidal hypotonus which may change with growth to abnormal athetoid involuntary movements and increased tonus under emotional stimuli.

Mixed type

The mixed type of neuromuscular disorder is a relatively common form. Most frequently spasticity is associated with athetosis and is characterized by a combination of hypertonus and abnormal movements. Reconstructive surgery through soft tissues techniques may be indicated in the mixed type of neuromuscular disorder if hypertonicity and, consequently, the overactive stretch reflex are present and dominant.

Extent of limb involvement

Cerebral palsy can involve all four extremities as follows:

- *Tetraplegia* (both arms and both legs); rarely reconstructive surgery is indicated in infantile tetraplegia since these cases are frequently associated with severe neurological defects such as learning disability, extrapyramidal neuromuscular disorder, emotional instability, deficiency in motivation and co-operation, etc.
- *Hemiplegia* (one side of the body, usually with greater involvement of the upper limb); this is the ideal condition for upper limb reconstructive surgery when spasticity is dominant; these cases usually offer the best local and general conditions for improving hand function and muscular balance and for correcting a pronator–flexor deformity
- *Diplegia* (all four limbs, with the lower limbs much more severely involved than the upper limbs).

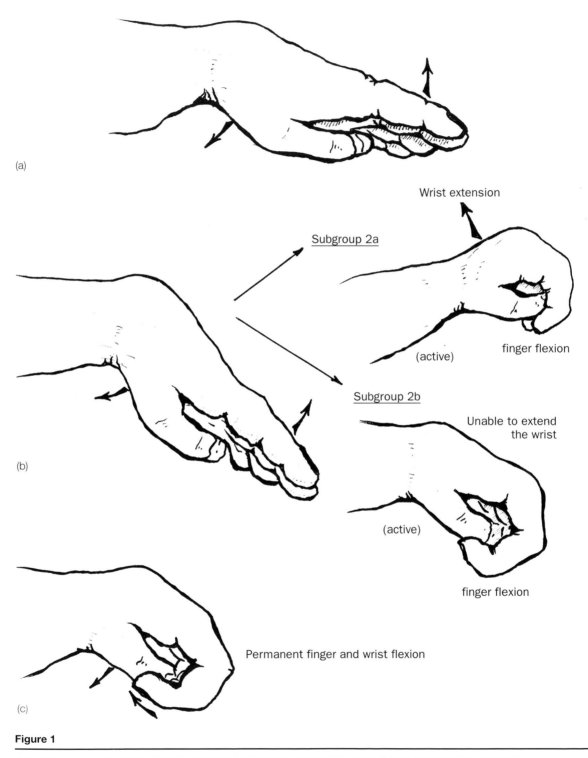

(a)

Subgroup 2a

Wrist extension

(active)   finger flexion

(b)

Subgroup 2b

Unable to extend
the wrist

(active)

finger flexion

(c)

Permanent finger and wrist flexion

Figure 1

Grouping of hand deformities (infantile spastic hemiplegia): a, group 1; b, group 2 (and subgroups); c, group 3

- *Triplegia* (three extremities, usually with both legs and one arm being affected)
- *Monoplegia* (single limb involvement).

Age

Surgical correction of spastic upper limb deformities is usually indicated after 5–6 years of age. Maturation of the central nervous system has occurred by this age, and the child is old enough to co-operate during postoperative rehabilitation. After adolescence, patients are not, in general, good candidates for reconstructive surgery since they have usually accepted their cosmetic and functional problems.

Hand sensory impairment

Based on our experience (Zancolli and Zancolli 1987) all patients with a pure spastic neuromuscular disorder who are candidates for reconstructive surgery have *some deficit of sensibility in proprioception* (conscious control of position, motion and power) and *stereognosia* (ability to recognize objects by touch only). In the classical infantile hemiplegia with a pure spastic neuromuscular disorder the affected hand preserves the ability to recognize the physical characteristics of objects (shape, size, texture) or protective sensations (hot, cold, pain, pressure), but the patient is unable to name the objects because of cortical involvement. This is the typical condition in these cases.

Defects in stereognosis (Twitchell 1966) is not a contraindication for attempting to improve hand motor function and appearance by surgery.

Only in cases where spasticity is combined with some athetoid component may hand sensibility be completely preserved.

Sensibility tests used in these patients are:

- *pinprick test* (protective sensation)
- *recognition of size and shape of objects* (differentiation of cubes from marbles in small children)
- *Seddon's coin test* (tactile gnosis); this is our preferred test during patient examination
- *two-point discrimination* (Moberg's paper clip test; tactile gnosis)
- *position sense* (proprioception or body position movement recognition).

Spastic hemiplegic children with stereognosis defects prefer to use the normal hand. They will use the affected hand only when necessary for bimanual activities and always as an assistant limb. When sensibility is not affected (mixed group), better function can be obtained and independent function of the affected hand can be expected.

In patients presenting with severe sensory defects, with loss of even touch and pain sensations and permanently flexed digits, any attempt at functional restoration through surgery is ineffective. This is the situation of some stroke patients.

Upper limb deformity (pronator–flexor spastic contracture)

The typical flexion–pronation deformity of the spastic upper limb in cerebral palsy is characterized by:

- shoulder: unusual and very mild internal rotation contracture
- elbow: flexion contracture
- forearm: pronation contracture
- hand:
  - wrist and fingers; flexion contracture of wrist and fingers, with occasional flexible swan-neck deformity
  - thumb; two types of deformities may be present (Fig. 2):
  - adduction (adduction of the first metacarpal)
  - flexion–adduction (thumb-in-palm deformity).

All these deformities are variable in severity.

Classification of hand deformity (voluntary grasp and release patterns of the hand, wrist and fingers)

Since earlier publications on hand deformity (Zancolli 1968 and 1979) we have classified hand deformity into three groups (see also Zancolli and Zancolli 1981, Zancolli et al 1983). The classification (Zancolli 1979, Zancolli and Zancolli 1987) is based on the voluntary ability of the patient to exhibit grasp and release patterns of the wrist and fingers (Fig. 1). The surgical programme is closely related to this classification.

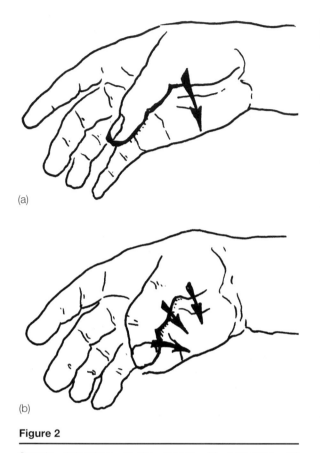

(a)

(b)

Figure 2

Spastic deformities of the thumb. (a) Adduction. (b) Flexion–adduction

It is important for the patient and the surgeon to have some type of voluntary control of the spastic muscles and some voluntary release and closure of the fingers for satisfactory results to be achieved through reconstructive surgery. Experience has shown that the most favourable cases for surgery are those in which it is possible to open the fingers by active flexion of the wrist. For this reason wrist arthrodesis should not be a primary option in typical spastic infantile hemiplegia if the patient has the ability to extend the fingers through wrist flexion. *Synergism between wrist and fingers should be preserved whenever possible.* We only consider wrist fusion in atypical spastic conditions – residual deformities of failed previous operations – where tendon transfers or other soft tissues procedures

are impossible to perform or contraindicated, and in some extrapyramidal neuromuscular disorders (Zancolli 1968).

Group 1

In this group flexion spasticity is minimal (Zancolli 1979). The patient can completely extend the fingers with a neutral position of the wrist or with less than 20° of flexion. Spasticity is basically localized at the FCU muscle. The principal deficits in this group are the lack of complete active wrist dorsiflexion when the fingers are totally extended and thumb deformity (Zancolli and Zancolli 1987). The general appearance of the upper limb is satisfactory and the emotional influence on spasticity is mild or almost absent.

Group 2

In these patients, the fingers can also be actively extended, as in group 1, but only with more than 20° of wrist flexion (Zancolli and Zancolli 1987). Spasticity is localized at the wrist and finger flexors. In severe cases the wrist needs to flex completely to permit complete or partial finger extension. Group 2 has two subgroups according to the functional condition of the extensor muscles of the wrist. In *subgroup 2a* the patient can actively extend – partially or totally – the wrist with the fingers flexed. This means that the extensor muscles of the wrist are active and voluntarily controlled and that the main spasticity is localized in the wrist and finger flexor muscles. In these cases, obviously, it is unnecessary to indicate tendon transfers to extend the wrist. In *subgroup 2b* the patient cannot actively extend the wrist with the finger flexed because of flaccid paralysis of the wrist extensor muscles. Tendon transfers to extend the wrist will be necessary in these cases.

Group 3

Here the spasticity and deformity are severe and localized at the flexor–pronator mass as in the other groups. The extensor muscles of the wrist and fingers are totally paralysed. The patient cannot extend the fingers even with maximal flexion of the wrist. Synergism is lost. This condition is the most difficult one to improve by reconstructive surgery. Release of the spastic muscles of the upper limb is the principal goal in this group of patients (Zancolli 1979, Zancolli and Zancolli 1981 and 1987, Zancolli 1982).

These three groups usually may be associated with: thumb contracture, elbow flexion contracture and pronation contracture of the forearm, of variable degrees of severity. The degree of *sensory impairment* may vary from one group to another.

Surgical goals

The principal goals in surgical rehabilitation of the spastic hand are to improve: grasp and release patterns, hand appearance; and the psychological status of the patient and the family.

Prognosis

According to the classification previously described, basic hand functions in grasp (release and pinch functions) can be significantly improved in groups 1 and 2. In these cases it is possible to obtain: improved finger release with decreased flexion of the wrist; decreased flexion contracture of the elbow, wrist and fingers; decreased forearm pronation contracture and correction of thumb deformity to improve gripping and lateral pinch.

The main concept in surgical reconstruction of the spastic hand is that an improvement in the existing pattern of function can be achieved by *improving the balance between the spastic pronator and flexor muscles and the normal or paretic-paralyzed extensor and supinator muscles*. Attempts to modify radically the existing patterns of activity (synergism) or overcorrection will usually give a poor result. Only in very mild group 1 cases is it possible to obtain normal complete and simultaneous extension of the wrist and fingers.

In group 3, surgery is indicated primarily to improve appearance, hygiene and comfort. This can be achieved by reducing the spasticity of the flexor–pronator muscles without, however, obtaining a voluntary hand release.

Adults and older patients with hemiplegia – vascular origin – do not adapt well to hand reconstruction because voluntary control of the wrist and fingers is usually absent. These patients generally cannot voluntarily flex the wrist to open the fingers, and, consequently, the hand is permanently closed and useless.

Surgical indications

According to the preoperative evaluations studied, the *best candidates for reconstructive surgery* (Zancolli and Zancolli 1981, Zancolli et al 1983) are those with the following characteristics:

- spastic type of neuromuscular disorder
- sufficient IQ and emotional stability
- low emotional influence on spasticity
- infantile hemiplegia (especially perinatal)
- young patients (infantile or adolescence)
- basic sensibility (even with some impairment of proprioception and tactile gnosia)
- some voluntary control of the spastic muscles and voluntary ability to open the fingers in flexion (synergism) (groups 1 and 2)
- capacity to concentrate and co-operate during the postoperative period
- good motivation and family support
- adequate behavioural patterns
- good general neurological condition.

Spastic flexion–pronation deformity is the only condition adapted to peripheral surgical reconstructive procedures. The surgical programme will depend on the severity and the various types of deformity at the different levels of the upper limb.

The most common deformities that can be corrected by reconstructive surgery are: thumb deformities, flexion contracture of the wrist and fingers, flexion contracture of the elbow and pronation contracture of the forearm. Very seldom swan-neck deformities of the fingers need to be corrected.

Surgery of the thumb is indicated to hold the digit out of the palm during grasp. The surgical procedures indicated depend on the type of deformity present: adduction contracture or adduction–flexion contracture (thumb-in-palm deformity).

Flexion contracture of the elbow is common in the spastic upper limb and is frequently influenced by emotional stimuli. Correction of marked flexion contracture of the elbow improves the appearance and function of the upper limb.

Pronation contracture of the forearm is corrected

when severe and when the patient has difficulty carrying out activities of daily living due to lack of supination. A mildly pronated forearm is a relatively useful position for hand function and its correction is not essential.

Flexion contracture of the wrist and fingers is corrected through surgical techniques based on the classification of hand deformity groups (1, 2 and 3). This indicates that during the preoperative examination it is of great importance to note the degree of wrist flexion needed to enable the patient to extend the fingers completely or partially. It is also important to note if the wrist can be extended with the fingers flexed (group 2a or b). These tests demonstrate the degree of spasticity of the flexor muscles of the wrist and fingers, the functional condition of the wrist extensors, and the degree of voluntary control; this information is needed to correct the deformity. This evaluation allows selection of the patient and of the most appropriate surgical procedure for each patient.

It is of paramount importance to correct all the existing deformities of the upper limb – elbow, forearm and hand – *at the same surgical procedure.* A contracted thumb must be simultaneously corrected with the rest of the hand to allow better active extension of the fingers and lateral pinch grip.

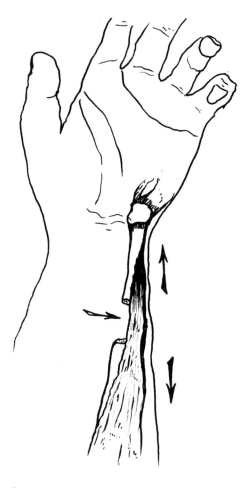

Figure 3

Flexor carpi ulnaris lengthening with muscular continuity (group 1 of spastic hand)

Surgical procedures

Surgical procedures which have been usually indicated in the spastic hand due to cerebral palsy include: muscle release, tenotomy, fasciotomy, tendon lengthening, tendon transfer, capsuloplasty, tenodesis, arthrodesis, osteotomy and neurotomies. The selection of the procedure depends basically on the type and severity of the deformity, the type of neuromuscular disorder, the functional deficiencies, the age of the patient and the surgeon's preferences.

Here we shall exclusively describe the operative procedure techniques of our preference.

Operative techniques

Flexion contracture of the wrist and fingers

This deformity basically results from the spasticity – occasional myostatic contracture – of the flexor muscles of the wrist and fingers. The goal of surgery is to improve the opening of the hand without affecting voluntary closure of the digits and grasping functions. This is achieved by reducing the muscular imbalance between the flexor and extensor muscles of the hand.

According to the grouping of cases previously presented, the surgical programme to correct flexion contracture of the wrist and fingers are as follows:

Group 1

As was said the principal muscular co-contraction is in the FCU. *Our aim is to lengthen the FCU through a tenotomy in continuity* (Zancolli 1979, Zancolli and Zancolli 1981 and 1987). In this type of tenotomy the tendinous part is sectioned or partially excised but the muscular fibres are preserved. After the release a passive stretching manoeuvre permits lengthening of the muscular unit. Tenotomy is located proximally to the distal end of the muscular belly (Fig. 3).

The *second aim is to reduce the spasticity of the medial epicondyle muscular mass by an ample aponeurotic release*, located 5 cm distally to the medial epicondyle. This technique is very effective for reducing flexion contracture of the wrist and fingers in this group of patients. The technique will be described in group 2 deformity.

The treatment of the thumb deformity and occasional elbow flexion or forearm pronation contractures, will be described in subgroup 2b.

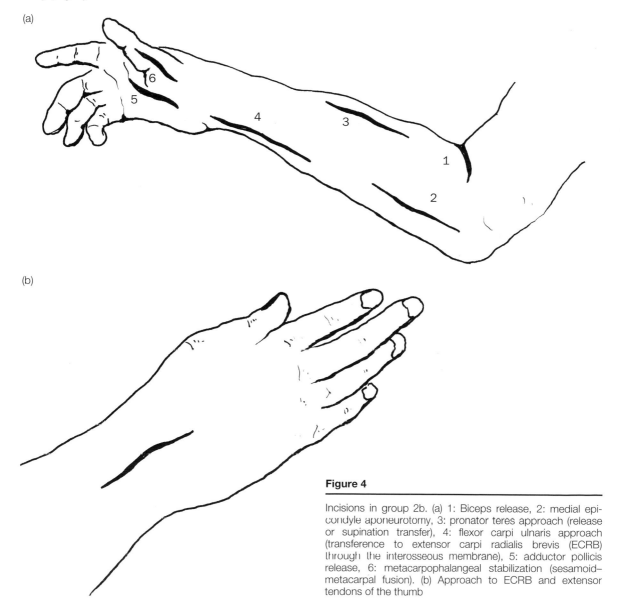

(a)

(b)

Figure 4

Incisions in group 2b. (a) 1: Biceps release, 2: medial epicondyle aponeurotomy, 3: pronator teres approach (release or supination transfer), 4: flexor carpi ulnaris approach (transference to extensor carpi radialis brevis (ECRB) through the interosseous membrane), 5: adductor pollicis release, 6: metacarpophalangeal stabilization (sesamoid–metacarpal fusion). (b) Approach to ECRB and extensor tendons of the thumb

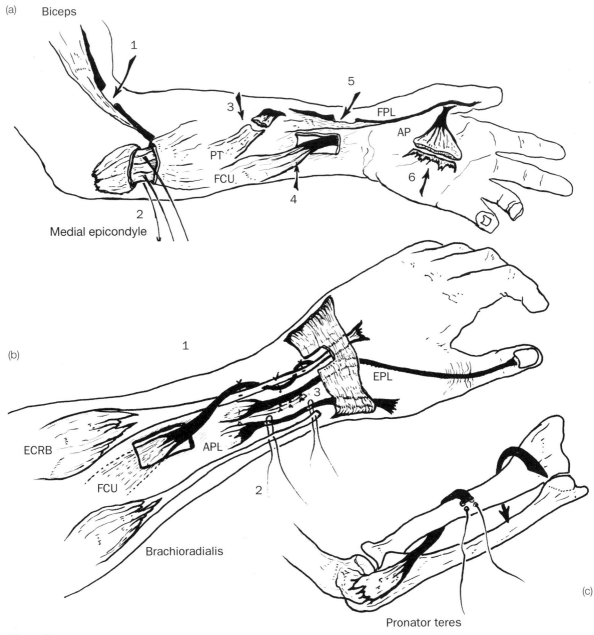

Figure 5

Surgical programme in subgroup *2b* of spastic hand with thumb-in-palm deformity. (a) 1: Biceps lengthening in continuity, 2: excision of superficial fascia and septae of medial epicondyle muscles, 3: pronator teres (PT) release in mild pronation contracture (pronator quadratus remains active), 4: transference of flexor carpi ulnaris (FCU) through the interosseous membrane to extensor carpi radialis brevis (ECRB), 5: lengthening in continuity of flexor pollicis longus (FPL) (avoid too much relaxation), 6: proximal adductor pollicis release. (b) 1: Transference of FCU to ECRB (partial excision of retinaculum cutis), 2: transference of brachioradialis to abductor pollicis longus (APL), 3: Transference to extensor pollicis longus (EPL) (too much tension should be prevented). Balance needs to be maintained between the lengthened FPL and the transferred EPL. Stabilization of the metacarpophalangeal joint of the thumb is frequently associated. In cases with adduction contracture of the thumb the FPL tendon is left unreleased and the EPL is translocated radially. (c) Transference of pronator teres through the interosseous membrane to obtain supination

Group 2

Surgical correction of flexion contracture of the fingers and wrist depends on their spasticity and the functional condition of the wrist extensor muscles (subgroups *2a* and *2b*) (Figs 4 and 5).

Correction of spastic wrist and finger muscles is obtained by our technique of *medial epicondyle aponeurotic release* (Zancolli 1968 and 1979, Zancolli and Zancolli 1987). *In subgroup 2b we add a tendon transfer to the extensor of the wrist.* Correction of spasticity producing flexion contracture of the elbow, pronation of the forearm and thumb deformities will be treated separately.

1 *Aponeurotic release of the medial epicondyle muscles.* This is a very effective technique in most cases – mild and median spasticity – of wrist and finger flexion contractures. In this procedure spasticity is reduced because all the deep attachments of the medial epicondyle muscles are released at the proximal third of the forearm. The muscular body proximal insertions are left intact. Mild and median cases are those in which preoperative voluntary finger extension is obtained with less than 70° of active wrist flexion.

In cases of severe spasticity or myostatic contracture of the wrist and finger muscles – finger extension is possible only with more than 70° of wrist flexion – we add release through selective tenotomies (preserving muscle continuity) of some retracted muscles (flexor digitorum superficialis and profundus and flexor carpi radialis). This complementary release is located distally to the proximal aponeurotic release, approximately at the level of the musculotendinous functions in the middle of the forearm. Myostatic contracture is recognized under anaesthesia: a passive extension manœuvre is unable to obtain complete and simultaneous extension of the wrist and fingers.

In the aponeurotic release of the medial epicondyle muscles a transverse excision of the superficial fascia is made around the whole muscular mass. This is followed by a complete excision of all the spate that divide the muscles. Each septa is followed up to its deep end where we can see the median and ulnar nerves under the muscles. The muscular bodies are left intact, particularly the FCU if this muscle is to be transferred to the extensor tendons of the wrist (subgroup *2b*).

We do not undertake the classical complete muscular slide technique as described by Page (1923; see also Inglis and Cooper 1966, White 1972). Using this technique we are unable to calculate the degree of muscular release and consequently overcorrection could be the result causing the fingers to lose their flex and grasp abilities. Another possible complication of an excessive muscular slide procedure is the loss of vascularization of the medial epicondyle muscular mass.

2 *Tendon transfer of the flexor carpi ulnaris to the extensor carpi radialis brevis.* This technique is indicated only when active wrist extensors are very weak or completely paralysed (subgroup *2b*). It is not indicated, obviously, in subgroup *2a* where active wrist extension is present. In the classic Green's procedure (Green 1942, Green and Banks 1962) the FCU tendon is passed around the ulnar border of the wrist and is fixed to the extensor carpi radialis brevis tendon, since this last muscle is the major dorsiflexor of the hand. The goal is to obtain wrist extension and supination of the forearm. The other wrist flexors, flexor carpi radialis and palmaris longus, must remain in place to avoid undesirable permanent wrist hyperextension postoperatively.

The present author has modified this procedure, preferring to pass the FCU through an ample window in the interosseus membrane – proximally to the pronator teres – and suture it to the extensor carpi radialis brevis tendon (see Fig. 5). The tension of the transfer is precisely calculated during surgery and is considered correct when the wrist maintains 20° of extension under the effect of gravity.

Group 3

This represents a hand with a permanent flexion contracture of the wrist and fingers particularly under emotional stimuli; it is impossible to voluntarily open the hand. The extensor muscles of the wrist and fingers are paralysed or in part reduced owing to the severe opposite flexor spasticity. Consequently, these patients do not have any kind of release and grasp pattern. Sensory function may be seriously affected. Myostatic contracture is very frequent due to the severity of the spasticity and permanent flexed position of the hand.

The best indication for these patients is to obtain

a released upper limb – elbow, forearm, wrist, fingers and thumb. This may be accomplished by multiple tenotomies with muscular continuity indicated in all the affected muscles.

If the tenotomies are insufficient because of the great severity of spasticity or myostatic contracture of the finger flexor muscles, then we employ a technique described previously (Zancolli 1957, Braun et al 1974). In this procedure the flexor superficialis tendons are divided distally, near the wrist, and the flexor digitorum profundus tendons are sectioned proximally at the mid-forearm level. The fingers are then extended to a median flexed position, and while maintaining this position, the proximal end of the flexor superficialis tendons is sutured to the distal end of the flexor digitorum profundus tendons with latero-lateral tenorraphies. The flexor tendons of the wrist are 'Z' lengthened. This procedure was initially performed by us to correct pronounced flexion contractures of the wrist and fingers in severe segmentary arthrogryposis, but this technique is also indicated in very severe group 3 cases of spastic hand in cerebral palsy.

Flexion contracture of the elbow

Flexion contracture of the elbow is a common finding in the spastic upper limb and is frequently influenced by emotional stimuli. Correction of marked flexion contracture of the elbow improves the appearance and function of the upper limb. Flexor muscle origin release or aponeurotic release of the medial epicondyle muscles usually produces a partial correction of the deformity. Correction is obtained by tenotomy in continuity or 'Z' lengthening of the biceps tendon. Occasionally the lacertus fibrosus may be sectioned.

Pronation contracture of the forearm

Mild cases of pronation, which reduce passively preoperatively are improved by simple division of the distal tendon of the pronator teres (see Fig. 5a). In severe contractures the distal tendon of the pronator teres is re-routed around the radius (procedure of Tubby, in Vulpius and Stoffel 1920) (see Fig. 5c).

In three cases of our series with severe and fixed pronation contracture, the distal end of the ulna was dorsally dislocated. In these cases it was necessary to add the complete release of the contracted interosseous membrane, the excision of the ulnar head and a distal radio-ulnar fusion – proximally to the distal growing cartilage of the radius. This technique fixed the forearm in 10° of pronation, which was a very useful position for the hand.

Thumb deformities

Surgery is indicated to hold the thumb out of the palm during grasp and to improve lateral pinch. The surgical technique depends on the type of deformity as pointed out before: adduction or adduction–flexion contracture (Fig. 2) (Zancolli 1979, Zancolli and Zancolli 1981 and 1987, Zancolli et al 1983).

Adduction contracture

The adduction contracture basically depends on spasticity of the adductor pollicis muscle. There is adduction contracture of the first metacarpal, but the metacarpophalangeal and interphalangeal joints are in extension. Correction is obtained by release of the adductor pollicis muscle and reinforcement of the abductor pollicis longus.

Release of the adductor pollicis is obtained by division of its origin from the third metacarpal through a palmar incision parallel to the proximal palmar crease (Matev 1963) (Fig. 5a).

It is not necessary to release the origin of the lateral thenar muscles in a pure or predominant spastic thumb deformity. Spasticity of the lateral thenar muscles in pure spastic neuromuscular disorder is not present. This only occurs in athetoid or other extrapyramidal hands.

Reinforcement of the adductor pollicis longus is usually accomplished by transfer of the brachioradialis (McCue et al 1970). Reinforcement of this tendon can be obtained by tendon plication (Matev 1963) or tenodesis of the abductor pollicis longus. In the latter, the proximal end of the abductor pollicis longus is fixed to the radius or to the distal tendon of the brachioradialis. The best results are obtained by tendon transfers.

Adduction–flexion contracture (thumb-in-palm deformity)

The main deforming forces are related to the spas-

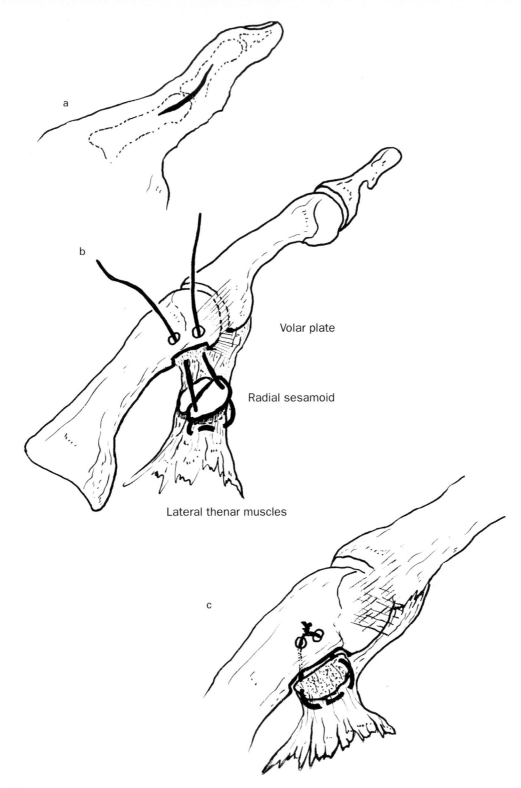

a

b

Volar plate

Radial sesamoid

Lateral thenar muscles

c

Figure 6

(a) Metacarpophalangeal hyperextension of the thumb. Radial incision. Sesamoid–metacarpal stabilization (synostosis). (b) A strong suture fixes the radial sesamoid to the metacarpal neck. Sesamoid cartilage and cortical bone of the metacarpal neck are excised. (c) Sesamoid–metacarpal fusion with 5° of joint flexion

ticity of the adductor pollicis and flexor pollicis longus muscles (Keats 1964). The most frequently used and effective reconstructive procedures are: 1, release of the origin of the adductor pollicis from the third metacarpal; 2, lengthening of the flexor pollicis longus at its musculotendinous junction in the forearm preserving the muscular continuity; 3, releasing and relocating the tendon of the extensor pollicis longus toward the radial aspect of the wrist; 4, reinforcement of the abductor pollicis longus and extensor pollicis longus by tendon transfers (motors: brachioradialis, palmaris longus, etc.).

It is very important to maintain some function of the flexor pollicis longus; overcorrection should be avoided.

When reinforcement of the extensor pollicis longus is indicated, but spasticity of the flexor pollicis longus is not evident, the latter tendon is not lengthened. Stabilization of the metacarpophalangeal joint of the thumb, through arthrodesis or capsuloplasty, is indicated when the joint is hypermobile in hyperextension (more than 20°).

In arthrodesis in children, damage to the epiphyseal line can be avoided by use of thin fixation pins. Arthrodesis alone, without proper release of contractures and diminution of spasticity and without reinforcement of the abductor and extensor muscles, will not in itself eliminate the thumb-in-palm deformity.

Metacarpophalangeal capsuloplasty (Zancolli 1968 and 1979, Filler et al 1976) is an excellent procedure for correction of hyperextension deformity of the joint. To accomplish a good joint stabilization the radial sesamoid is fixed to the neck of the first metacarpal in 10° of flexion (sesamoid–metacarpal synostosis) (Fig. 6).

Swan-neck deformity

Swan-neck deformity is relatively common in the hands of patients with cerebral palsy (Swanson 1960 and 1982). The classic spastic flexion–pronation deformity is the result of a muscle imbalance caused by the permanent flexion of the wrist but the patient has the ability to extend the fingers. Stretching of the volar plate of the proximal interphalangeal (PIP) joint results in its hyperextension and in flexion of the distal interphalangeal joint (dysfunction of the extensor apparatus). The fingers frequently lock in extension, and the ability and force

of pinch and grasp are impaired. When the fingers develop permanent and pronounced swan-neck deformities, surgical treatment is indicated, but surgical treatment of swan-neck in cerebral palsy is common (Filler et al 1976).

Mild swan-neck deformities can improve spontaneously with correction of flexion contracture of the wrist because this decreases the traction of the digital extensor tendons over the middle phalanx. In severe deformities correction is obtained by a procedure described by us and called the *'sling' operation* (Braun 1974, Zancolli 1975, 1982, 1986 and 1991, Zancolli and Zancolli 1987). The deformities are corrected during the same surgical procedure as correction of the flexor–pronation deformity.

The sling procedure is achieved by re-routing the entire lateral extensor tendon of the extensor apparatus through the flexor tendon sheath. The deformity and the incision used for the operation is shown in Fig. 7a. The first step of the operation consists of freeing the extrinsic lateral extensor tendon of the affected fingers (radial side) between the middle third of the proximal and middle phalanges (Fig. 7) The distal end of this tendinous sling remains attached to the extensor apparatus, and the proximal end remains attached to the central extrinsic extensor tendon and the intrinsic muscles (radial interosseous and lumbrical). The second step consists of opening the flexor tendon sheath between A2 and A4 pulleys and exposing the flexor

Figure 7

(a) Mid-lateral longitudinal incision on the radial side of the finger. (b) The lateral band (1) is dissected between the middle of the proximal and middle phalanges (arrows X–X'). The proximal end of the dissected band is in continuity with the lateral slip of the extensor tendon and the intrinsic tendons. The flexor tendon sheath is opened at the proximal interphalangeal PIP joint level (2). (c) The dissected lateral band (3) is translocated to the volar part of the finger and placed between the volar plate (5) and the flexor superficialis (6). Two strong stitches (4) join the volar plate and the chiasma of Camper, distally to the PIP joint level. These sutures maintain the lateral band volarly to the joint. (d) After the procedure, the finger must extend passively or actively up to the neutral extension. The suture of the volar plate to the flexor superficialis represents a pulley for the transferred lateral band (7). During active finger extension the transferred band produces an active stabilization of the PIP joint and extension of the distal interphalangeal (DIP) joint. The lateral band in its new position is relatively shortened. The normal use of the finger produces a relocation of the opposite lateral band to its normal course

(a)

(b)

(c)

(d)

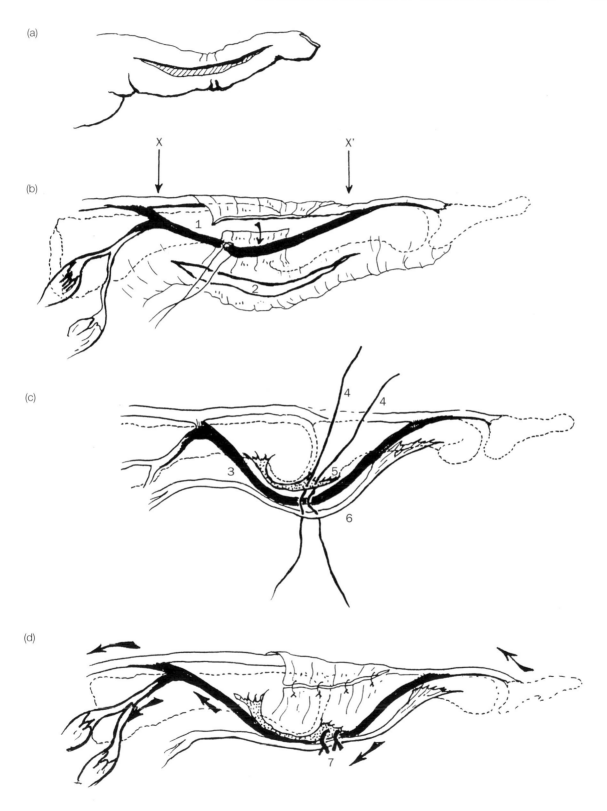

tendons at the PIP joint level. In a third step the tendinous sling, formed by the lateral tendon, is re-routed volar to the joint, and introduced between the volar plate and the flexor superficialis tendon (Camper's chiasma). The lateral tendon is maintained in this position by two strong separate sutures – with the finger in 5° of PIP flexion – that unite the lateral borders of the chiasma and the volar plate (Fig. 7c). These sutures are located distal to the joint at the middle phalanx base level. The tendon sheath is then closed. If the tension of the tendinous sling is correct (Fig. 7d) the attitude of the fingers, passively extended, should be with 5° of flexion of the middle joint and neutral extension of the distal joint. If the attitude of flexion of the middle joint is greater then the freeing of the lateral tendon is continued at its proximal and distal ends to arrive at the correct flexion position of the joint. If there is still some swan-neck deformity, stitches are applied at either end to tighten the sling. Flexion greater than 5° of the PIP joint may produce a boutonnière deformity.

This technique represents the reconstruction of an *active retinacular ligament*. The activation of the tendinous sling by the action of the extensor tendons and the intrinsic muscles produces complete finger extension and corrects the hyperextension of the PIP joint. The finger is immobilized in slight flexion for 1 week before active exercises begin. The results of this procedure have been encouraging. The procedure cannot be used in cases of claw-hand due to intrinsic paralysis (this is a complementary comment on the procedure indications).

Assessment of hand motor function

Grouping of the patients is achieved by a precise examination of upper limb function. This enables grouping of the results after surgery (Zancolli and Zancolli 1987).

1 *Study of the ability to open the hand.* This is evaluated by measuring with wood discs of graduated sizes (6, 8, 10, 12, 14, 16 and 18 cm); determining hand placement over the table; and measuring the degrees of wrist flexion that will enable the patient to extend the fingers.
2 *Grasp and pinch patterns.* The ability to grasp is evaluated though the use of spherical balls of graduated sizes (5, 8, 10 and 12 cm) and cylin-

ders of graduated sizes (3, 5, 8, 10 and 12 cm). Pinch patterns including tip, pulp and lateral pinches, and chuck or three-digit pinch are evaluated with the use of different objects.
3 *Speed, skill, voluntary control and co-ordination for prehension* are functions that are evaluated by the pick-up test and by manipulation of different objects. The use of manipulative toys in evaluating children can help the surgeon to make decisions on the indication for reconstructive procedures to improve both function and cosmesis. Co-ordination between both hands is observed and recorded.

Other evaluations include:

1 *Grasp and pinch strength.* The grip strength is evaluated with a dynamometer. (A sphygmomanometer may be used to record grip strength in weak hands.) A pinch meter is used to evaluate pinch strength.
2 *Activities of daily living.* These involve hygiene, dressing, writing and feeding.
3 *Active and passive range of motion of all the joints.* Shoulder, elbow, forearm, wrist, fingers and thumb are evaluated. The range of motion should be recorded on the principle that the neutral position equals 0°. The patient is asked to straighten the fingers and to make a fist to obtain a general idea of motion of all digits and to note any limited motion or abnormal attitudes.

Results

Results after surgery can be grouped as good, fair and poor according to the function of the hand.

- Good
  – complete digital extension with less than 20° wrist flexion
  – complete elbow extension and partial supination of the forearm
  – good lateral pinch and grasping (thumb-in-palm deformity corrected)
  – good voluntary control of muscles
- Fair
  – complete digital extension with more than 20° of wrist flexion
  – partial elbow extension and forearm supination
  – weak and partial lateral pinch and grasping

• Poor
  – hand function and deformities not improved
    (passive hand)

In the present author's series of 91 operated cases (selected patients), only 47 cases were evaluated in the final result (29 were females). The average age at operation was 7 years. According to the classification presented earlier the number of patients was: group 1, 8 cases; group 2, 31 cases; and group 3, 8 cases.

The results were group 1–7 good and 1 poor; group 2 – 19 good, 10 fair and 2 poor; group 3 – 1 fair and 7 poor.

Three athetoid cases operated using soft tissues procedures had a very poor result. The initial deformities were transformed into other uncontrolled deformities.

Conclusions

Selected patients with cerebral palsy can be helped by reconstructive surgery of the upper limb. The principal evaluations for the selection of patients are: aetiology, general neurological conditions, type of neuromuscular disorder, topographic involvement, age, hand sensibility, type of deformity, motivation, co-operation, voluntary control of muscles, emotional influence on spastic muscle, and voluntary grasp and release patterns of the hand.

Although surgery cannot make a limb which was functionally poor into a perfect one, it can greatly improve on the initial condition. Most poor surgical results are due to poor selection of patients or incorrect execution of the surgical procedures. The worst mistake is to perform soft tissue procedures – tendinous release or tendinous transfers – on patients with athetosis.

The surgical programme is organized according to the type and severity of the deformity.

The goal is to correct the deformities and to improve the muscular balance of the hand. It must be remembered that spastic muscle cannot be used for tendon transfer with the same efficiency as muscle in patients with exclusive flaccid paralysis.

References

Blumel I, Eggers GWN, Evans EB (1960) Genetic metabolic and clinical study on one hundred cerebral palsied patients, *JAMA* **174:**860.

Braun RM, Guy TV, Roper B (1974) Preliminary experience with superficialis-to-profundus tendon transfer in the hemiplegic upper extremity, *J Bone Joint Surg* **52A:**466–72.

Filler BC, Stark HH, Boyes J (1976) Capsulodesis of metacarpophalangeal joint of the thumb in children with cerebral palsy, *J Bone Joint Surg* **58A:**667–70.

Goldner JL (1955) Reconstructive surgery of the hand in cerebral palsy and spastic paralysis resulting from injury to the spinal cord, *J Bone Joint Surg* **37A:**1141.

Goldner JL (1975) The upper extremity in cerebral palsy. In: Samilson RL, ed. *Orthopaedic Aspects of Cerebral Palsy.* Harper & Row: New York: 221–57.

Green WT (1942) Tendon transplantation of the flexor carpi ulnaris for pronation–flexion deformity of the wrist, *Surg Gynecol Obstet* **75:**337–42.

Green WT, Banks HH (1962) Flexor carpi ulnaris transplant its use in cerebral palsy, *J Bone Joint Surg* **44A:**1343–52.

Inglis AE, Cooper W (1966) Release of the flexor pronator origin for flexion deformities of the hand and wrist in spastic paralysis, *J Bone Joint Surg* **48A:**847–57.

Keats S (1964) Surgical treatment of the hand in cerebral palsy: correction of thumb-in-palm and other deformities, *J Bone Joint Surg* **47A:**274.

McCue FC, Honner R, Chapman WC (1970) Transfer of the brachioradialis for hands deformed by cerebral palsy, *J Bone Joint Surg* **52A:**1171–80.

Matev I (1963) Surgical treatment of the spastic 'thumb-in-palm' deformity, *J Bone Joint Surg* **45B:**703–8.

Page CM (1923) An operation for the relief of flexion contracture in the forearm, *J Bone Joint Surg* **5A:**233–4.

Samilson SL, Morris JM (1964) Surgical improvement of the cerebral-palsied upper limb, *J Bone Joint Surg* **46A:**1203–16.

Swanson AB (1960) Surgery of the hand in cerebral palsy and the swan-neck deformity, *J Bone Joint Surg* **42A:**951–64.

Swanson AB (1968) Surgery of the hand in cerebral palsy and muscle origin release procedures, *Surg Clin North Am* **48:**1129–38.

Swanson AB (1982) Surgery of the hand in cerebral palsy. In: Flynn JE, ed. *Hand Surgery*, 3rd edn. Williams & Wilkins: Baltimore: 476–88.

Twitchell TE (1966) Sensation and the motor deficit in cerebral palsy, *Clin Orthop* **46:**55–62.

Vulpius O, Stoffel A (1920) *Orthopädische Operations Lehre*. Ferdinang Enke: Stuttgart.

White WF (1972) Flexor muscle slide in the spastic hand. The Max Page operation, *J Bone Joint Surg* **54B:**453–9.

Zancolli EA (1957) Un nuevo método de corrección de las contracturas congenitas de los musculos flexores digitales (alargamiento intertendinoso), *Prensa Med Argentina* **44:**279–81.

Zancolli EA (1968) *Structural and Dynamic Bases of Hand Surgery*. JB Lippincott: Philadelphia.

Zancolli EA (1975) La operación del 'asa' en la corrección de la deformidado en 'cuello de cisne'. *1st National Congress of the Spanish Society for Surgery of the Hand, 17–19 October 1975, Bilbao, Spain* (not published).

Zancolli EA (1979) *Structural and Dynamic Bases of Hand Surgery*. JB Lippincott: Philadelphia.

Zancolli EA (1982) Management of boutonnière and swan-neck deformities, *25th Congress of the Japanese Society for Surgery of the Hand, 7–9 May 1982, Tokyo, Japan*.

Zancolli EA (1986) Panel on soft tissue reconstruction in rheumatoid arthritis, *41st Annual Meeting of the American Society for Surgery of the Hand, New Orleans*.

Zancolli EA (1991) Surgical correction of flexible swan-neck deformity – volar translocation of the radial lateral band, *Curr Orthop* **5:**230–2.

Zancolli EA, Goldner LJ, Swanson AB (1983) Surgery of the spastic hand in cerebral palsy: report of the Committee on Spastic Hand Evaluation, *J Hand Surg* **8:**766–72.

Zancolli EA, Zancolli ER (1981) Surgical management of the hemiplegic spastic hand in cerebral palsy, *Surg Clin North Am* **61:**395–406.

Zancolli EA, Zancolli ER (1987) Surgical rehabilitation of the spastic upper limb in cerebral palsy. *The Paralysed Hand*. Churchill Livingstone: New York: 153–8.

49
Neuro-rehabilitation of the spastic upper limb

M Antonietta Vannini

A lesion in the neural structures between the cortical layer and the pyramidal decussation, in the anatomical space devoted to the activation of the upper limb, causes the loss of useful motor activity. The same lesion also allows the onset of attitudes and movements which oppose the independent aims of the patient (Fig. 1). In fact, in human beings, the upper limb not only maintains equilibrium by virtue of the hands' support and hold capabilities, but also co-operates with the legs in spatial movement acting as either a balancing, support or traction tool. Furthermore, the upper limb is suitable for defensive and offensive purposes when personal integrity is under possible threat. The arms also explore and manipulate the environment in a remarkable operative and cognitive productivity. The arms also enable expressive gestures to be made.

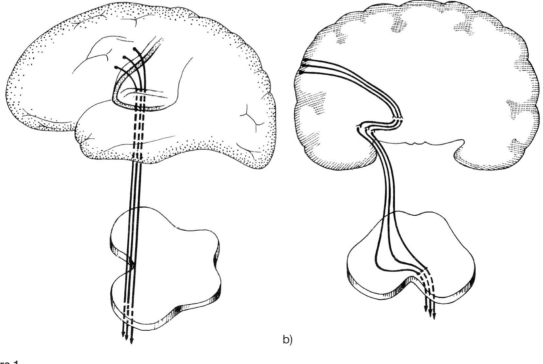

a)   b)

Figure 1

(a,b) Anatomical space where the 'central lesion' of the upper limb occurs: cortex: direct and indirect motor ways, pyramidal and extrapyramidal, of the shoulder, arm, forearm and hand.

A central lesion, depending on its depth and extension, may prevent useful movements of the arm. The arm takes stiff positions from which it frees itself by spontaneous reflex either with changes in general body posture or in conjunction with coenaesthetic disturbances.

The rigid posture of the upper limb can be removed either during autonomic disreflexia (i.e. the hand opening when yawning deeply) or during arm extension when the shoulder undergoes a passive front elevation. Furthermore, the spastic arm changes its basic attitude when motions are performed in other areas, in a non-productive synergy which jeopardizes the motion being performed.

The upper limb, affected by a central lesion, grows incapable of useful movements, in contrast with limbs affected by peripheral lesions which cause a real paralysis leaving the arm totally inert.

The most common pathological attitudes of the arm change depending on the central lesion which induced them; these attitudes are an essential clinical sign not only for diagnosis, but also for designing a rehabilitation programme.

In child cerebropathy, there are frequent observations of the arm's massive abduction, extension and intrarotation with extreme pronation of the forearm. The latter position recalls the swimming attitude of reptiles, which swim with the forearm close to the body to achieve better water penetration under the tail propulsion force. This attitude indicates a depth of central lesion which allows only the expression of a primordial pattern deeply rooted in the central nervous system (CNS) genetic memory (Fig. 2a).

In coma decerebration syndromes, equally frequent are observations of the arm elevated and in shoulder retropulsion, with the elbow and forearm in an extreme flexopronation with a closed hand. This position reproduces the final stage of an escape gesture in a futile attempt to avert serious danger when under threat (Fig. 3a).

Thus, the ictus-induced hemiplegia shows an arm adducted to the body, while the forearm and hand are flexed in a gesture which reproduces the pattern of grasping something to keep the body balanced (Fig. 4a).

These common spastic arm attitudes leads us to suggest how different central lesions destroy the most recent motor experience, depending on their depth. Consequently, archaic motion patterns appear with no consistent purpose, hence the origin of the definition of the central lesion as the 'loss of purposeful movement'.

To be useful, gestures must meet a necessary and demanded requirement. They must be prompt,

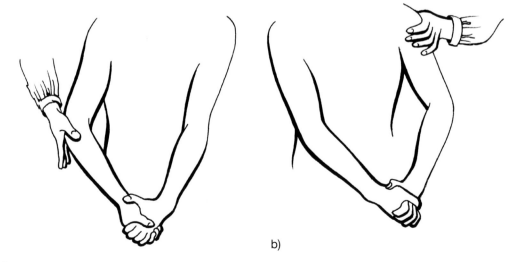

a)   b)

Figure 2

(a,b) Every gesture of the upper limb corresponds to consequent dynamics of the trunk, scapular belt and contralateral arm. Therefore, all rehabilitation procedures treat rotations and derotations of the trunk and scapular belt.

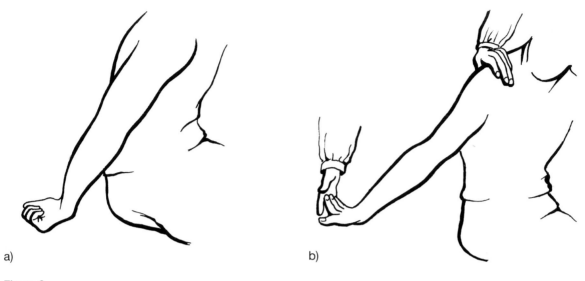

a)   b)

Figure 3

Starting from the pathological posture which prevents statical and dynamical functions of the arm (a), the therapist performs a slow flexopronation stretching and guides the upper limb in a loading position, in support of the trunk (b). Functional surgery can remove the stiffness of the flexopronatory system making the rehabilitation procedure easier.

suitably strong and precise; should be repeated with swinging and rhythmic movements with the necessary fluidity and economy; should use the most effective trajectories, the available muscular or gravitational strengths in the different steps of the gesture, in a controlled drive of the arm.

A deep central lesion requires rehabilitation programmes aimed at learning movement anew. The re-education procedures designed to pursue the functional recovery of the upper limb are based on the following neurobiological beliefs: the patterns of the different-purpose movements of the arm are acquired at different times in a specialization process leading the arm, especially the dominant one, to become the servo system of the psychointellectual apparatus of humans. At the same time, however, specialization rules the basic motions concerning defence, offence, statics and walking. In central lesions, most damage occurs to the most recently acquired, most specialist and most selective motions. Conversely, the most massive and most ancient attitudes and behaviours, concerning either defence or statics/walking, remain with an enhanced spastic/hypertonic expressivity.

This clinical pattern is caused by the imbalance

between enhancing and inhibiting effects – which jeopardizes the latter – as a result of the central lesion. In fact, due to the inhibitory system, motor activity can evolve and specialize into new behavioural patterns by selectively sedating and inhibiting neural system hyperactivity, thus producing differentiated activity.

The most evolved motion behaviours are not produced by a neuronal silence in which special neuromuscular chains are involved and activated. These evolved behaviours stem from the neuromuscular chaos where the inhibitory system prevents excessive and purposeless activities while preserving essential motions only. Useful and purposeful motor activity expresses itself through a process of denial of activity rather than by the addition of new motions. Gazzaniga (1990) likened this process to the sculptor's activity. The artist removes material by milling and chiselling the shapeless marble chunk thus revealing the figure that he has in mind.

For this reason, re-education procedures have different purposes. They promote the intervention of the inhibitory systems over the selected gesture to prevent purposeless neuromuscular hyperactivity. Re-education procedures also allow the flexible

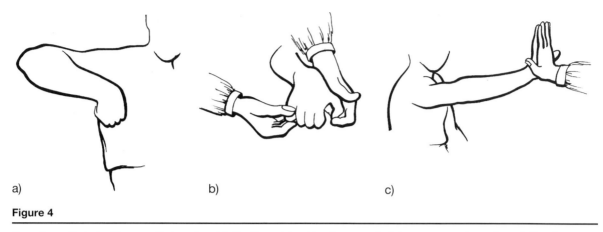

a)   b)   c)

Figure 4

From the pathological 'escape-like' posture (a), the therapist guides the upper limb to reverse gestures, by soliciting the zones which trigger the hand opening reflex (b), and subsequently providing pressure inputs to stabilize the gesture (c). Functional surgery makes the procedure easier by changing the tension of the flexopronatory system.

intervention of the inhibitory system with the consequent functional rhythmic alternation of gestures and swinging movements. To achieve this goal, re-education procedures make use of several selected inputs to the CNS which are capable of promoting inhibition. These inputs have varying spatial/temporal combinations, enabling the goal to be reached. These include: slow and extended stretching of the muscles to obtain the Golgi's lengthening reaction; fast and ballistic stretching to produce the 'gamma' shortening reaction; the use of postural top safety decubitus to prevent postural alarm reactions; the stimulation of trigger zones causing the spontaneous reaction reflex consequent to the gesture to be evoked; the constant offer of an object or a target consistent with the gesture to be solicited; the constant repetition of the gestures' rhythmic alternation such as hold and drop, press and lift, move forward and backward.

These basic re-education concepts are articulated in various times and ways, depending on definite protocols concerning the different types of patients and diseases.

Rehabilitation aims at obtaining purposeful gestures by submitting consistent inputs: information on the expected gesture; order to perform the gesture; positioning of the patient in a decubitus consistent with the solicited gesture; positioning of the arm in an attitude which is contrary and opposite to the direction of the expected gesture; contemporary

involvement of possible trigger zones; simplification of the kinetic execution chain; use of a target for the execution of the solicited gesture; repetition of the procedure for a minimum of 30 times each treatment session (three sessions a day).

Example 1: patient with an arm kept in a massive hold attitude. The therapist aims at evoking the extension of the supported arm. When the patient is comfortably seated, the therapist: a, performs preliminary stretching of the flexor/pronatory system; b, uses the trigger area controlling hand opening; c, leads the hand to the support surface and moves the trunk and the scapular belt in side torsion, to transfer the weight to the supported paralysed arm. Subsequently the therapist brings the trunk and scapular belt back, thus discharging the arm, and requests the patient to lift and flex the arm. This procedure must be repeated 30 times until the arm is left engaged for about 15 min.

Example 2: the arm of the patient is kept in the escape position. The therapist wants to evoke the gesture of attack push. Thus, with the patient comfortably seated with the contralateral arm resting against the surface, the therapist invites the patient to rotate the scapular belt and trunk toward the contralateral side; he forces the contrary flexion of the shoulder and stimulates the trigger zone for hand opening by guiding extension and pronation of the elbow/forearm with return to the starting position after each cycle.

The acquisition of less specialist motor behaviours which are more deeply rooted in the CNS, also when damaged, allows the subsequent introduction of re-educational procedures capable of evoking purposeful motor patterns for environmental exploration and manipulation gestures, in those cases where the forearm/hand dynamic fluidity is the premise to a successful outcome.

Only in this second stage do re-education techniques treat pronation/supination associated with hand opening and closing to simplifying the overall movement.

Example: patient seated with the elbow fully rested against the table surface; prolonged preliminary stretching; solicitation of trigger zones for hand opening and closing with the contemporary introduction of a target to either explore or grasp. These gestures solicited by the therapist, must be repeated at least 30 times per session.

The neural rehabilitation of the spastic arm restores the purposeful motor synergies step-by-step: starting from the basic gestures concerning posture, support and walking to gradually obtaining the recovery of more specialized manual gestures aimed at environmental exploration and manipulation.

Functional surgery releases the various muscular/articular districts from their pathological attitudes. This makes the spastic upper limb more accessible to neuro-rehabilitation procedures, thus increasing the latter's efficiency and producing faster results.

It is possible that functional surgery has not only a mechanical role, which is based on the readjustment of the various muscular/articular districts. It is therefore likely that the rearrangement of both the elastic tension and the self-image promoted by surgery corresponds to the rearrangement of the information inputs sent to the CNS, with the consequent correction of the latter's response, while acting on the tone and behaviour of the upper limb. Functional surgery, therefore, is not only a co-operation tool for the therapist's work, but a re-education procedure capable of intervening in the upper limb's motor restoration and control.

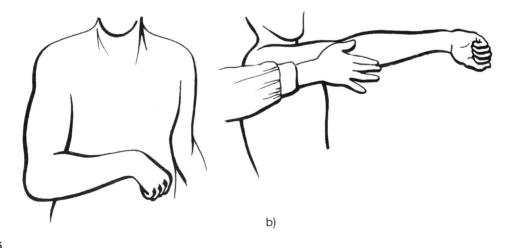

a)   b)

Figure 5

From the pathological posture of maximum 'hold' (a), the therapist guides the upper limb in a front elevation at 90°, thus simulating the support position of the foreleg in a quadruped (b). Forearm and hand keep a flexed position, pronated in a 'hoof-like' gesture: a position which can be removed by functional surgery while permitting the therapist to change this attitude in an open-handed exploration gesture.

References

Adams RD, Victor M (1985) *Principles of Neurology*, 3rd edn. New York: McGraw Hill.

Bach-y-Rita P (1982) Sensory substitution in rehabilitation. In: Illis J, Sedgwick M, Granville H, eds. *Rehabilitation of Neurological Patient*. Oxford: Blackwell Press: 361–83.

Bobath B, Bobath K (1978) *Adult Hemiplegia Evaluation and Treatment*. London: Heinemann.

Brewer CV (1961) *The Organization of the Central Nervous System*. London: Heinemann.

Brunnstrom S (1970) *Movement Therapy in Hemiplegia: A Neurophysiological Approach*. New York: Harper & Row.

Cooper PR, ed. (1982) *Head Injury*. Baltimore: Williams & Wilkins.

Eccles J, ed. (1966) *Brain and Conscious Experience*. Berlin: Springer.

Gazzaniga MS (1990) *La Mente Umana*, 5th Conference Internationale Citta del Vatico. November 15–17.

Griffin JW (1974) Use of proprioceptive stimuli in therapeutic exercise, *Phys Ther* 54:1072–9.

Harris FA (1978) Facilitation techniques in therapeutic exercise. In: Basmajian JV, ed. *Therapeutic Exercise*, 3rd edn. Baltimore: Williams & Wilkins.

Katz B (1966) *Nerve, Muscle and Synapse*. New York: McGraw Hill.

Konorski J (1967) *Integrative Activity of the Brain. An Interdisciplinary Approach*. Chicago: University of Chicago Press.

Rosemberg RM, ed. (1983) *The Clinical Neurosciences*. New York: Churchill Livingstone.

Ryerson DS (1985) Hemiplegia resulting from vascular insult or disease. In: Umphred DA, ed. *Neurological Rehabilitation*. St Louis: CV Mosby: 474–514.

Shapiro DC, Schmidt RE (1982) The schema theory: recent evidence and developmental implications. In: Kelso JAS, Clark JE, eds. *The Development of Movement Control and Coordination*. New York: John Wiley: 113–50.

Toole JF (1984) *Cerebrovascular Disorders*, 3rd edn. New York: Raven Press.

Young JZ (1964) *A Model of the Brain*. Oxford: Clarendon Press.

50

Arthrogryposis multiplex congenita of the elbow

Loris Valdiserri, Stefano Stilli and Raffaele Pascarella

Arthrogryposis multiplex congenita (AMC) is characterized by non-progressive multiple joint stiffness and deformity present at birth, muscle weakness and normal sensation. The cause of this disorder has been attributed to a reduction of foetal intrauterine movement primary or secondary to loss of anterior horn cells with a picture similar to intrauterine poliomyelitis. Whatever the aetiopathogenesis, the final result is that muscles are replaced by fibrous tissue with loss of movement, stiffness and fixed deformities.

There are several clinical forms of arthrogryposis, the most common being amyoplasia (43%) (Sarwark et al 1986, Sarwark and MacEwen 1990) in which the limbs are affected symmetrically. Sarwark and MacEwen (1990) reported an involvement of all four limbs in 63% of cases, only lower limbs in 24% and only upper limbs in 13%.

The most common clinical picture is classically characterized by adducted and intrarotated shoulders, extended elbows (rarely flexed), flexion and ulnar deviation of the wrist and thumb-in-palm deformity. Frog-like flexion, abduction and external rotation or dislocation of the hip may occur. Extension contractures are seen in the knees (sometimes dislocation), while flexion contractures are rare. The feet are in an equinovarus supine position. Varying degrees of stiffness can be found in every part of the body. Scoliosis is also often present.

Conservative treatment

Passive range of motion (ROM) exercises, begun immediately after birth, can improve the shoulder and wrist/hand, while the elbow responds much less if it is fixed in extension with less than 30° ROM. If passive flexion of the elbow is forced, fractures, necrosis and chondrolysis of the articular heads may occur, resulting in further stiffness. The mother is taught passive ROM exercises to perform at home four to five times a day for at least 10–15 minutes. The little gain achieved is supported and maintained by the use of positional orthoses at night and when resting during the day. The orthoses should be applied with the shoulders abducted and externally rotated, elbows flexed at about 90°, forearm in intermediate pronosupination, wrist and fingers slightly flexed and thumb abducted. For economic reasons, the orthoses and splints will be made of plaster or fibre glass or polyurethane bandages. As the child gets older and grows less quickly it is better to use lighter factory manufactured devices. The results of conservative treatment are good in the first year of life, fair in the following year and practically nil after age 3 or 4 years. Gradually, as the child starts to co-operate, the exercises should be made into a game so that they are less boring. Design construction and adaptation of special toys or daily instruments (forks, spoons, combs, etc.) are very useful. Swimming is usually liked and helps to develop muscular tone and ROM, so the child should be accustomed to the water at an early age. Team work (physiotherapist, paediatrician, psychologist, orthopaedist, neurologist, social worker, etc.) is fundamental. It should be explained to the parents that the deformities present at birth are bound to improve, intelligence is normal and that good function can be recovered with help from the medical team and the family environment (Thompson and Bilenker 1985). Thompson and Bilenker (1985) define this concept with the term 'comprehensive care program'.

Surgical treatment

Despite the deformity, the child with AMC manages to invent ingenious ways of carrying out the three basic tasks of daily life, eating, dressing and toiletting. It is therefore best, before embarking on a surgical adventure with an uncertain outcome, to carefully study what compensation mechanisms the child is developing or has already adopted. Surgery must be exclusively 'functional' and aimed at improving the autonomy of the patient and not only the aesthetic aspect. A child with arthrogryposis quickly learns movements or tricks (leaning the head forward, putting his elbows on the table, working with two hands, etc.) to handle objects, drink and later to draw and write. It can be difficult for him to dress by himself, so he needs to be helped by having clothes or accessories with minor modifications such as a zip instead of buttons, velcro instead of shoe laces and belts without holes. Independent toilet care, especially in the genital region, should never be neglected. This problem is a minor one when the child is young, increases as the child gets older and is prominent during puberty. The predominant limb should be identified in the first years of life. This will be the 'feeding limb', while the contralateral limb will be used for hygiene of the perineal area.

Another equally important element to consider for correct surgical indication is the functional correlation between upper limbs and lower limbs. If a patient needs sticks to walk or has to use a wheelchair (and therefore to move from the bed to the wheelchair), the strength of at least one triceps muscle must be maintained. Therefore bilateral and contemporary correction of elbows fixed in extension should be avoided. The mode and capability of walking have to be assessed first, then the surgical strategy and the procedure for the upper limbs can be planned (Fig. 1).

Even the functional correlations between shoulder, elbow and wrist on the same limb have to be carefully considered. It would be a mistake, for example, to correct a flexed wrist before knowing the destiny of the homolateral elbow fixed in extension. In fact wrist flexion can be very useful for reaching the perineum, the torso and, possibly (with special movements), the mouth if the elbow extension cannot or need not be corrected.

In conclusion, surgery is one, but not the only, tool available for treatment. Any surgical intervention on any of the three joints (shoulder, elbow,

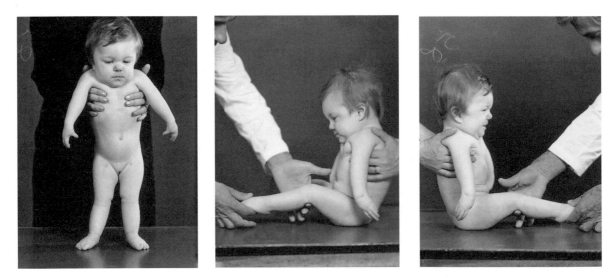

Figure 1

One-year-old female. AMC involving four limbs which are extended and stiff. No decision for surgery should be taken before identifying the predominant upper limb and walking pattern.

wrist/hand) should be part of a precise plan, made-to-measure for each individual and for the function of nearby joints. With regards to timing, it is best to wait until the child's voluntary and controlled muscular activity begins to develop, and see how he behaves standing up and walking. Performing surgery before 2–3 years of age may be risky and cause disappointment. We are therefore opposed to 'early one-stage' corrective surgery on the wrist and elbow according to Mennen (1993).

Surgery of each joint

The shoulder

It is almost always stiff with adduction and internal rotation. The deltoid muscle is often very weak. Despite this, the shoulder joint makes only a small contribution to the total functional damage of the upper limb.

Among the rare surgical indications are patients who, with the elbow extended, may reach the perineum only with the back of the hand or who, despite having an active contraction of the elbow up to 90°, cannot reach the mouth and head with the hand because of a marked internal rotation of the scapulohumeral joint. Surgery can also be indicated when both shoulders are so internally rotated as to produce back to back hand contact, thus making it impossible or difficult to use a walking frame, sticks or to grasp objects. The latter problem, however, can be overcome by the crossover style when careful consideration must be given to whether it is desirable to surgically alter the functional balance so laboriously achieved.

Surgical technique

Due to recurrence, intervention on the soft tissue is unanimously considered insufficient. Derotation osteotomy gives better results. It can be performed at the upper third, just below the deltoid insertion (Lloyd-Roberts and Lettin 1970), or at the lower third. Plates or staples can be used for fixation. A 'low' osteotomy (supracondylar) avoids the use of a bust cast and allows a certain amount of flexion or extension to be combined with the derotation, sometimes useful for improving elbow function.

The elbow

This is the key joint in the upper arm for the patient with arthrogryposis.

Extension deformity in both elbows

The joints are almost always completely extended and stiff or have a few degrees of passive ROM. The flexor muscles (biceps and brachialis) are absent and fibrotic. The aim is to obtain a self-feeding limb around a right angle position and the contralateral limb extended as a self-toiletting limb. Generally the noble limb (the one that reaches the head) is the predominant one, and is identified by studying the child for some time. This observation period can also be exploited to solve any combined problems of the lower limbs (hip dislocation, stiffness and knee and foot deformities).

The fixed extended elbow

This is treated in two stages. The first is compulsory and the second is optional: 1, correction of the deformity trying to give the elbow as much passive ROM as possible around a right angle; 2, creation of a muscular motor to reanimate the flexor muscles.

1 *The correction of the fixed extension deformity* is achieved by triceps lengthening and posterior capsulotomy, which almost always enable the elbow to be positioned at 90°. If this position is hard to achieve, the wing ligaments can be sectioned, taking care not to weaken them too much or an unstable joint may result.

2 *Muscular transfer*
   a *Anterior transfer of the triceps.* This is generally done at the same time as the triceps tendon lengthening, which – according to Bunnel's technique modified by Carrol – (Bunnell 1951, Carrol 1952, Carrol and Hill 1970) is totally or partially transferred onto the biceps tendon or onto the radial tuberosity passing it through a lateral subcutaneous tunnel. After re-examining his patients at the end of growth, Williams (1978) noticed that nearly all the initial good results had deteriorated due to progressive flexion deformity and loss of ROM (which was only 20°). In some cases

he was even compelled to perform an extension osteotomy of the elbow to improve function.

b *Pectoralis major transfer*. Clark (1946) transferred the sternal head and Schottstaedt et al (1955) the entire pectoralis major rotated on its neurovascular pedicle, as did Brooks and Seddon (1959) who attached the tendon of the pectoralis major to the proximal end of the long head of the biceps. Atkins et al (1985) mobilize the muscle by detaching it from its upper sternal and clavicular insertions and fixing its distal tendon (opportunely lengthened also using the fascia) to the distal insertion of the dissected and mobilized biceps. They obtained good results in six cases with preservation of elbow extension.

Tachdjian (1990) proximally detaches the long head of the biceps, mobilizes it distally together with the muscle and passes it through a buttonhole in the tendon of the pectoralis major detached from the humerus, finally lowering it to be reinserted onto the bicipital tuberosity of the radius.

c *Transfer of the epitrochlear muscles* according to Steindler (1949). The muscular bulk is detached together with a bony bract and fixed to the lower fourth of the humerus, medially and anteriorly, with a screw, pins or simply using reabsorbable sutures.

It is a criticized and controversial operation. Tachdjian (1990) and Drummond et al (1974) maintain the flexion force is insufficient (due to the primary deterioration of the muscles) and, in time, a progressive flexion deformity of the wrist, fingers and even the elbow is produced. Conversely, Carrol and Hill (1970) report good long-term results, with a 20° flexion deformity and 70° useful flexion motion.

Whatever technique is used to provide a muscular motor to the elbow flexion, it is advisable not to perform surgery before the patient is 5–6 years old: first, because the functional interconnections between the joints of the upper limbs and between these and the lower limbs have to be carefully evaluated; second, because often, at least in our experience, 'reanimation' surgery of the flexors

Table 1   Surgical experience concerning the shoulder

Operation	Cases	Male	Female	Age	Mean follow-up (years)	Result
Derotational osteotomy of proximal humerus	2	1	1	6	6	fair
Derotational supracondylar osteotomy of distal humerus	4	1	3	8	6	fair

Table 2   Surgical experience concerning the elbow

Operation	Cases	Male	Female	Age (years)	Pre-op ROM passive (degrees)	Follow-up (years)	Active ROM (degrees)
Arthromyolysis	27 (11 bil)	9	7	5 mean	0–20	7	30–90 passive
Triceps pro biceps Pectoralis major pro biceps	1	0	1	14	10–90	6	70–90
Clark (1946)	1	0	1	5	30–110	6	20–45
Clark (1946)	1	1	0	8	0–120	6	25–50
Tsu-Min Tsai (1983)	1	0	1	6	5–120	6	45–90
Steindler (1949)	1	0	1	11	0–30 active	3	5–90
	1	0	1	9	30	5	50–140

becomes superfluous (and sometimes refused) due to the motor and function acquisitions following the simple triceps lengthening and posterior capsulotomy. These patients, in fact, learn to bring the hand to the head with an active push forwards by the shoulder, 'throwing' the limb and possibly using the help of the other hand or avoiding the effect of gravity by leaning the elbows on a table top. The best functional results and the acquisition of greater autonomy are achieved when the deltoid is working.

Flexion deformity in both elbows

This is rare. Physiotherapy may improve ROM. When there are problems reaching the genitourinary area, an extension osteotomy of the elbow of the non-dominant limb may be indicated.

Case report

From 1975 to 1994, 168 patients with AMC were treated at Rizzoli Orthopaedic institute: 85 males and 83 females. Of these, 113 cases had four limb involvement, while 55 had only upper limb involvement. The age at which the patients were first examined was between 10 days and 14 years. Forty patients started treatment in the first month of life, and 100 patients started within the first 12 months. Mean follow-up was 8 years 7 months, with a range of 1–20 years.

Table 1 shows our surgical experience concerning the shoulder and Table 2 concerning the elbow. With regards to the latter joint, 86% of the 113 patients examined had the elbow *extended or flexed a few degrees* and often the triceps were strong while the flexors were absent or considerably weak. In 14% of the cases the elbow was flexed and ROM was fair around a right angle. The biceps were generally good and the triceps were insufficient. This deformity required surgical treatment (extension on the soft tissues) in one case.

References

Atkins RM, Bell MJ, Sherrand WJ (1985) Pectoralis major transfer for paralysis of elbow flexion in children, *J Bone Joint Surg* **67B**:640–4.

Brooks DM, Seddon HJ (1959) Pectoral transplantation for paralysis of the flexors of the elbow: a new technique, *J Bone Joint Surg* **41B**:36–43.

Bunnel S (1951) Restoring flexion to the paralysed elbow, *J Bone Joint Surg* **33A**:566.

Carrol RE (1952) Restoration of flexor power to the flail elbow by transplantation of the triceps tendon, *Surg Gynecol Obstet* **95**:685.

Carrol RE, Hill NA (1970) Triceps transfer to restore elbow flexion, *J Bone Joint Surg* **52A**:239–44.

Clark JMP (1946) Reconstruction of biceps brachii by pectoral muscle transplantation, *Br J Surg* **34**:180–1.

Drummond DS, Siller TN, Cniess RL (1974) Management of arthrogryposis multiplex congenita, *AADS Instr Course Lect* **23**:79–95.

Lloyd-Roberts GC, Lettin AWF (1970) Arthrogryposis multiplex congenita, *J Bone Joint Surg* **52B**:494–508.

Mennen U (1993) Early corrective surgery of the wrist and elbow in arthrogryposis multiplex congenita, *J Hand Surg* **18B**:304–7.

Sarwark JF, MacEwen GD (1990) Current concepts review amyoplasia (a common form of arthrogryposis), *J Bone Joint Surg* **72A**:465–9.

Sarwark JF, MacEwen GD, Scott CI Jr (1986) A multidisciplinary approach to amyoplasia congenita ('classic arthrogryposis'), *Orthop Trans* **10**:130.

Schottstaedt ER, Larsen LJ, Bost FC (1955) Complete muscle transposition, *J Bone Joint Surg* **37**:897–919.

Steindler A (1949) Arthrogryposis, *J Int Coll Surg* **12**:21–5.

Tachdjian MO (1990) *Pediatric Orthopedics*, 2nd edn. Philadelphia: WB Saunders.

Thompson GH, Bilenker RM (1985) Comprehensive management of arthrogryposis multiplex congenita, *Clin Orthop Rel Res* **194**:6–14.

Tsu-Min Tsai (1983) Restoration of elbow flexion by pectoralis major and pectoralis minor transfer, *J Hand Surg* **8**:186–90.

Williams PF (1978) The management of arthrogryposis, *Orthop Clin North Am* **9**(2):67.

51

Arthrogryposis multiplex congenita of the hand and wrist

Paul J Smith and Adriaan O Grobbelaar

Introduction

Arthrogryposis multiplex congenita (AMC) is a congenital syndrome characterized by multiple joint contractures present at birth. It is non-progressive and the muscles are smaller, fewer and may be replaced by fibrous tissue. The sensory system is intact. It is a manifestation of a neurogenic or myopathic disorder of unknown aetiology and involves the upper and lower extremities. This disorder has been classified as a failure of differentiation (Yonenobu et al 1984).

The evaluation of the hand in patients with arthrogryposis should begin with assessment of the mobility of the joints, the position of the contractures and determination of functional motor elements. This disease involves contracture of joints and musculotendinous structures, with frequent aplasias and abnormal insertions of muscles. Mennen (1993) classifies patients into two groups: the 'loose' type with an optimistic prognosis for a good range of motion after surgery and the 'stiff' type with a predictably reduced range of motion.

The most pressing problem with these children is their inability to perform the activities of daily living, particularly feeding and attention to toilet requirements (Williams 1985). The inability to achieve these goals becomes of paramount importance as these children approach adolescence, and the most important contribution of treatment is to achieve this goal. Treatment includes physiotherapy and splintage with a move towards surgery if conservative measures are inadequate (Bayne 1985). The timing of surgery is a controversial issue. Earlier surgery produces better results because deformities often become severe with growth, and joints become fixed in the abnormal position, even though arthrogryposis multiplex congenita is not a progressive disease (Yonenobu et al 1984, Bayne 1985,

Thompson and Bilenker 1985, Mennen 1993). Treatment in the infant or very young child usually begins with cast stretching of the various contractures followed by splintage. Frequently, mobilization of contractures is not possible, and after an adequate trial of 6 months to 1 year without progress, it is appropriate to consider surgical correction (Bayne 1985).

The wrist

One of three types of deformities are usually seen:

- pronation contracture of the forearm
- dorsiflexion with radial deviation
- palmar flexion with ulnar deviation (Yonenobu et al 1984, Bayne 1985).

Pronation contracture of the forearm

Isolated pronation contractures of the forearm are rare and exceedingly resistant to passive stretching (Palmer et al 1985). The pronation contracture is primarily caused by a shortened pronator teres that arises from the medial epicondyl and inserts on the radial border of the radius (Bayne 1985). It can easily be corrected by release of the insertion of the pronator teres to the radius. When the pronator teres is functional the tendon is step-cut and the distal segment is de-rotated around the radius and re-attached to the proximal portion of the pronator teres (Bayne 1985).

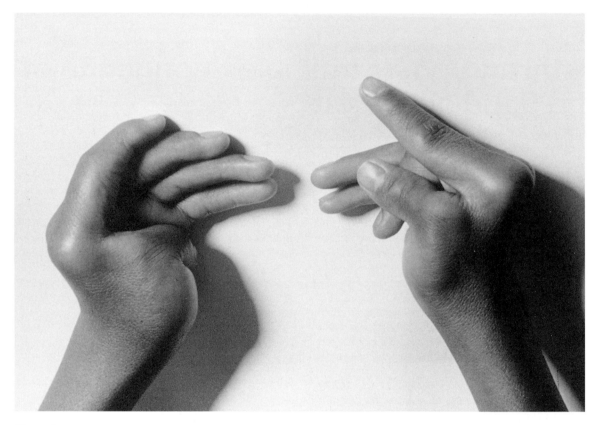

Figure 1

Dorsiflexion with radial deviation.

Dorsiflexion with radial deviation (Fig. 1)

With dorsiflexion deformities, wrist stabilization or arthrodesis is the procedure of choice. The optimum position for wrist fusion varies from case to case, but is usually in the range of 5–20° of palmar flexion (Yonenobu et al 1984, Williams 1985).

Palmar flexion with ulnar deviation (Fig. 2)

This is the most typical deformity of the wrist (Bennett et al 1985). In cases with palmar flexion, the wrist extensors are often absent and the flexors weak (Williams 1985). Treatment by volar capsular

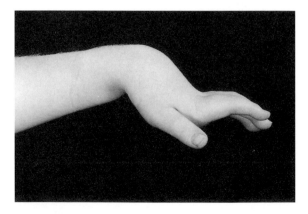

Figure 2

Palmar flexion with ulnar deviation.

release only, proximal row carpectomy with tendon transfer or dorsal wedge osteotomy of the distal radius have been advocated for the palmar flexed and ulnar deviated wrist (Yonenobu et al 1984, Bennett et al 1985, Wenner and Saperia 1987, Mennen 1993). It is important to transfer any functional volar wrist flexors dorsally to decrease deforming forces across the wrist and in doing so prevent recurrence (Bennett et al 1985, Mennen 1993). Forearm shortening has been advocated in severe cases with a rigidly flexed wrist to avoid damage to the shortened median and ulnar nerves (Weeks 1965). We prefer one-step carpectomy with transfer of the flexor carpi ulnaris to the extensor carpi radialis brevis in these cases. In young children volar wrist release only may be sufficient.

The hand

Deformities of the thumb and fingers vary with each case. Yonenobu et al (1984) clearly identified two types. Type I is a thumb-in-palm deformity (Fig. 3) with the fingers in the intrinsic plus position. The thumb is flexed at the metacarpophalangeal joint and adducted at the carpometacarpal joint with the fingers flexed and deviated ulnarly to various degrees at the metacarpophalangeal joint. The grade of impairment of the fingers advances from radial to ulnar. Type II is less common and present with fixed flexion contracture at the interphalangeal joints and the metacarpophalangeal joint in an extension contracture. The thumb is relatively normal in type II hands.

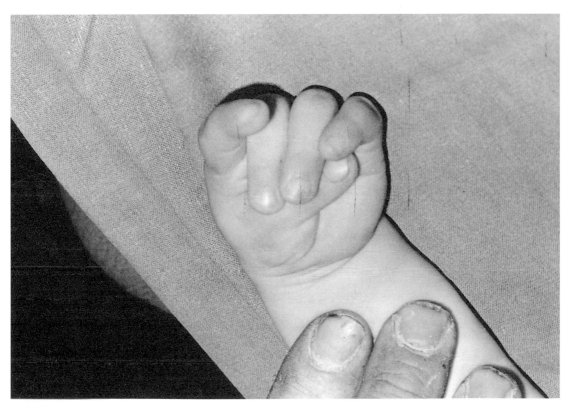

Figure 3

Thumb-in-palm deformity.

Correction of the thumb in palm deformity depends on the severity. The skin deficiency can be remedied by 'Z' plasty, rotational flap and/or skin grafts (Yonenobu et al 1984, Bayne 1985, Bennett et al 1985). Deficiency of the extensor mechanism is best corrected by a tendon transfer: either flexor digitorum sublimis or the extensor indicis proprius (Bayne 1985). Release of the adductor pollicis, flexor pollicis brevis and first dorsal interosseous may be necessary. Contracture of the flexor pollicis longus may require lengthening to achieve adequate correction (Weeks 1965, Bayne 1985).

Various procedures, including skin grafting of the palm, release of the ulnar lateral bands, tendon transfers of the ulnar intrinsic muscles to the radial aspect and osteotomy of the metacarpals have been advocated to correct flexion contracture and ulnar drift of the fingers at the metacarpophalangeal joints (Yonenobu et al 1984, Bayne 1985, Bennett et al 1985). In mild cases when the deformity is composed primarily of ulnar deviation, the extensor tendons will be displaced in an ulnar direction and will produce an extensor lag of the metacarpophalangeal joints. Correction of this deformity can be achieved by centralizing the extensor tendons and cross intrinsic transfers. In more severe cases a more extensive release will be necessary. Release of the volar plate, the transverse retinacular fibres of the extensor mechanism and lengthening of the flexor tendons may be necessary. When the palmar skin is deficient, skin grafts may be used. Wood and Biondi (1990) recommended shortening of the metacarpals in older children to achieve adequate function and Smith (1973) recommended metacarpophalangeal arthroplasties to restore adequate function.

Proximal interphalangeal joint contracture may initially be treated by soft tissue release and skin grafting. Shortening osteotomies of the proximal phalanges, release of the volar plate and sublimis tendon transfer to the digital extensor hood have been recommended, but no cases have reported an improved active motion (Yonenobu et al 1984, Bayne 1985, Bennett et al 1985). An isolated camptodactyly type deformity may benefit from systematic release of all structures involved from the palmar to the dorsal surface. Abnormal lumbrical attachments with absent or abnormal insertions of interossei muscles have been implicated in this deformity.

Proximal interphalangeal fusion may improve function in cases with severe flexion contracture (Bennett et al 1985).

Arthrogryposis is a disease of persistent contracture. Even after correction of the deformity has been accomplished surgically, further splintage at night until maturity is essential to prevent recurrence (Wenner and Saperia 1987). Early surgery significantly improves not only the cosmetic appearance, but also the range of active motion. It alleviates the patient's dependency on parents and relatives and, in doing so, decreases their overall level of disability.

References

Bayne LG (1985) Hand assessment and management of arthrogryposis multiplex congenita, *Clin Orthop Rel Res* **194**:68–73.

Bennett JB, Hansen PE, Granberry WM, Cain TE (1985) Surgical management of arthrogryposis in the upper extremity, *J Ped Orthop* **5**:281–6.

Mennen U (1993) Early corrective surgery of the wrist and elbow in arthrogryposis multiplex congenita, *J Hand Surg* **18B**:304–7.

Palmer PM, MacEwen GD, Bowen JR, Mathews PA (1985) Passive motion therapy for infants with arthrogryposis, *Clin Orthop Rel Res* **194**:54–9.

Smith R (1973) Hand deformities with arthrogryposis multiplex congenita. *J Bone Joint Surg* **55A**:883.

Thompson GH, Bilenker RM (1985) Comprehensive management of arthrogryposis multiplex congenita, *Clin Orthop Related Res* **194**:6–13.

Weeks PM (1965) Surgical correction of upper extremity deformities in arthrogryposis, *Plastic Reconstructive Surg* **36**:459–65.

Wenner SM, Saperia BS (1987) Proximal row carpectomy in arthrogrypotic wrist deformity, *J Hand Surg* **12A**:523–5.

Williams PF (1985) Management of upper limb problems in arthrogryposis, *Clin Orthop Rel Res* **194**:60–7.

Wood VE, Biondi J (1990) Treatment of windblown hand, *J Hand Surg* **15A**:431–8.

Yonenobu K, Tada K, Swanson AB (1984) Arthrogryposis of the hand, *J Ped Orthop* **4**:599–603.

52
Atypical compartment syndromes of the upper limb

Antonio Landi, Giuseppe Caserta, Antonio Saracino and Marco Esposito

Introduction

The effects of an unrecognized compartment syndrome (CS) are often produced by polyarticular muscles, and all the joints crossed will therefore be affected to some extent. It is therefore essential, when dealing with an established muscle contracture, that the negative repercussions on each joint should be analysed and dealt with in order to achieve a good functional outcome.

In this chapter we examine some aspects not strictly related to the usual post-traumatic origin of this syndrome, and try to classify the atypical CSs, which have a multidisciplinary interest and therefore require a particular approach since these forms often cannot be treated by the conservative and surgical procedures usually indicated for this syndrome. Even within the post-traumatic CS group, there are peculiar features based on the aetiology and site of manifestation.

A CS occurs when the increase of pressure in an osteofascial space reduces capillary perfusion of the tissues below the vitality level. The Volkmann ischemic contracture represents, in the majority of cases, the outcome of an unrecognized, and therefore not adequately treated, CS which ultimately can be considered a failure of the capillary system. The CSs have been codified in terms of their pathogenesis and guidelines of treatment (Mubarak and Hargens 1981).

The muscular ischaemic lesion

Acute muscular ischemia reveals itself with the typical signs of the CS. The stabilized picture leads to the Volkmann ischaemic contracture. The common pathogenesis of these aspects of the same phe-nomenon is due to two main causes already described by Perricone in 1958 and Holden in 1975: lesion of a major blood vessel proximal to the site of muscular ischaemia or local multifactorial pathologies. We have modified this classification as follows: type 1a consists of a lesion of a major artery proximal to the region of muscular ischaemia; type 1b is the revascularization syndrome; and muscular ischaemia can occur even after an isolated lesion of the vascular pedicle when this is unique (type 1c). In the upper limb, even if much less frequent than in the lower, it is possible to encounter a CS due to massive venous congestion (flegmasia cerulea-dolens, type 1d) (Landi et al 1991, 1996, Celli et al 1995).

Within Type II, we have subdivided local isolated lesions (type 2a) from the ones associated with aggravating systemic factors (type 2b), because these (heroin and other drugs, haemophilia, carbon monoxide poisoning, barbiturates, crush syndrome etc) condition the overall treatment.

General assessments of CS

The CS may occur because of reduction of the compartment's dimensions (from plaster casts or tension sutures of the fascia) or because of an increase in its contents. This latter, much more frequent, situation may be caused by haemorrhage, or oedema or in association with both, as typically occurs in fractures.

The clinical diagnosis of CS is based on the presence of pain often related to the basic pathology (Royle 1990), the presence of tension within the muscular compartment, pain during passive stretching of the muscles, sensory impairment in the territory of any nerves crossing it and paralysis of the muscles of the affected compartment. The peripheral pulses are usually present in the usual CS and, if not, the reason might be due to local spasm or proximal arterial lesion.

Instrumental examination

The study of the intratissue pressure within a compartment is recognized as a fundamental benchmark that must be considered even in the presence of clear clinical symptoms (Barca et al 1996), both for an accurate diagnosis of acute CS and for correct evaluation of the severity of muscle ischaemia. This examination becomes compulsory in uncooperative patients (i.e. those with altered mental status, children, etc), or when the CS occurs in an atypical anatomical site or derives from atypical aetiologies; in these cases it represents the only easily available diagnostic tool.

The measurement of the pressure levels performed through insertion of a needle catheter in the muscle compartments represents a relatively non-invasive procedure that can give very reliable data within a few seconds. The measurement techniques are well codified in terms of the anatomical site; only the methods of recording vary, but these always require the introduction of an 18-gauge guide needle followed by insertion of the catheter. These are usually thin plastic (polyethylene or Teflon) tubes with different tips that are filled, when introduced, with saline (Esposito et al 1996). The STIC Catheter (Solid State Transducer Catheter) (Stryker) and a silicon transducer enables us to use the guide needle as a catheter, directly connected to the transducer, which is excellent for quick emergency measurements or the introduction of a slot catheter (SLIT catheter) for short continuous monitorings. The reading appears on a liquid crystal display a few seconds after the introduction of 1 or 1.5 ml of saline solution. The Camino catheter 720 uses a fibreoptic reader connected to an external computerized unit provided with monitor. This system enables the reading of the data according to 5 different scales, and allows long-term monitoring. The Horizon system has a pocket size and also uses a silicon transducer, and it is particularly useful in emergency situations (Esposito et al 1996).

The pressure in a healthy and resting muscular tissue measured with these instruments is usually 7 ± 2 mmHg and coincides with the data obtained with other catheters (2–10 mmHg). An increase in intracompartmental pressure progressively reduces perfusion. At 20 mmHg there is already an appreciable fall in capillary perfusion, and the critical pressure level at which blood flow is interrupted in normotensive patients with a diastolic blood pressure of 70–80 mmHg is 40–50 mmHg. However, these values may vary greatly depending on the presence of hyper- or hypotension due to associated pathologies, and it is therefore necessary to relate the intratissue pressure to the systemic pressure. The literature considers intracompartmental values of 30–35 mmHg still compatible with adequate perfusion (Matsen III FA et al 1980, McDermott AGP et al 1984, Whitesides TE 1975). These borderline values drop progressively with the reduction of systemic blood pressure, requiring fasciotomy even with compartmental pressures of 15–20 mmHg when systemic hypotension is present.

In addition to compartmental pressure measurements, P^{31} spectroscopy can also be performed, through an analysis of the Pcr/Pi ratio (where Pcr = phosphocreatine; Pi = inorganic phosphate) using a bioenergetic index of cellular and tissue vitality, contributing to the identification of reversible muscle lesions. This test used by us for the definition of CS at the scapula (Landi et al 1992) is, however, not easily performed nor routinely available.

In established forms when muscle contracture has developed, computerized tomography scans (CT) can reliably define hypodensity of the affected muscles in both planes (Landi et al 1989a, b, 1991, 1992 and MRI has recently been established as the most accurate measuring technique in this field (Cerofolini E et al 1996).

Indications for fasciotomy

The clinical signs (swelling, spontaneous pain and pain on stretching of the muscles, neurological symptoms, etc) (Landi et al 1991) and instrumental studies help us decide whether fasciotomy is required; this procedure must be preceded, in case of external compression, by removal of the dressing and by opening of a plaster cast that reduces the local pressure by 30% and 50%, respectively (Garfin et al 1981). Fasciotomy is routinely performed after revascularization of large segments, when ischaemia has lasted more than 6 hours. In fact, after revascularization, the reperfusion of ischaemic tissues with oxygen leads to the production of toxic metabolites (H_2O_2 and free hydroxylic radicals, •OH), which are responsible for the oedema that triggers CS. The administration of superoxide dismutase (SOD) in the first ten minutes of revascularization appears, experimentally, to ward off the need for fasciotomy (Perler et al 1990).

Late fasciotomies, carried out after the third or fourth day, must be performed with caution owing to the possibility of infection of the necrotic muscle tissue. The main reasons for failure of fasciotomy are in fact delay and incompleteness. The different fasciotomy techniques for each compartment have been extensively codified and well described (Mubarak and Hargens 1981; Rowland 1982, Landi et al 1996).

Site of manifestation

The entire upper limb, at the level of the various anatomical compartments, is a potential site of CS, which is usually encountered in our practice as a sequela of trauma (Mubarak and Carroll 1979).

Shoulder

The compartments of the shoulder and pelvic girdles have received only scant attention, with the exception of the gluteal region. In 1932 Comolli first described a clinical sign which he considered specific for fracture of the scapula: in a series of 8 cases, he demonstrated a discrete triangular swelling corresponding to the shape of the underlying scapula, easily visible on clinical examination. Comolli's sign came to be considered pathognomonic with fracture of the scapula, and is thought to be caused by increased pressure and swelling in the three osteofascial compartments of the scapula, containing the supraspinatus, infraspinatus and subscapularis. These muscles are enclosed in a thick fascia which is firmly attached to the upper third of the humerus. The subscapularis compartment, on the anterior surface of the scapula, is the largest. It is covered by the weakest aponeurosis; the triangular swelling following scapular fracture is largely due to elevation of the scapula caused by the anterior haematoma (Fig. 1).

These features in our experience suggest that Comolli's sign is indicative of an underlying CS. In the case that we described (Landi et al 1992), the intracompartmental pressure in the infraspinatus compartment was 75 mmHg 22 hrs after trauma, well above the cut-off of 40–50 mmHg. The observed early conduction block recovered partially when spontaneous gradual reabsorption of the haematoma allowed the pressure to decrease from 75 to 39 mmHg, making surgical decompression unnecessary.

The diagnosis of a CS on Comolli's sign may be supported by the standard methods of evaluation of compartment pressures (Landi et al 1991).

The rarity of this syndrome does not allow us to suggest a standardized treatment. The spontaneous drainage which occurred after measurement of the compartment pressure in our case would suggest that when a post-traumatic haematoma is associated with fracture of the scapula in the presence of an impending CS, its localization by ultrasound sonography could help percutaneous drainage.

Arm

Presentation of a CS in the arm is more uncommon (Rigings and Gault 1994) than at the thigh, where its large circumference makes the site very compliant, and might lead to delayed treatment. At this level a CS is usually of post-traumatic origin, as in the case reported above where a man working under a automobile, due to a collapse of the jack, had his arm compressed between the floor and thoracic cage. The clinical features were swelling of the arm, severe pain on passive extension and flexion of the elbow, elevation of the compartmental pressure and the presence of an area of necrotic skin (a 'kissing' lesion) which has been reported to be an indicator of severe crush injury.

A medial fasciotomy which allows direct decompression of the main vessels and nerves was indicated.

Forearm

Unusual presentations of a CS have been encountered in our experience when operative procedures have been undertaken for treatment of traumatic or surgical events in association with congenital deformities of the upper limb. We have seen two cases: a congenital proximal radioulnar synostosis and a Madelung deformity. The CS was established after a rotation osteotomy was performed in the first case

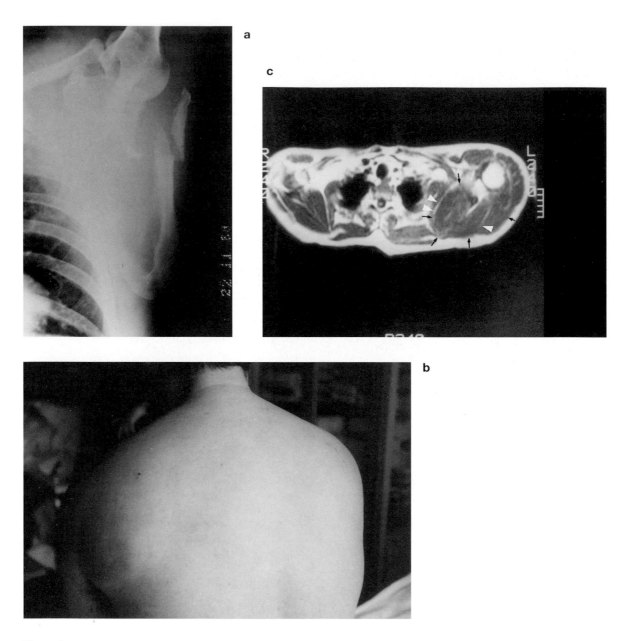

Figure 1

(a) A 45-year-old school janitor sustained a lateral impact which fractured the neck and body of the left scapula. (b) The next day he developed marked tenderness at the fracture site with an obvious, positive Comolli sign. Compartment pressures for the infraspiratus muscles were recorded 22.5 hrs after trauma with a STIC catheter; 75 mmHg (left) and 20 mmHg (right). Pressure measurement were repeated 65.5 hrs after trauma: 39 mmHg (left) and 19 mmHg (right). (c) MRI and spectroscopy were performed 68 hrs after trauma. On T1-weighted MRI axial scans, the subscapularis (double arrows) and infraspinatus (single arrow) muscles appeared grossly enlarged without significant intensity changes on the affected side. A large intramuscular haematoma was identified by the characteristic signal pattern evolution on follow-up MRI examination (black arrows)

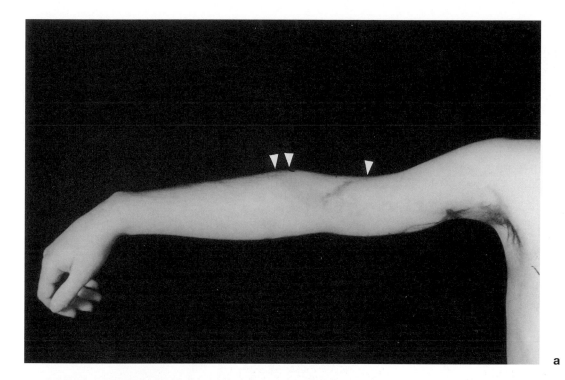

a

b

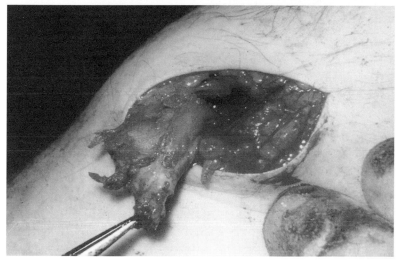

Figure 2

(a) A 35-year-old male patient affected by infraclavicular brachial plexus lesion associated with fracture of humerus and local swelling at forearm (double arrows), due to proximal rupture of the biceps muscle and its retraction (single arrow). (b) Intraoperative exploration of the forearm lump revealed a clear ischaemic nature to the mass

and after a post-traumatic fracture of the radius had been internally fixed with a dynamic compression plate (DCP) plate in the second.

The affected compartment was confined to the deep dorsal aspect of the forearm affecting the abductor pollicis longus (APL). The most relevant clinical manifestation was stiffness of the trapeziometacarpal joint leading to retroposition of the first metacarpal. Surgical exploration in the established clinical forms revealed a frank ischemic contracture of the dorsal distal extensor muscles (APL, extensor pollicis longus, extensor pollicis brevis), which was hypothetically related to a vascular anomaly associated with congenital deformities.

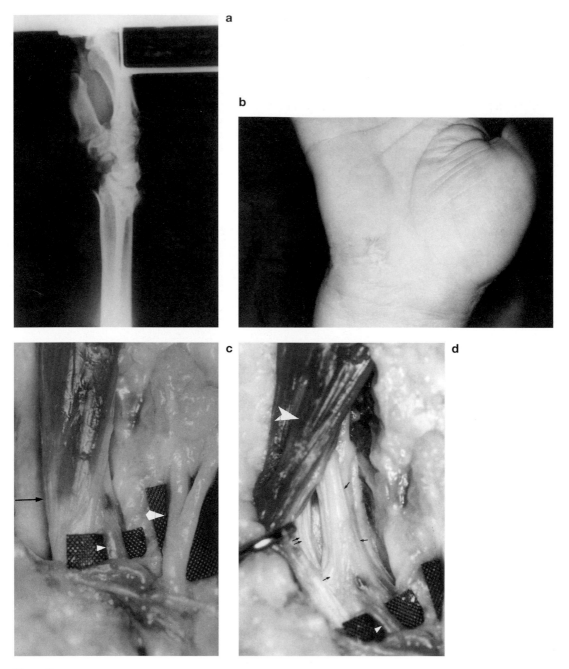

Figure 3

(a,b) A 58-year-old male truck-driver, affected by a right wrist fracture, treated by plaster cast. When the cast was removed, hyperabduction of the little finger was present. MRI and EMG showed compression of ulnar nerve at the Guyon canal. A Volkmann contracture of ADM was clearly visible. (c) Biopsy of the hypothenar muscles confirmed the ischaemic lesion of the muscle, detected at surgery (ADM, black arrow; vascular pedicle of the flexor brevis of the little finger, small white arrow; sensitive branches of the ulnar nerve, large white arrow). (d) Biopsy (ADM, large white arrow; partially ischaemic ADM, double black arrows; ischaemic and retracted flexor brevis of the little finger, single black arrows; vascular pedicle of the flexor brevis of the little finger, small white arrow)

Another unexpected complication was post-traumatic proximal displacement at the forearm level of the biceps muscle that was observed following an infraclavicular lesion of the brachial plexus associated with fracture of the humerus. Due to the violence of the trauma the biceps, deprived of its neurovascular bundle, recoiled and disguised itself as a 'mysterious lump' in the forearm (Fig. 2).

Surgical exploration revealed that the lump consisted of a typical necrotic muscle which would assign this lesion to type Ic of the presented classification. Once the nature of the lump became obvious, the direct repair of the musculocutaneous nerve was no longer indicated.

Hand

Isolated CS of each single volar and dorsal compartment is very rare. In the literature a vast review of isolated contracture of the hypothenar muscles has been reported by Monteleone (Monteleone et al 1985), and the prevailing cause of the established contracture was observed to be related to a distal radius fracture treated by a plaster cast. Direct pressure on the hypothenar base is responsible for a type Ic lesion, as the vascular supply of this group of muscles is proximally located and basically unique. An occasional vascular contribution might arise from the posterior interosseous artery (Becker and Gilbert 1988). The clinical manifestation is a hyperabduction of the little finger, whether associated or not with flexion and supination deformity of this digit.

In some cases (2 out of 5 in our personal experience) active abduction might be preserved, and this may be explained by the different contributions of the vascular supply to the abductor digiti minimi (ADM) (Fig. 3) or the presence of an accessory muscle originating proximal to the wrist (Luethke and Dellon 1992).

The established contracture of the hypothenar muscle causes various functional impairments, the most relevant being the difficulty of placing one's hand in one's pocket. Simple tenotomies are required to overcome this problem. Very rarely an isolated contracture of the second, third and fourth compartment can be observed as a consequence of isolated trauma.

We have seen a single case where a constrained lateral deviation of the middle finger was the result of a post-traumatic contracture of the muscles of the second compartment. In this case the fingers were crossed without being passively correctable, in the absence of a metacarpal fracture; this was not easy to interpret, but since the Bouvier sign was positive, a simple tenotomy and release of the extensor hood finally corrected the deformity.

Isolated contracture of the first web is a more frequent event and guidelines on how to treat this deformity have been presented in Chapter 42.

Aetiology

Unusual traumatic events and the perioperative CS

Posterior CS following the rupture of a Baker's cyst often presents dramatically and might mimic deep vein thrombophlebitis (Petros et al 1990). Furthermore, anterior dissection of a popliteal cyst has been reported to cause anterior CS in the leg (Hammoudeh et al 1995), but these forms of atypical CS are confined to the lower limb and do not have an equivalent in the upper limb. In both cases the challenge was to establish the diagnosis, but successful treatment was achieved by the standard fasciotomies.

Rare aetiologies reported at the upper limb comprise extravasation injuries, suction injuries, fracture of the neck of the radial head in children and CS following epidural anaesthesia and analgesia for postoperative pain.

Extravasation injuries are often associated with antiblastic agents, but they are not usually accompanied by a CS as the drugs concentrate in the subcutaneous tissue due to their lipophilic nature. However, in drug addicts, CS might follow heroin extravasation, when white spirit (which causes a powerful vasoconstriction) has been used as a solvent (Maladay et al 1991).

In critically ill hypotensive patients treated with high doses of dopamine, prolonged treatment may produce ischaemia at the hand and digits (Simpson 1994). Following increased perfusion, a progressive CS might show up, characterized by a blue swollen hand. This condition is aggravated when administration of high doses or extravasation of dopamine occurs. Under those circumstances prompt fasciotomy is required. A different picture is recorded when iron extravasation follows intravenous infu-

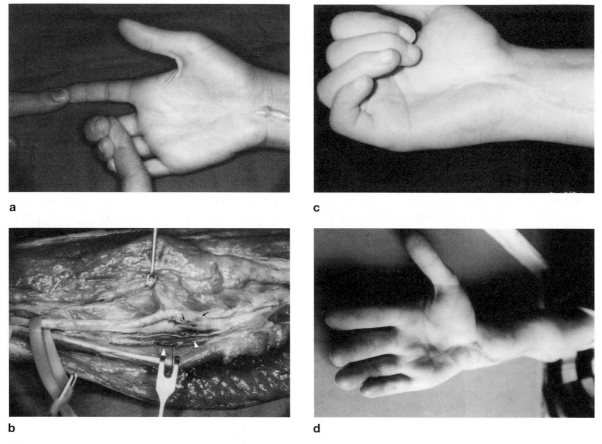

Figure 4

(a) A 24-year-old female was affected by chemical myositis with retraction of the superficialis and profundus flexor tendons of the third, fourth and fifth fingers following accidental extravasation of intravenous injection of iron for iron-deficiency anaemia. The patient underwent, in another hospital, neurolysis of the ulnar nerve. (b) One year later neurolysis of the ulnar nerve was repeated and the nerve appeared to be compressed (black arrows) by a local accumulation of iron which infiltrated the superficialis and profundus flexor muscles of the third, fourth and fifth fingers (white arrows). A muscle sliding and distal tenotomy were performed. (c,d) Good intermediate functional outcomes were obtained

sion. We have seen one case where recurrent inflammatory reaction occurred and settled only after wide excision of the affected forearm muscles which had, over time, produced a flexion contracture of the long fingers (Fig. 4).

In the medical literature two cases have been reported in children of suction injuries to the upper extremity when the hands were caught in a swimming-pool intake-pipe filtration system (Shin et al 1996). The maximum vacuum or suction generated at the intake by a 2-horse-power filter is approximately 760 mmHg. The favourable outcome was

related to a prompt surgical decompression and early post-operative rehabilitation.

A volar compartment syndrome of the forearm was identified following a minimally displaced fracture of the radial head or neck. These cases have to be added to the classic CS following a supracondylar fracture. Guidelines for treatment were the generally accepted ones, and as intracompartmental pressure was elevated, the reported cases were all managed as emergencies with fasciotomy. A minimally displaced fracture of the proximal radius in a skeletally immature patient might produce a CS in spite of limited haemorrhage or oedema, possibly because of the low compliance of the small fibro-osseous space of the antecubital region (Royle 1990, Peters and Scott 1995).

Perioperative CS

A very unusual case of CS has been reported following implantation of a neuromuscular stimulator in the tetraplegic hand (Keith et al 1989). During the early post-implantation period CS developed as a consequence of the extensive exercise programme and settled soon after reducing the workload. A more frequent aetiology is linked to epidural anaesthesia and analgesia which have recently been extensively adopted for control of post-operative pain (Strecker et al 1986; Price et al 1996).

Continuous epidural infusion of bupivacaine offers excellent relief of post-operative pain and provides a chemical sympathectomy (Strecker et al 1986), whereas epidural administration of morphine does not alter the vasoconstriction or vasodilatation reflexes.

This practice is more extensively used at the level of the lower limb. An unrecognized CS might therefore develop, and it has been reported in a patient who underwent an osteocutaneous free fibular transfer (Strecker et al 1986). We had a similar experience (Landi et al 1996), and we have therefore become much more cautious in utilizing this method for controlling post-operative pain. It appears more appropriate and less risky to resort to analgesic pumps for pain control in the post-operative phase.

Perioperative CS has also been described at the upper limb when a potentially contaminated wound was irrigated with a pressurized pulsatile irrigation system; this should therefore be used with extreme caution, especially when dealing with small wounds.

Fasciotomy has been performed with success in such cases but prevention of this kind of complication obviously needs to be carefully kept in mind (Seiler et al 1996).

Perinatal CS and thrombosis of the brachial artery in the newborn

Several definitions regarding this pathology have been proposed in the past, basically because differ-ent degrees of severity of the same process have been described separately: subcutaneous fat necrosis (Lightwood 1951), sclerema neonatorum or radial nerve palsy of the newborn (Feldman 1957), neonatal Volkmann's ischemic contracture of the forearm (Caouette-Laberge et al 1992) or gangrene in the newborn (Hensinger and Delaware 1975).

It would appear that in pregnancies associated with spontaneous rupture of the amniotic sac, particularly if there is a delay in delivery or a difficult labour, the extremities might become trapped and compressed. Indeed, the fetus is particularly vulnerable to compression after the thirty-seventh week of gestation, when the volume of amniotic fluid starts to fall (Caouette-Laberge et al 1992). In the most prominent areas (frontal area, chest wall, deltoid region, lateral aspect of the arm) a bruise might be present at birth, and when compression of this last area has lasted several hours, paralysis of the underlying radial nerve might appear. Involvement of the entire dorsal compartment might be the next step in clinical severity.

Overall, local compression might pass through the phases of simple bruise and subcutaneous fat necrosis to frank skin necrosis present at birth. Circumferential contracture due to the skin eschar and persistent underlying intrauterine hyperpression might be associated, at delivery, with a clear picture of CS with diffuse swelling and oedema. This clinical condition benefits from a simple escharectomy (Fig. 5). Skin necrosis may be so diffuse as to consider necrotizing fasciitis in the differential diagnosis. The underlying muscular and neural deficit is strictly proportional to the duration and severity of compression.

Radial nerve paralysis associated with subcutaneous fat necrosis carries a good prognosis, and full recovery is usually achieved within days or months (Hensinger and Delaware 1975, Lightwood 1951, Rombouts et al 1993). However, if CS was already established during intrauterine life, and the various compartments but especially the dorsal one had been more severely affected (Rombouts et al 1993), the outcome is less favourable. In very severe cases the volar and dorsal compartments might be equally affected with only the ulnar nerve preserved. This is in fact contained in the 'watershed' between the two compartments, whereas the median nerve, located in the centre of the volar compartment, is often irreversibly damaged (see Fig. 5).

Real gangrene in the newborn has a different

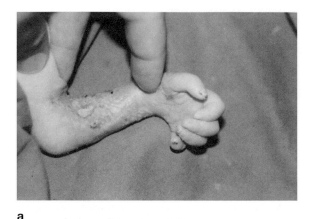

a

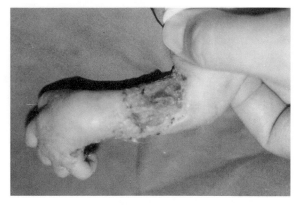

b

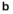

c

Figure 5

Perinatal Volkmann contracture: escharectomy was performed 48 hrs after birth in order to relieve the associated vascular symptoms of venous congestion and swelling of the hand. (a,b) One month later severe ischaemic retraction of the extrinsic muscles on a stiff claw hand deformity were present. Neurolysis and superficialization of the median and ulnar nerves, tenotomy of the flexors of the wrist, thumb and long fingers and removal of infarcted flexor tendons were performed. (c) The appearance of the ulnar nerve (white arrows) suggests a mild lesion, whereas the median nerve presents a pseudo-continuity with a distal shrunken appearance (black arrows). Full recovery of the adductor muscle occurred after 6 months

pathogenesis and carries a different prognosis (Heinsinger et al 1975), Ricciardelli et al 1995). In utero brachial artery thrombosis leads to neonatal gangrene of the extremity. Possible causes include umbilical artery catheterization, polycytaemia, dehydration and paradoxal venous embolism. This last possibility might arise from a thrombus from the renal vein or inferior vena cava passing to the arterial side via a patent foramen ovale. Placental emboli or a state of maternal hypercoagulability is usually present at birth and indicates an in utero rather than a birth-related thrombosis.

Once the diagnosis has been made, systemic urokinase therapy should begin soon after the angiogram at a dose of 5000 U/kg bolus followed by a 5000 U/kg per hour infusion. This might lead to a complete or partial salvage of the upper limb (Ricciardelli et al 1995).

Drug-induced rabdomyolysis, primitive malignant tumours and muscular metastases

Theophylline overdose has been noted to cause bilateral CS of the lower limbs (Lloyd et al 1990) requiring dialysis in addition to local surgical decompression. The picture might be exacerbated by hypocalcaemia, a recognized feature of rabdomyolysis. In spite of early fasciotomy complete muscle necrosis may develop.

In patients with a history of alcohol and heroin abuse receiving benzodiazepines to overcome their addiction, fulminant rabdomyolysis usually affecting the lower limbs can occur. Only in one case reported by Rutgers et al (1991) was the upper limb affected, requiring fasciotomy at the deltoid and

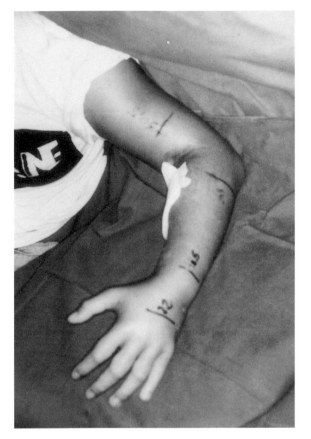

a

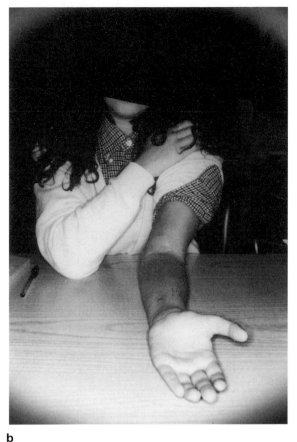

b

Figure 6

A 22-year-old female affected by a promyelocytic leukaemia was treated with all-*trans*-retinoic acid 1500 mg/day. (a) On the left arm a CS apparently triggered by an initial extravasation of the antiblastic drugs was immediately recognized and interrupted. The muscle-stretching test was positive, ulnar and radial pulses were absent, and anaesthesia in the median nerve distribution was recorded. (b) The patient underwent medical treatment with steroids, and full recovery from the local manifestation of 'retinoic acid syndrome' was observed 6 months later. Nevertheless, death occurred 2 years later following bone marrow transplantation

forearm compartments. These patients should be admitted to the Intensive Care Unit because of frequent associated renal failure. The pathogenesis of CS linked with non-traumatic rabdomyolysis is related to both prolonged coma and immobility, which might cause localized CS (besides the direct myotoxic effects of alcohol and heroin). In fact, post-mortem studies have shown that myonecrosis can become widespread, affecting the pharyngeal, sternocleidomastoid and pectoral muscles (Rutgers et al 1991).

Primitive malignant tumours, localized metastases and local manifestations of leukaemia

Synovial sarcoma presenting as an acute CS has been described in the lower limb as a manifestation of a synovial sarcoma (Shapiro and Brindley 1995), as a result of a traumatized vascular hamartoma (Joseph et al 1984) and as a presentation of a non-Hodgkin's lymphoma (Southworth et al 1990).

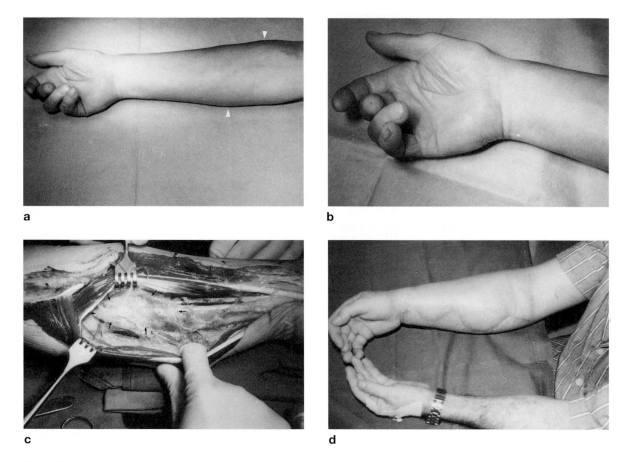

a   b

c   d

Figure 7

(a,b) A 63-year-old male presented with an apparently subacute swelling of the right forearm and retraction of the flexor tendons of the 3rd, 4th and 5th finger (white arrows). He underwent local fasciotomy in a local hospital for an impending CS. (c) Intraoperatively, 'muscular necrosis' of the 3rd, 4th, and 5th deep flexors were found, associated with extension of the area of necrosis to the flexor superficialis muscles (black arrows). (d) When admitted to our unit, local biopsies showed, at the axillary lymph-nodes, metastases of adenocarcinoma. Intramuscular swelling also became apparent in the adductor area of the thigh, and biopsy of this area showed fibrocystic reactive hyperplasia and intravascular isolated atypical epithelial nests, indicating infiltration from carcinoma. A final diagnosis of adenocarcinoma of the cardias was finally established but the patient died 4 months later

More frequently forearm CS is secondary to leukaemic infiltrates (Trumble 1987, Frankel et al 1992). The clinical presentation raises no doubts as to the diagnosis of CS, but treatment should not follow the established guidelines of post-traumatic CS. In the case of an acute lymphocytic leukaemia, CS should not be treated with fasciotomy, since symptomatic treatment is often ineffective and wound management can make the overall care more difficult and uncomfortable due to the risks of local haemorrhage and infections. However, early diagnosis should be made and treatment by chemotherapy and local radiation undertaken. In the case of promyelocytic leukaemia treated with all-*trans*-retinoic acid in order to induce haematologic remission, we have observed CS at the forearm as part of the 'retinoic acid syndrome' (Frankel et al 1992).

This syndrome is characterized primarily by fever, dyspnoea, pleural and pericardial effusions and is frequently associated with leucocytosis. The cause of this syndrome is speculative and suggests that drug-induced maturation of previously undifferentiated cells, although still dysfunctional, could confer certain functional properties of mature neutrophiles including migratory capacity. Migration of these cells into tissue such as lung, kidney and forearm muscles could explain the respiratory distress, occasional renal impairment and the CS observed in some cases (Fig. 7). Early intervention with corticosteroids may decrease morbidity and mortality associated with this syndrome.

CS can also resolve following other medical treatment (Fig. 6).

In conclusion, in similar cases, where platelets during chemotherapy are very low, surgical treatment of the underlying CS should be avoided by all means.

Intramuscular metastases

Intramuscular metastases are a rare presentation of carcinoma (Porile et al 1990, Sudo et al 1993). Even more rarely do these sites of metastasis ossify (Allen et al 1992). We are not aware of muscular metastases originating from a gastric carcinoma and presenting as a CS. There is only one case reported in the literature where Volkmann's contracture of the forearm muscles was the presentation of a breast carcinoma (Hazeltine et al 1990). We observed a patient in whom a metastasis localized in the forearm muscles was the atypical primary manifestation of gastric carcinoma. The acute signs were initially related to an acute thrombophlebitis as a possible cause of the underlying CS Fasciotomy was therefore carried out (see Fig. 7), but it must be stressed once again that the rules regarding assessment of tumours, even in the presence of a very unusual presentation such as an impending CS, should be followed and the appropriate investigations carried out according to the generally accepted protocols.

Conclusions

A pathogenetic classification, as outlined above, is very useful in order to frame the different possibilities which might lead to CS.

The ultimate result of an unrecognized CS is

necrosis of the affected muscles, and this event might follow arterial insufficiency, massive venous thrombosis or a pathology confined to a single or multiple muscle compartments. The overall assessment of a CS is described in detail for the most common features, which are linked to a traumatic origin usually considered the typical aetiology of a CS. The atypical forms are distinguished according to the site of manifestation and aetiology, and the treatment might substantially differ from the ones adopted for the typical forms.

We have tried to group the former into four main categories:

- atypical CS of post-traumatic origin
- perinatal CS
- CS associated with drug-induced rabdomyolysis,
- CS associated with primitive malignant tumours and localized muscular metastases.

General guidelines for treatment do not differ when clinical symptoms and intracompartmental measurements warrant surgical fasciotomy in both typical and atypical post-traumatic cases but the atypical CS of non-traumatic origin should be considered separately as regards treatment.

In the atypical localization at the scapula when CS is produced by haematoma, resolution might be spontaneous or, after a more precise localization, drainage may be considered.

In perinatal CS severity will vary from a simple mild CS localized in the lateral compartment of the forearm to massive muscle necrosis and, finally, to gangrene of the hand. The last may be caused by embolism of the humeral artery, which requires specific treatment.

CS associated with drug-induced rabdomyolysis, almost invariably observed in drug addicts, belongs to type IIb of the proposed classification. Adverse effects on renal function, which must be carefully monitored, deserve equal attention in treatment.

When a CS represents a local manifestation of leukaemia, surgical decompression must be avoided, and radiotherapy or chemotherapy in association with steroids should be adopted on an individual basis according to the underlying neoplasia. When confronted with an enlarging mass confined to a muscular compartment threatening a CS of the upper limb, the basic steps of oncological staging should be carried out. Fasciotomy should never be undertaken lightly but eventually performed as a palliative procedure only in a subcutaneous fashion.

Acknowledgements

The authors wish to acknowledge Dr J Pradelli and J Bemporad for their assistance with the English translation.

References

Allen A, Wetzel L, Borek D (1992) Malignant myositis ossificans. A case report, *Tumori* **78:**55–8.

Barca F, Busa R, Landi A, Saracino A (1996) Sindromi compartmentali acute della gamba e del piede: quadri clinici. In: Gaggi A, ed. *Progressi in Medicina e Chirurgia del Piede*. Vol. 5, Bologna: 45–54.

Becker C, Gilbert A (1988) Le lambeau cubital, *Ann Chir Main* **7:**136–42.

Caouette-Laberge L, Bortoluzzi P, Egerszegi EP, Marton D (1992) Neonatal Volkmann's ischemic contracture of the forearm: a report of five cases, *Plast Reconstr Surg* **90:**621–8.

Celli L, Mingione A, Maleti O, Tassi A (1995) In la trombosi profonda in ortopedia e traumatologia, *Giorn Ital Ortop Traum* **21:**S53–65

Cerofolini E, Guicciardi L, Burani A (1996) La diagnostica per immagini della sindrome compartimentale stabilizzata dell'arto inferiore. In: Gaggi A, ed. *Progressi in Medicina e Chirurgia del Piede*. Vol. 5, Bologna: 109–15.

Comolli A (1932) Uber ein deutliches Zeichen bei geswissen Schulterbruchen, *Zbl Chir* **15:**937–40.

Esposito M, Caserta G, Saracino A, Barca F, Landi A (1996) La misurazione della pressione intracompartmentale nella sindrome compartmentale acuta. In: Gaggi A, ed. *Progressi in Medicina e Chirurgia del Piede*. Vol. 5, Bologna: 55–62.

Feldman GV (1957) Radial nerve palsies in the newborn, *Arch Dis Childh* **32:**469–71.

Frankel SR, Eardley A, Lauwers G, Weiss M, Warrell RP (1992) The retinoic acid syndrome in acute promyelocytic leukemia, *Ann Internal Med* **117:**292–6.

Garfin SR, Tipton CM, Mubarak SJ, Savio L-Y Woo, Hargens AR, Akeson WH (1981) Role of fascia in maintenance of muscle tension and pressure, *J Applied Physiol* **51:**317–20.

Hammoudeh M, Siam AR, Khanjar I (1995) Anterior dissection of popliteal cyst causing anterior compartment syndrome, *J Rheum* **22:**1377–9.

Hazeltine M, Duranceau L, Gariepy G (1990) Presentation of breast carcinoma as Volkmann's contracture due to skeletal muscle metastases, *J Rheumatol* **17:**1097–9.

Hensinger RN, Delaware W (1975) Gangrene of newborn, *J Bone Joint Surg* **57A:** 121–3.

Holden CEA (1975) Compartment syndromes following trauma, *Clin Orthop Rel Res* **113:**95–102.

Joseph FR, Posner MA, Terzakis JA (1984) Compartmental syndrome caused by a traumatized vascular hamartoma, *J Hand Surg* **9A:** 904–7.

Keith WM, Peckham PH, Thrope GB, Stroh KC, Smith B, Buckett JR, Kilgore KL, Jatich W (1989) Implantable functional neuromuscular stimulation in the tetraplegic hand, *J Hand Surg* **14A:**524–30.

Landi A, De Santis G, Torricelli P, Colombo A, Bedeschi P (1989a) CT in established Volkmann's contracture in forearm muscles, *J Hand Surg* **14B:**49–52.

Landi A, De Santis G, Sacchetti GL, Ciuccarelli C, Luchetti R, Bedeschi P (1989b) The use of CT scan in evaluating Volkmann's syndrome in the limbs, *Giorn Ital Ortop Traum* **15:**521–33.

Landi A, Esposito M, Caserta G, Alfarano M, Cavana R (1991) Valutazione clinica e strumentale della sindromi compartmentali degli arti e degli esiti del trattamento, *Giorn Ital Ortop Traum* (76th SIOT Congress):169–77.

Landi A, Schoenhuber R, Funicello R, Rasio G, Esposito M (1992) Compartment syndrome of the scapula: definition on clinical data, neurophysiological and magnetic resonance data, *Ann Hand Surg* **11:**383–8.

Landi A, Caserta G, Tcherkes-Zade T, Barca F, Esposito M, Saracino A (1996) Terapia chirurgia della sindromi di Volkmann stabilizzate: indicazioni e tecniche. In: Gaggi A, ed.: *Progressi in Medicina e Chirurgia del Piede*. Vol. 5, Bologna: 130–42.

Lightwood R (1951) Radial nerve palsy associated with localized subcutaneous fat necrosis in the newborn, *Arch Dis Childh* **26:**436–37.

Lloyd DM, Payne SPK, Tomson CRV, Barnes MR, Allen MJ (1990) Acute compartment syndrome secondary to theophylline overdose, *Lancet* **336**:312.

Luethke R, Dellon AL (1992) Accessory abductor digiti minimi muscle originating proximal to the wrist causing symptomatic ulnar nerve compression, *Ann Plast Surg* **28:**307–8.

Maladay D, Fahed I, Zinabidine M, Kullhann JM, Ninoun N, Baux S (1991) Syndrome de Volkmann par injection, *XXVII Congress of Société Française de Chirurgie de la Main*: 41.

Matsen III FA, Winquist RA, Krugmire RB (1980) Diagnosis and management of compartmental syndromes, *J Bone Joint Surg* **62A:**286–91.

McDermott AGP, Marble AE, Yabsley RH (1984) Monitoring acute compartment pressure with the STIC catheter, *Clin Orth Res* **190:**192–8.

Monteleone M, Montorsi A, Luchetti R, Rovesta C (1985) Ischaemic isolated retraction of the abductor digiti minimi, *J Hand Surg* **10B:**57–9.

Mubarak SJ, Carroll NC (1979) Volkmann's contracture in children: aetiology and prevention, *J Bone Joint Surg* **61B:**285–93.

Mubarak SJ, Hargens AR (1981) *Compartment Syndromes and Volkmann's Contracture.* WB Saunders: London.

Perler PA, Tohmeh AG, Bulkley GB (1990) Inhibition of the compartment syndrome by the ablation of free radical-mediated perfusion injury, *Surgery* **108:**40–7.

Perricone G (1958) Sindrome ischemica di Volkmann dell'arto inferiore, *Atti SERTOT* **III:**1–51.

Peters CL, Scott SM (1995) Compartment syndrome in the forearm following fracture of the radial head or neck in children, *J Bone Joint Surg* **77A:**1070–4.

Petros DP, Hanley JF, Gilbreath P, Toon RD (1990) Posterior compartment syndrome following ruptured Baker's cyst, *Ann Rheum Dis* **49:**944–5.

Porile JL, Olopade OI, Hoffman PC (1990) Gastric adenocarcinoma presenting with soft tissue masses, *Am J Gastroent* **85:**76–7.

Price C, Ribeiro J, Kinnebrew T (1996) Compartment syndrome associated with postoperative epidural anesthesia, *J Bone Joint Surg* **78A:**597–9.

Ricciardelli E, Morgan RF, Lin KY (1995) In utero brachial artery thrombosis: limb salvage with postnatal urokinase infusion, *Ann Plast Surg* **34:**81–3.

Rigings P, Gault D (1994) Compartment syndrome of the arm, *J Hand Surg* **19B:**147–8.

Rombouts JJ, Debauche C, Verellen G, Lyon G (1993) Paralysies congénital par compression. A propose de quatre observations, *Ann Chir Main* **12:**39–44.

Royle SG (1990) Compartment syndrome following forearm fracture in children, *Injury* **21:**73–6.

Rowland SA (1982) Fasciotomy. In: Green DP, ed. *Operative Hand Surgery.* Vol 1. Churchill Livingstone: London: 565–81.

Rutgers PH, Van der Harst E, Koumans RKJ (1991) Surgical implications of drug-induced rhabdomyolysis, *Br J Surg* **78:**490–2.

Seiler JG, Valadie AR, Drvaric DM, Frederick RW, Whitesides T (1996) Perioperative compartment syndrome, *J Bone Joint Surg* **78A:**600–2.

Shapiro SA, Brindley GW (1995) Synovial sarcoma presenting as an acute compartment syndrome, *J Bone Joint Surg* **77A:**1249–50.

Shin AY, Chambers H, Wilkins KE, Bucknell A (1996) Suction injuries in children leading to acute compartment syndrome of the interosseous muscles of the hand: case report, *J Hand Surg* **24:**675–8.

Simpson RL (1994) Fasciotomy of the hand: revisited, *Corresp Newsletter* ASSH Feb 25.

Southworth SR, O'Malley NP, Ebraheim NA, Zeff L, Cummings V (1990) Compartment syndrome as a presentation of non-Hodgkin's lymphoma, *J Orthop Trauma* **4:**470–3.

Strecker WB, Wood MB, Bieber JE (1986) Compartment syndrome masked by epidural anesthesia for postoperative pain, *J Bone Joint Surg* **68A:**1447–8.

Sudo A, Ogihara Y, Shiokawa Y, Fujinami S, Sekiguchi S (1993) Intramuscular metastasis of carcinoma, *Clin Orthop Rel Res* **296:**213–17.

Trumble T (1987) Forearm compartment syndrome secondary to leukemic infiltrates, *J Hand Surg* **12A:**563–5.

Whitesides TE (1975) Tissue pressure measurement as a determinant for the need for fasciotomy, *Clin Orthop Rel Res* **113:**43–51.

53
Reflex sympathetic dystrophy: an overview

CB Wynn Parry

Introduction

One of the most devastating problems that confronts the hand surgeon is the frozen painful hand in the late stages of reflex sympathetic dystrophy (RSD) or causalgia. As in so many situations, prevention is the best cure. Now that RSD is being more frequently recognized there is some hope that patients can be cured or at least substantially relieved if seen early enough. With late presentation however, rehabilitation is a complex, prolonged and often unsatisfactory procedure. This chapter will highlight the early manifestations of the disorder review theories of causation, draw attention to the disorders that can be associated with RSD and discuss specific and general management.

The late stages of reconstruction to provide movement in grossly stiff joints is the province of the surgeon and will be discussed elsewhere. The definition of RSD is confused. There are almost as many terms as there are claimed cures. The consensus of opinion in the world literature is that reflex sympathetic dystrophy is the preferred term for what used to be termed Sudeck's atrophy and causalgia for the painful state arising from damaged peripheral nerves. The term sympathetically dependent pain implies a pain that is relieved by sympathetic block and can cover both conditions. It also implies that there are painful disorders that do not respond to sympathetic block.

It used to be believed that if sympathetic block cured the pain then the sympathetic nervous system must be at fault. However, it is well recognized that severe painful states can follow sympathectomy. Moreover Wallin et al (1976) showed by microelectrode recording in sympathetic fibres in patients whose pain responded to sympathetic blockade, that discharges from the sympathetic nerves remain unaltered. As will be seen later the physiology is highly complex, and both central and peripheral factors are involved.

It is customary to divide the evolution of RSD into three stages. First, the acute or so-called warm stage in which there is severe burning pain – the affected part of the limb cannot bear to be touched and there is marked swelling with obvious circulatory changes such that the part feels warm. Classically this is followed by the second subacute so-called cool stage in which the skin is cool, there is increased sweating, hair loss is now obvious with ridged and cracked nails. Osteoporosis may develop at this stage, and pain is usually constant. In the chronic or final stage pain may spread proximally, the skin becomes shiny, there is wasting of the soft tissues of the affected part, the fascia in the hand or the foot may be thickened and marked osteoporosis seen. It is at this stage that marked stiffness and deformity of the joints may develop. Pain is usually considerably diminished compared with the previous stages. These three stages may well run into each other.

Perhaps the most impressive signs are the allodynia and hyperpathia. Allodynia is used to describe a painful response to stimuli that are normally not nociceptive and hyperpathia is an enhanced response to a painful stimulus which may outlast the stimulus by many seconds or even minutes. Classically the condition follows trivial injuries or a relatively minor strain, although there is a significant incidence of RSD after Colles' fractures of the wrist.

The condition is commonest in the hand and the wrist, but is not uncommon in the foot, ankle and knee. A variant or more severe version of the condition is the so-called shoulder hand syndrome in which the hand, wrist, elbow and shoulder become very stiff – the stiffness of the shoulder being out of all proportion to the loss of movement that commonly occurs with restricted activity of a painful hand. A great variety of antecedent events have been described and these include venepuncture, renal transplants, carcinoma of the lung, following bone marrow transplant, lumbar spinal surgery, electric shock and herpes zoster. Most of the cases in our series followed relatively trivial injuries without fracture.

A particularly interesting aspect of this condition is that it can be related to central nervous conditions. Some of the most severe cases we have had to treat have followed stroke or brain injury.

RSD can also follow systemic disorders particularly of the cardiac and gastrointestinal system such as peptic ulcer, cardiac infarction and cholecystitis. Schott (1991) in a comprehensive account of the central causes of RSD includes epilepsy, Parkinson's disease, cervical cord disease, spinal tumours, syringomyelia and multiple sclerosis. The condition also occurs in children when there is usually no obvious antecedent event.

Wilder et al (1992) reported on 70 patients who were younger than 18 years old, with an average age of 12.5 years. They were predominately girls and the lower extremity was most often involved. The average time from onset to the diagnosis was 1 year. They suggest that the syndrome is often unrecognized in children. They report that the standard multidisciplinary approach was effective with sympathetic blockade, transcutaneous stimulation antidepressants and intensive rehabilitation, but that 38 of the 70 patients continued to have some degree of residual pain and dysfunction years later.

The association with Colles' fracture is obviously of great importance to hand surgeons and there have been a number of publications recently on this topic.

Atkins et al (1990) reported a prospective study of the incidence of RSD following Colles' fracture in 60 patients. Nine weeks after fracture, 24 patients had vasomotor instability, 23 had significant tenderness of the fingers and 23 had actually lost movement. Warwick et al (1993) studied 100 consecutive patients with displaced Colles' fracture reviewed 10 years after injury. Of those with an unsatisfactory result, 62% had objective features of reflex sympathetic dystrophy compared with only 6% of those with a satisfactory result. Atkins et al (1989) determined the prevalence of RSD at 9 weeks and 6 months after Colles' fracture. At 9 weeks, 27 of 109 patients showed signs with more than one feature of the disorder. At 6 months, 62% of the previously affected patients showed some residual abnormali-

ties and in two-thirds of these there was evidence of continuing vasomotor instability or swelling.

Ten years after Colles' fracture Field et al (1992) reported that 26% of 55 cases showed features of the syndrome. Poor finger function three months after a fracture correlated significantly with the presence of RSD after 10 years. Sarangi et al (1993) made a prospective study of the incidence and natural history of RSD in the ankles and feet of 60 consecutive patients who had suffered unilateral fracture of the tibial shaft. At bone union, 18 patients showed signs of RSD independent of the type of management and severity of injury. Fortunately in only four patients were there significant symptoms and signs at 1 year after injury. Although most patients lose their pain and recover reasonable function within months of the developed condition, there is unfortunately a significant number who progress to chronic disability.

Subbarao and Stillwell (1981) followed up 86 patients and found that after some years 17% had significant disability with stiffness, pain and lack of function.

There is universal agreement in the world literature that the long-term results depend greatly on the speed with which intensive treatment can be introduced. The later the condition is diagnosed and treatment started, the worse is the prognosis.

Running through the literature over the last century is the suggestion that there is such an entity, 'Sudeck's diathesis', making a patient with a certain type of psychological profile more vulnerable to the condition.

We have never subscribed to this view and there have been several recent reports indicating that after exhaustive psychological testing, there is no evidence at all for such a diathesis (Bruehl and Carlson 1992, Lynch 1992). Patients with the florid condition suffer severe pain which affects their life and it is to be expected that they will be miserable and depressed. Once successful treatment is instituted, these patients return to a normal psychological profile.

Many authors in reviews of this condition emphasize that the diagnosis is primarily clinical, as the classical osteoporosis with changes on scintinography and blood flow studies are not present in the early stages.

Such bone studies are helpful in distinguishing true RSD from the disuse wasting that can follow immobilization with fractures. But functional results depend upon the early institution of treatment in the early stages before obvious X-ray changes appear (Bickerstaff and Kanis 1994). Thermography, skin blood flow and temperature measurements are useful in assessing the effectiveness of treatment such as sympathetic blockade but have no real place in the day-to-day management of this condition.

Causalgia has some historical references. In the French wars of the 17th century it is recorded that a Monsieur Portail damaged a nerve whilst bleeding King Charles IX. The king apparently let out a great cry of pain and for many days afterwards the part was extremely painful with a burning sensation, but as time went on the pain subsided and neither the king nor Monsieur Portail suffered any long-term consequences. Guthrie (1820) gave a graphic description of severe causalgia in the Peninsular campaign of the Napoleonic Wars following damage to peripheral nerves. He also described a soldier (at the battle of Waterloo) who received a wound in the back of the thigh which was shortly followed by considerable pain not in the part actually injured but on the outside of the leg below the knee, on the sole of the foot and the toes. The pain gradually increased rather than diminished, became intolerable and rendered the sufferer's life miserable. It increased by paroxysms during which the man was in agony. The pain not only being permanently intense in the foot, but shooting down to it accompanied by severe spasms. No treatment had any effect and the only relief he got was by putting his foot on a cold stone or soaking his footwear in water. He was discharged without having attained any evident benefit although he eventually became less aware of the pain and accustomed to the necessity of protecting it.

The classical description of causalgia was by Weir Mitchell (repr. 1982) in the American Civil War. He opened a special ward for gunshot wounds of peripheral nerves and made a special study of the severe pain that so often accompanied these injuries, coining the term causalgia (burning pain) which is such a characteristic feature of this condition. The pain occurred often immediately on injury, but sometimes hours or even days later. He described the pain as burning, developing in the hand or foot according to which nerve was involved. He described hyperaesthesia which we would now call allodynia. He noted marked circulatory changes, a cyanosis and mottling of the skin, often eruptions mimicking a number of skin diseases, swelling of joints, severe changes in the nails with pitting, coarseness and overgrowth, loss of

hair, atrophy of the soft tissues of the affected part and eventually spread to other nerves so that, for example, after damage to the median nerve some months later the patient would notice severe pain and allodynia in the distribution of the ulnar nerve. In severe cases it might spread to the whole arm.

Later a fine tremor or even complex spontaneous movements would develop in the affected limb, and after a time could spread to the contralateral limb. Often the condition could become chronic. Weir Mitchell's son was a neurologist and 27 years after the publication of his father's classical book he was able to locate 22 of those patients and found that half of them were still suffering very severe pain (Mitchell, repr. 1985).

A whole variety of treatments were used including local injections of morphine into the painful part which, surprisingly, seems to have been quite effective. Multiple nerve resections were often carried out. Weir Mitchell pointed out that the early results of nerve resection were very encouraging, but at long-term follow up a significant proportion had relapsed. Since Weir Mitchell's report, workers in this field have been well aware of the problems of pain following damage to peripheral nerves and the term causalgia has been retained.

It is generally agreed that about 5% of patients who suffer injuries to peripheral nerves affecting particularly the median or sciatic nerve can develop this condition. There seems no rhyme or reason why some people should suffer and not others, although there is a possible clue in the fact that certain strains of rat do not develop autotomy (self mutilation after nerve damage) while others do; suggesting a genetic background. The clinical features of RSD and causalgia, as can be seen, are remarkably similar and there is a general consensus that both conditions are similar in nature. Causalgia resulting from damage to major nerve trunks and RSD from damage to fine nerve terminals. Both conditions are associated with severe pain, swelling, trophic changes, involuntary movements, gradual spread to other parts of the limb and osteoporosis. In both conditions, there is a significant incidence of long-term chronicity.

The first breakthrough in the management of this condition was in 1916 when Leriche noted that periarterial sympathectomy often relieved the pain of RSD. Barnes (1954) showed the spectacular effect of sympathetic block by stellate ganglion injections in several patients with severe causalgia following peripheral nerve damage. He enlarged the original clinical description of Weir Mitchell noting that noise, high notes and low flying aeroplanes or even a child's cry could provoke severe spasms of pain and that excitement and worry often exacerbated it. Some of his patients were unable to enjoy exciting films or dramatic novels. A painter by trade complained that he had to skip pages of books where there were mentions of cliffs, heights or ladders and whenever he saw someone high up on a ladder it caused him severe pain. We have a patient with classical causalgia of the finger following trivial skin trauma whose pain is greatly exacerbated whenever her husband knocks his pipe out on a glass ash tray. Barnes' paper shows photographs of patients with extreme pain holding their hand in a bowl of water to gain relief, but following sympathetic block, they are observed smiling and being able to do up their shoelaces thus having function restored to their painful hand.

The next breakthrough was the work of Hannington-Kiff in the early 1970s who showed that guanethidine block was a more efficient and simpler way of obtaining sympathetic blockade than stellate blocks Hannington-Kiff (1974). It is now generally agreed that the sympathetic nervous symptom plays an important role in this condition, but its exact nature is still far from clear.

The relation of this condition to the sympathetic nervous system is strongly suggested by these facts:

1 The pain can be relieved by blocking a sympathetic nerve either by guanethidine or a similar substance or stellate block.
2 The pain is increased by alpha adrenergic stimuli applied locally.
3 Guanethidine elicits pain and then abolishes the pain generated by noradrenalin release.
4 Electrical stimulation to the decentralized thoracic sympathetic ganglia for causalgia in conscious patients reproduces the burning pain.

Pathophysiology

The pioneering work of Wall and Devor (1978) has shed a great deal of light on the results of the consequences of nerve damage. They showed that after nerve damage, spontaneous discharges arise from the neuroma and that these spontaneous discharges incite increased activity from the resting discharge of the dorsal root ganglion. They also showed that these discharges were highly sensitive to circulating noradrenalin. Subsequently both Wall and Woolf (1983) have showed that there are profound central changes that follow even quite trivial peripheral damage. Woolf showed that acute thermal injury caused a heightened flexion reflex to natural electrical stimulation that persisted after local anaesthesia at the site of injury indicating an alteration of the excitability of the spinal cord. It is now known that activation of peripheral nociceptors by tissue damage or chemical or electrical stimulation can lead to hyperexcitability in the spinal dorsal horn. There are a growing number of chemical mediators that appear to be responsible for this condition and the subject is well reviewed by Dubner (1991).

Woolf has pointed out that there are three types of peripherally produced pain: 1, nociceptive, the physiological response to potentially damaging stimuli; 2, inflammatory, a reparative phenomenon; 3, neuropathic, with damage to nervous system of no value to the organism.

In inflammation a variety of chemical compounds sensitize the nociceptors changing their properties such that their transductive sensitivity is altered and can now be activated by non-noxious stimuli. In the post-injury hypersensitivity/or hyperalgesia, sensitivity spreads and hyperalgesia is mainly mediated by low threshold A fibres.

In neuropathic pain, ectopic activity with damaged terminal fibres in a neuroma produces central sensitization. C fibres terminate in very specific areas of the dorsal horn (lamina 2). A fibres terminate in different areas. After nerve damage A fibres invade the area of C fibres with marked reorganization of nervous pathways. A fibres now contact C fibre territories thus explaining allodynia. There are thus functional chemical and structural changes in the central nervous system, and this is why pain can be so intractable. Sympathetic fibres now affect A fibre cells and sensitize them. Adrenergic receptors develop in C fibre territory and the scene is set for ongoing central and peripheral hypersensitivity. That hyperalgesia in causalgia is signalled by activity in myelinated fibres and not in unmyelinated nociceptive fibres is shown by the fact that an ischaemic block of A beta fibres when C and A delta fibres were functional eliminated the hyperalgesia. Local anaesthetic block of C and delta fibres did not affect hyperalgesia. Roberts (1986) has argued cogently for the spreading sensitivity of the wide range dynamic (WD) neurones in the cord and their affection by normal sympathetic activity. These WD neurones are known to receive excitatory input from low threshold mechanoreceptors and from nociceptors. These theories not only explain why pain is so chronic, they also explain why pain can be so immediate. Weir Mitchell's patients would often feel pain almost as the bullet struck the brachial plexus or peripheral nerves – central sensitization occurring very rapidly. Presumably central lesions act by reducing inhibition in dorsal horn neurones and rendering them sensitive to central sympathetic activity. Interestingly Loh Nathan and Schott (1981) showed that such centrally determined pain could respond to peripheral sympathetic blockade.

The more rapid excitatory events in dorsal horn neurones are mediated by excitatory amino acids such as glutamic acid and aspartic acid which act at NMDA receptor sites. Dubner (1991) points out that development of clinically effective NMD antagonists is an exciting challenge for future relief of symptoms. Janig (1991) has suggested a hypothesis to explain the development of RSD and pain after causalgia. He points out that there are four interconnected components. The lesions of peripheral nerves are followed by abnormal activity and by changes of other slower processes such as ortho and retrograde axoplasmic flow of the primary afferent neurones. Secondly, changes in the primary afferent neurones induce alterations in the synaptic processing of information in the spinal cord. This affects the thoracolumbar sympathetic outflow and results in a change of the discharge pattern of sympathetic neurones to the lesioned extremity and thus abnormal regulation of blood flow and sweating.

The sympathetic post-ganglionic activity influences activity in primary afferent neurones from the lesioned territory. The pathological discharge pattern in sympathetic neurones, possibly in connection with the changes of the primary afferent neurones, produces the trophic changes and a vicious cycle may develop.

There is now general agreement among hand surgeons that repeated resection of the nerve is likely to be disastrous often exacerbating pain. It is now clear from the work of Wall and Devor (1981) why this is – further damage to the nerve produces further ectopic discharges, further hypersensitivity to noradrenaline and further central effects of deafferentation. In a series that we published in 1989 we noted that in a group of patients in whom 71 opera-

tions had been carried out specifically to relieve pain, such as neurolysis, nerve resection and nerve grafting, pain was only relieved in one patient (Wynn Parry and Girgis 1989).

Birch and Wynn Parry (Wynn Parry 1991) take the view that if one attempt to restore continuity of the nerve to relieve pain fails, then further surgical attempts are to be abandoned. When confronted with a patient with a very severe painful neuroma in front of the wrist following unsuccessful nerve suture, it is reasonable to excise the neuroma and put in a graft on the grounds that there is no prospect of further recovery of the nerve and that the condition cannot be made worse. If however resection of the neuroma and grafting does not produce pain relief, no further surgery should be considered. The backbone of our treatment has been serial guanethidine blocks.

In the early days we were too timid in our approach and would only use one block a week for up to three blocks and would abandon further attempts if unsuccessful. However, we have learnt by experience that repeated sympathetic blocks produces a cumulative effect and that after six blocks there may be a marked improvement, even though the first two or three blocks were ineffective. We admit all out patients whenever possible to our in-patient rehabilitation unit. The patients are given guanethidine blocks on alternate days. Immediately after intensive care each session is followed by an intensive rehabilitation programme involving desensitization of the affected part by rubbing and pressure and the encouragement of maximum use of the limb, both to desensitize the painful part and to restore power to weak muscles and movement to stiff joints. This is carried out both in the physiotherapy and the occupational therapy department with activities commensurate with the patient's interest and experience.

This programme is carried out on a full-time basis interspersed with general exercises and games. General fitness is important because there is evidence that physical fitness increases the level of circulating endorphins. It also helps to take the patients out of themselves and to become more involved with other people. If after six blocks there is no response then this method of treatment is abandoned. It is worth trying stellate blocks because some patients respond to one and not the other. Where the nerve is accessible we have tried the effect of long-term local anaesthetic perfusion, e.g. in the case of severe causalgia of the ulnar nerve at the elbow or median nerve at the wrist. The patient can attend the various therapy departments for intensive rehabilitation. Following 10 days of this treatment, several patients have shown substantial relief, but the technique in our experience seems less effective in the lower limb.

Indeed the prognosis for low limb causalgia is less good than for the upper limb. A multidisciplinary approach is all important with the integrated contributions of physiotherapists, occupational therapist, rehabilitation nurse, anaesthetists when indicated and clinical psychologists. By far the best results are obtained on an in-patient progressive intensive programme. Follow-up is essential because patients with severe pain have an unfortunate habit of relapsing. Our experience showed that those in which good but not perfect results were obtained after our regime were more likely to relapse months or years later. It is important therefore to be able to resume an intensive programme of rehabilitation in the early stages of relapse. Wynn Parry and Girgis (1989) reported on 78 patients with severe causalgia among which there were 25 median nerve lesions of the wrist, 21 digital nerve, 12 ulnar nerve lesions at the elbow, eight nerve lesions involving the foot, three ulnar nerve lesions of the wrist and three at the knee.

Sympathetic blockade with this or similar agents is now standard therapy. The maximum number of blocks given to a single patient on admission was 31. In total, 700 guanethidine blocks were administered during 1979–1986. All the patients had temporary relief of pain for a few minutes, presumably through the effect of ischaemia or local anaesthetic, and thereafter patients either showed relief for some hours or an increasing period of relief after subsequent blocks.

Of our patients 30% had excellent relief with complete abolition of symptoms and restoration of normal function, 30% had good results with some residual discomfort, 20% had moderate results in which pain was substantially reduced but was still somewhat of a problem and in 20% there was no effect. In general, we find that lesions on the foot do not do as well as in the upper limb and that median nerve lesions respond well, but ulnar nerve lesions are the most recalcitrant. There seems to be no relation between the length of time of symptoms and the response to treatment and therefore one need not be deterred by the chronicity of the symptoms from instituting a full-scale rehabilitation programme. There have been many reports of the

successful use of guanethidine in RSD (Eulry et al 1991).

As a last resort some surgeons carry out surgical sympathectomy, although pain can return some weeks or months later and in occasional cases may be exacerbated – the so-called post-sympathectomy pain described, for instance, after sympathectomy for hyperidrosis. Olcott et al (1991) report on 35 patients with RSD who were so treated. All patients had at least one positive diagnostic sympathetic block before surgery was commenced. Excellent results were obtained in 74%, good results in 17%, poor results in 9%. Three patients required repeat surgery. The best results were obtained in those treated early in the course of the disorder.

There have been sporadic reports of satisfactory results from the use of oral steroids in large doses for RSD, but this approach seems now to have been abandoned. Calcitonin, either by snuff or orally, has been reported as helpful in some cases and is certainly worth trying. The standard analgesic preparations are singularly unhelpful although the antidepressants can be effective. Tryptophan which is a combination of an antihistamine and an antidepressant was the most effective in our hands. It must be explained that these drugs are being used for their serotonin sparing effect and not because the patients are believed to be depressed. Transcutaneous electrical stimulation is more valuable in causalgia than it is in the classical RSD. It is certainly worth trying but in our experience was only effective in a few cases.

As in so many fields of chronic pain, pain coping strategies and involvement in progressive functional activity encouraging use of the hand and reinstatement in the community are the most effective means of treatment. There have been reports of the use of dorsal column stimulation by Tasker and his group (Tasker 1990) who showed that 50% of 14 patients with causalgia obtained relief and Levy et al (1987) reported that 75% of 16 patients with neuropathic pain were relieved. Chronic brain stimulation was used for a while but has been abandoned by most people because of complications. In very severe cases, the dorsal root entry zone operation has been used and has been effective in a few cases. However, there are complications from this procedure and in a significant number of patients there is a return of pain in the years following surgery.

Electrical perineural stimulation with electrodes

around or near the nerve was used for a time but the long-term results were disappointing and there was a significant incidence of scarring and infection.

A small but significant group of patients will present with chronic pain and severe deformity with a frozen hand and a frozen shoulder. Here all the resources of the rehabilitation team need to be used. Specialized physiotherapy using corrective splintage followed by dynamic splintage is particularly valuable and has been well described by Thomas (1997).

Physiotherapy and rehabilitation

In the acute stage the physiotherapist evaluates the degree of pain with a visual analogue scale noting area, intensity, quality and duration. This is reassessed weekly in the early stages and at 2-weekly intervals thereafter. Passive and active joint ranges are recorded noting when limits are reached because of pain and response to pressure over joints and the palmar plate. At every evaluation ranges in all upper limbs are measured, noting particularly any limitation of internal rotation of the shoulders. Sensation is evaluated in standard ways noting areas of allodynia and hyperpathia and any actual sensory loss. Tinel's sign is used to pick up any median nerve involvement. Oedema is measured by tape. Colour and temperature changes are noted. Any evidence of irritation or pain due to casts is noted and reported immediately.

Splinting is vital at this stage to maintain the hand in the optimal position for maximum function and for maintaining digital extension. Splinting must not constrict tissues and must accommodate variable swelling. Active exercises combined with elevation are the cornerstones of therapy. Continuous passive movement is of great value in recalcitrant cases, but it is remarkable how even severe oedema can resolve with a religiously applied programme of elevation. Pressure can be applied by wrapping digits with Coreban or custom-made pressure garments. Effleurage is helpful to assist fluid dispersion. Intensive progressive active exercises for individual joints and general hand activity are vital elements of therapy. Home exercises are insisted upon with bouncing, putty and squash balls used as helpful adjuncts. The patient must become constantly conscious of the need to use the hand.

Many therapists, particularly in France, Italy and Germany, use electrical stimulation as an adjunct to active exercise. Although it has rather gone out of fashion in the UK, it can certainly act as a reinforcer when pain inhibits active exercise. Gentle Maitland's-type movements are used to encourage an increased passive range, but never to the point of pain. Any stiffness of the shoulder is treated with active assisted movements and PNF (proprioceptive neuromuscular facilitation) techniques particularly the hold, relax and slow reversals.

Once pain has been relieved, attempts can be made to desensitize the area of allodynia by rubbing, pressure and intense active use. Occupational therapy activities are of particular value as they encourage use of the hand in absorbing, meaningful activities. Where stiffness of joints has supervened it is important to use techniques that demand active flexion of the wrist and fingers. Many occupational therapy techniques can use only generalized grip but this is insufficient for this purpose. The use of secateurs, pliers and other activities requiring progressive wrist and finger movements through a significant range are helpful. Adjustments can be made to conventional occupational therapy activities by using spring-loaded grips, the power varying according to the patient's weakness of grip and can be increased as recovery occurs. Constant use of spring grips and balls, stiff putty, etc. is encouraged throughout the day. If hyperaesthesia or allodynia are difficult to eradicate by sympathetic blockade, a custom-made pressure glove (Jobst type) can be useful. Constant firm pressure stimulates the large diameter afferent touch and pressure fibres which selectively inhibit C fibre traffic at the spinal level. It is well worth making a well-fitting Jobst-type glove and the patient is more likely to use his hand for everyday activities. Splinting is a valuable adjunct to active exercises in helping to restore movement to stiff joints. In the acute stage when pain is overriding and the condition is akin to acute inflammation, a splint is made in which the wrist and fingers are rested, and most likely will need to be well padded to allow firm continuous overall pressure. Thomas (1997) has emphasized the importance of splinting the wrist in some dorsiflexion and slight ulnar deviation and the metacarpopharyngeal (MCP) joints in 70° flexion and proximal interphalangeal (PIP) joints in 30° flexion. Later when activity becomes possible, several plasters can be used to restore passive range little by little. These plasters are not active stretch plasters but maintain the correction obtained by the physiotherapists slow gentle stretches at each session. If in-patient facilities exist, which we favour for such patients with such severe disabilities, four sessions a day can be used. Every few days a plaster is kept and dated and prognosis can be well seen over the weeks. Finger stiffness is probably better treated by the use of spring wire ('lively splints') as first described by Capener (1949), though if the MCP or PIP joints of all the fingers are affected, this is not feasible and plaster splints must be used. We are unhappy with the use of spring-loaded traction extensions for the small joints of the hand as it is almost impossible to avoid causing deformity at the joint distal to that being corrected. With intensive progressive physiotherapy using slow stretches, resting plasters, intensive active exercises and occupational therapy, even severe contractures can be relieved. The secret is little and often throughout the day, consistently over a period of weeks. Any sign of swelling must immediately be treated with elevation in a sling, if necessary also at night. The shoulder easily becomes stiff in RSD, quite apart from the true shoulder hand syndrome, and exercises to maintain full range in all the upper limb joints are vital.

Thomas (1997) favours well-ventilated elastic thermoplastic material which is remodelled as movement increases. Double finger stalls are useful to help the better finger mobilize its stiff neighbour. Bunnel block splints are used to support the MCP joints and focus long muscle action on the stiff interphalangeal (IP) joint. Dynamic splints using pulleys and elastics come into their own. Only one level should be corrected at a time. Four mechanisms are noted by Thomas: 1, dynamic; 2, serial static as with serial casting; 3, progressive static using the same splint but replacing traction with an adjustable static force; 4, dynastatic in which traction pulls the digit against an adjustable block.

There are clear indications for reconstructive surgery for ligament resection and volar plate arthroplasty, but this is the province of the hand surgeon, as discussed in Chapter 36. Above all, the management of these painful conditions is multidisciplinary. As indicated in the description of the pathophysiology of these conditions, there are many factors involved and therefore a multipronged approach has to be taken. The condition must be explained very carefully to the patient so that there is as much understanding as possible of the pathophysiology and the means by which the team hope to relieve pain and improve function.

We believe that in severe cases there is no alternative to an in-patient intensive rehabilitation programme. The approach that is often adopted of carrying out a single guanethidine block as an outpatient and not following this up with an intensive rehabilitation programme is not approved. Sympathetic blockade is, after all, merely an attempt to relieve pain so that a subsequent rehabilitation programme can be made possible. Patients cannot involve themselves in such a programme if their extremity is painful with allodynia and hyperpathia. Finally, we wish to emphasize the great importance of long-term follow-up to detect relapses and to institute a rehabilitation programme as soon as possible.

A comprehensive review of RSD is to be found in Schwartzman and McLellan (1987).

References

Atkins RM, Duckworth T, Kanis JA (1989) Algodystrophy following Colles fracture, *Br J Hand Surg* **14B**:161–4.

Atkins RM, Duckworth T, Kanis JA (1990) Features of algodystrophy after Colles fracture, *J Bone Joint Surg* **72**:105–10.

Barnes R (1954) Causalgia. A Review of 48 Cases. *Peripheral Nerve Injuries, Medical Research Council Special Report HMSO*: 156–85.

Bickerstaff DR, Kanis JA (1994) Algodystrophy, an under recognised complication of minor trauma, *Br J Rheumatol* **33**:240–8.

Bruehl S, Carlson CR (1992) Predisposing psychological factors in the development of reflex sympathetic dystrophy. A review of the empirical evidence, *Clin J Pain* **8**:278–99.

Capener N (1949) The use of orthopaedic appliances in the treatment of anterior poliomyelitis. *J Bone Joint Surg* **37B**:591–7.

Dubner R (1991) Pain and hyperalgesia following tissue injury new mechanisms and new treatments, *Pain* **44**:213–14.

Eulry F, Lechavalier D, Pats B, Alliaurne C, Crozes P, Vasseum P, Coutant G, Fetten D, Pattin S (1991) Regional intravenous guanethidine blocks in algodystrophy, *Clin Rheumatol* **10**:377–83.

Field J, Warwick D, Bannister GC (1992) Features of algodystrophy 10 years after Colles fracture, *J Hand Surg* **17**:318–20.

Guthrie GJ (1820) *Treatise of Gunshot Wounds on Injuries of*

Nerves and of Wounds of the Extremities. Burgess & Hill: London.

Hannington-Kiff JG (1974) Intravenous regional sympathetic block with guanethidine, *Lancet* **i**:1019–20.

Hannington-Kiff JG (1990) Intravenous regional sympathetic blocks. In: Stanton-Hicks M, Janig W, Boas RA, eds. *Reflex Sympathetic Dystrophy*. Massachusetts: Kluwer Academic: 113–24.

Janig W (1991) The generation of reflex sympathetic dystrophy, a hypothesis. Paper read to an invited symposium, London 1991.

Leriche R (1916) *The Surgery of Pain*. 1939, trans A Young. Baltimore: Williams & Wilkins: 48–52.

Levy RM, Lamb S, Adams JE (1987) Treatment of chronic pain by deep brain stimulation, long term follow up and review of literature, *Neurosurgery* **21**:885–93.

Loh Nathan PW, Schott GD (1981) Pain due to lesions of central nervous system removed by sympathetic block, *BMJ* **282**:1026–7.

Lynch ME (1992) Psychological aspects of reflex sympathetic dystrophy, a review of the adult and paediatric literature, *Pain* **49**:337–47.

Mitchell JK (repr. 1985) *Remote Consequence of Injuries of Nerve and their Treatment*. Philadelphia: JP Lippincott.

Mitchell Weir S (repr. 1982) *Injuries of Nerves and Their Consequences*. New York: Dover.

Olcott CE, Therington LG, Wilcosky BR, Shoor PM, Zimmerman J, Fogarty TJ et al (1991) Reflex sympathetic dystrophy, the surgeon's role in management, *J Vasc Surg* **14**:488–92.

Roberts WJ (1986) A hypothesis on the physiological basis for causalgia and related pains, *Pain* **24**:297–312.

Sarangi PP, Ward AJ, Smith EJ, Staddon GE, Atkins RM (1993) Algodystrophy and osteoporosis after tibial fractures, *J Bone Joint Surg* **75**:450–2.

Schott G (1991) Central causes of peripheral pain. In: CB Wynn Parry, ed. *Management of Pain in the Hand and Wrist*. New York: Churchill Livingstone: 34–47.

Schwartzman RJ, McLellan TL (1987) Reflex sympathetic dystrophy, a review, *Arch Neuro* **44**:535–61.

Schwartzman RJ, Toni L, McLellan TL (1987) *Articles Neurol* **44**:555–60.

Subbarao J, Stillwell GK (1981) Reflex sympathetic dystrophy syndrome of the upper extremity, analysis of total outcome of management of 125 cases, *Arch Phys Med* **62**:549–54.

Tasker R (1990) Management of nociceptive deafferentation and central pain by surgical intervention. In: Fields C, ed. *Pain Syndromes in Neurology*. Butterworth: Oxford: 143–200.

Thomas D (1997) Physiotherapy and Splinting. In: Moutet F, ed. *Algodystrophie: Cahiers Kinésothérapie*. Masson: Paris.

Wall PD, Devor M (1978) Physiology of sensation after peripheral nerve injury. Regeneration and neuroma formation. In: Waxman SG, ed. *Physiology and Pathobiology of Axons*. Raven Press, New York: 377–88.

Wall PD, Devor M (1981) The effect of peripheral nerve injury on dorsal root potentials and on transmission of afferent signals into the spinal cord, *Brain Res* **209**:95–III.

Wall PD, Gutnick M (1974) Ongoing activity in peripheral nerves. The physiology and pharmacology of impulses originating from a neuroma, *Exp Neurol* **43**:580–93.

Wallin G, Torebjork E, Hallin R (1976) Preliminary observations on the pathophysiology of hyperalgesia in the causalgic pain syndrome. In: Zotteman Y, ed. *Sensory Function of the Skin in Primates*, Pergamon Press: Oxford: 489.

Warwick D, Field J, Prothero D, Gibson A, Bannister GC (1993) Function 10 years after Colles fracture. *Clin Orthop* **295**:270–4.

Wilder RT, Berde CB, Woldhan M, Vieyra MA, Masek BJ, Michell LJ (1992) Reflex sympathetic dystrophy in children. Clinical characteristics and follow up of 70 patients, *J Bone Joint Surgery* **74**:910–9.

Woolf C (1983) Evidence for a central component of post injury pain hypersensitivity. *Nature* **306**:686–8.

Wynn Parry CB, Girgis F (1989) Management of causalgia after peripheral nerve injury, *Int Disability Stud* **11**:15–20.

Wynn Parry CB (1991) Management of painful peripheral nerve disorders In: Wynn Parry CB, ed. *Management of Pain in the Hand and Wrist*. Churchill Livingstone: New York: 69–99.

Index

adductor pollicis, denervation 315–17
adhesions
  between tendon and synovium, prevention by
      inhibiting transforming growth factor-β
      21–3
  shoulder 15, 56
    biological molecules implicated 18–23
    clinical causes 15–18
adhesive capsulitis *see* frozen shoulder
adoption phenomenon, denervation in spastic palsy
    315–16, 317
algodystrophy 216
alkaptonuria 262
allodynia 381, 383, 384
amyloidosis 262
analgesics
  osteoarthritis 28
  rheumatoid arthritis 27
ankylosing spondylitis, wrist stiffness 172
ankylosis *see under individual joints*
apatite-associated destructive arthritis of shoulder
    29
arm
  compartment syndrome 367
  see also forearm
arthritis
  crystal-induced 172–3
  degenerative *see* osteoarthritis
  destructive, shoulder 29
  infective, elbow stiffness after 79
  juvenile chronic, elbow replacement arthroplasty
      113, 114–16
  post-traumatic, elbow replacement arthroplasty
      115, 116–17
  psoriatic 172, 262
  shoulder 4
    medical management 25–30
  wrist 166, 172–3
  see also osteoarthritis; rheumatoid arthritis

arthrodesis
  distal ulnar joint see Sauv-Kapandji procedure
  elbow, angle of fusion 83
  four-corner, radiocarpal joint 187–9
  metacarpophalangeal joint 244
  proximal interphalangeal joint 268
  radiocarpal joint
    limited 185–9
    total 190–1
  shoulder 63–6
    complications 66
    contraindications 64
    indications 63–4
    position 64
    postoperative management 66
    technique 65
arthrography
  distension 50
  radiocarpal stiffness 153, 155, 162
  shoulder stiffness
    diagnosis 5, 48, 55, 56
    treatment 50
arthrogryposis multiplex congenita 212, 355, 361
  clinical presentation 355
  elbow 78, 355–9
    conservative treatment 355
    surgical treatment 356–9
  hand 361, 363–4
  shoulder 355, 357
    surgical treatment 357, 358
  wrist 361–3
arthrolysis
  elbow joint
    arthroscopic arthrolysis 86–9
    choice of procedure 99–101
    elementary surgical procedures 99
    open arthrolysis 95–8
    open arthrolysis with distraction 91–4
  proximal interphalangeal joint 267–8

open arthrolysis *contd*
    wrist, arthroscopic arthrolysis 193–4
arthroplasty
    distal radioulnar joint 214, 216, 217–18, 221–5
    elbow
        distraction 108–9, 111
        excision 108, 111
        replacement 103–29
    metacarpophalangeal joint 244–5
    proximal interphalangeal joint 268–70
        Eaton Malerich 269
        Modified Tupper 269–70
    shoulder 67–70
    thumb
        interpositional resection techniques 290,
            291–5, 297
        replacement 295–6, 297
    see also replacement arthroplasty
Arthroscan (arthrography followed by CT scan),
    radiocarpal stiffness 155, 162
arthroscopy
    elbow 86
        postoperative rehabilitation 88
        results 88–9
        technique 86–8
    glenohumeral joint, manipulation under
        anaesthesia 44–5
    radiocarpal joint 155, 156, 162
arthrolysis 193–4
    shoulder
        anatomical factors 9, 12
        diagnostic use 35
        frozen shoulder 56
        management of stiffness 57–60
aspirin, rheumatoid arthritis 27
ataxia 333
athetosis 333

Bakhach flap 238
bandages, Biflex 274, 275
benorylate 27
biceps brachii muscle 12
Biflex bandages 274, 275
bone formation *see* ossification
bone scanning, shoulder 35
bony disorders, shoulder stiffness and 4
botulinum toxin, focal dystonia 322
boutonnire deformity 253, 267, 286
Bowers' hemi-interpositional tendon arthroplasty
    214, 218, 221, 223
    results 224–5
brachial plexus palsy 3–4

brain damage, severe, assessment of outcome
    320–1
Bunnell test 233
bupivacaine, suprascapular nerve block 30
burns
    elbow stiffness 79, 82
    proximal interphalangeal joint stiffness 253
    shoulder joint 16
    wrist stiffness 155–6, 157, 179, 181

calcitonin, reflex sympathetic dystrophy 386
calcium pyrophosphate dihydrate (CPPD) crystal
    deposition 172, 173, 262
Capener splint 302
capitate proximal migration 162
capitolunate arthrodesis 185–7
caprectomy, proximal row 194–5
capsulitis, adhesive *see* frozen shoulder
caput ulnae syndrome 216
carcinoma, intramuscular metastases 377
carpal arcs 153
carpal dislocations 160, 164
carpal height 153, 154
carpal instability 162
carpal synostosis 145
carpal tunnel syndrome 160
castle flap 238, 239, 240
causalgia 383, 384
    management 383–4, 385–7
    pathophysiology 384–5
Charcot joints 262–3
Chinese forearm flaps *see* radial forearm flaps
chloroquine, rheumatoid arthritis 28
chondrocalcinosis, wrist 167, 173
chondromatosis, synovial 78, 262
    elbow replacement arthroplasty 115
club hand
    radial 143–4, 211
        treatment 144
    ulnar 144–5, 211
        treatment 145
Colles' fracture, reflex sympathetic dystrophy after
    382
coma 319
    prolonged 319–20
        anaesthesiological guidelines 323
        clinical assessment of survivors 321–2
        functional assessment 322
        neurorehabilitation 319–20
        spasticity after 319–30
        surgical rehabilitation 322, 323–8
coma decerebration syndrome 350

compartment syndromes, atypical 365–79
  aetiology 371–7
  diagnosis 365–6
    instrumental examination 366
  indications for fasciotomy 366–7
  malignancy and 375–7
  muscle ischaemia 365, 366
  perinatal, and brachial artery thrombosis 373–4,
      377
  perioperative 373
  post-traumatic 371–3
  site 367–71
computed tomography (CT)
  radiocarpal joint 155, 162
  shoulder 5
congenital disorders
  distal radioulnar joint 210–12
  elbow 75
  radiocarpal joint 143–8
  shoulder 3–4
Constant shoulder functional score 35–6
continuous passive motion (CPM), postoperative
    rehabilitation of elbow 88, 96
coracoacromial ligament 9
coracohumeral ligament 9
  frozen shoulder 56
corticosteroid therapy
  frozen shoulder 49–50, 51
    manipulation and 51
  osteoarthritis 28
corticosteroids, oral, frozen shoulder 51
crush injuries, wrist stiffness 156, 158, 179, 181
cryotherapy, proximal interphalangeal joint 273
crystal arthropathies, shoulder 25
crystal-induced arthritis, wrist 172–3
cuff tear arthropathy 29
cytokines
  fibrogenic 15, 16, 17, 18
  see also names of specific cytokines

Darrach excisional arthroplasty 214, 217, 221, 223,
    224
  results 224–5
deltoid muscle 12
  abduction contractures 17–18
denervation
  spastic palsy 315
  wrist 189–90
dermatosclerosis 78
dextropropoxyphene, rheumatoid arthritis 27
diabetes, frozen shoulder and 51
discus articularis, wrist 135, 138

disease modifying anti-rheumatic drugs (DMARDs)
    28
distal radioulnar joint (DRUJ)
  alignment disturbance 214–15
  capsulectomy 215–16
  incongruency 214, 221
  osteology 203–6, 207
  soft tissues 206–10
distal radioulnar joint stiffness
  arthrodesis see Sauv-Kapandji procedure
  arthroplasty 214, 216, 217–18, 221–5
  causes 203–19
  congenital 210–12
  post-traumatic 212–16
  rehabilitation 227–8
  rheumatoid arthritis and 216–18
  surgical treatment 221–6
    complications 224
    operative techniques 223–4
    results 224–5
distraction surgery, elbow 91–4, 108–9, 111
distractor, elbow 91
  implantation 93
  Judet distractor 91–2, 94
dorsal instability of segment incalated (DISI) 160,
    168, 175, 198
dorsalis pedis flap plus extensor 181
Dupuytren's disease 254–5
dwarfism, diastrophic 147
dysosotosis multiplex 147
dystonia 309–10
  focal (writer's cramp) 307, 310

elbow joint
  ankylosis 78
    after juvenile chronic arthritis 113, 114–16
    in full extension 82
    replacement arthroplasty 103–29
  arthrodesis, angle of fusion 83
  arthrogryposis 78, 355–9
    conservative treatment 355
    surgical treatment 356–9
  functions 81
  movement(s) 73–4, 81
    activities of daily living 81–2
    loss 73
  spastic (flexion) contracture 335, 337
    surgical treatment 323, 326–7, 337, 342
  stabilizers 73
elbow stiffness
  aetiology 73–5
    arthrolysis

elbow stiffness *contd*
    choice of procedure 99–101
    elementary surgical procedures 99
    see also subheadings arthroscopic/open
      arthrolysis
    arthroplasty *see subheadings* arthroscopic/
      excision/replacement
  arthroplasty
  arthroscopic arthrolysis 85–9
    postoperative rehabilitation 88
    results 88–9
    technique 86–8
  articular (intra-articular)
    non-traumatic 78
    post-traumatic 75, 79–80
  assessment 77–80, 85
  classification 75, 77–80
  compensation by other joints 82–3
  definition 119
  distraction arthroplasty 108–9, 111
  effect on activities of daily living 82
  excision (resection) arthroplasty 108, 111
  extra-articular
    non-traumatic 77–8
    post-traumatic 75, 79
  incidence 74
  non-surgical management 85
  open arthrolysis 95–8
    indications 95
    postoperative management 96
    results 97
    technique 96
  open arthrolysis with distraction 91–4
  post-traumatic 73, 74, 79–80
    classification 75
  replacement arthroplasty
    complications 107, 117, 128
    GSB III prosthesis 119–29
    indications 119–20
    postoperative management 123
    results 103, 107, 113–17, 118, 123–8
    technique 105–7, 111–13, 123
electrical stimulation, reflex sympathetic dystrophy
  386, 387
electromyographic kinesiology (EK) 310
electromyography (EMG) 310–11, 312
electrotherapy, metacarpophalangeal joint stiffness
  248
enchondromas, radiocarpal joint 146
epicondyle, medial, aponeurotic release 339, 341
epidermolysis, bullous 78
ergotherapy, metacarpophalangeal joint 249

Essex-Lopresti injury 207, 213
exostoses
  multiple cartilaginous, radiocarpal joint 145–6
  ulna 210, 211
extensor retinaculum, wrist 208, 210
extensor tendon tenolysis 267

F wave recording 312–13
fasciotomy, compartment syndromes 366–7
fibroblasts, wound healing 20
fibromatosis 147
fibrosis
  pathogenesis 15
  shoulder 15
    biological molecules implicated 18–23
    clinical causes 15–18
fingers
  spastic (flexion) contracture 336–7
    surgery for 338–42
  splinting, wrist stiffness 180–1, 182
flail shoulder 63
flaps
  metacarpophalangeal joint stiffness 237–40
  radiocarpal joint stiffness 179–80, 181–2
flexor carpi ulnaris 138
  lengthening with muscular continuity 338, 339
  tendon transfer to extensor carpi radialis brevis
    340, 341
flexor tendons
  repair 255
    healing after 255–6
    joint stiffness after 256
  sheath anatomy 260–1
  tenolysis 265–7
focal dystonia (writer's cramp) 307, 310
forearm
  compartment syndrome 367, 369, 370
  fractures, distal radioulnar joint stiffness 212–13
  pronation contracture, arthrogryposis 361
  spastic (pronation) contracture 335, 337
    surgery for 327, 337–8, 340, 342
forearm flaps 179–80, 181, 238, 239
free radicals, role in fibrosis 18
frozen shoulder 4, 47–53, 56
  causes 33
  definition 47
  diagnosis 34–6, 48
  manipulation under anaesthesia 44–5
  natural history 47–8
  pathogenesis 51–2
  pulmonary disease and 52

secondary 37–8, 51
   treatment 48–51

gangrene, newborn 373–4
glenohumeral joint
   arthritis 25–6, 28
   arthroscopy
      manipulation under anaesthesia 44–5
      release of contractures 57–60
   mobility testing 41
glenohumeral ligaments 9
glenoid labrum 7–8
glove, pressure (Jobst type) 387
gold salts 28
gout 172–3, 262
grip strength 153
growth factors see cytokines; *names of specific*
      growth factors
guanethidine blocks, reflex sympathetic dystrophy
      384, 385, 386, 388

H reflex 311, 312
haemophilic arthropathy 79
hand
   arthrogryposis 361, 363–4
   compartment syndrome 370, 371
   denervation in spastic palsy 315–17
   immobilization
      interphalangeal joints 257, 260, 263
      position 257, 263
   spastic contractures 335–7
      assessment of motor function 346
      surgery for 327, 338–46
hemiarthroplasty, shoulder 69
humerus
   fornix 9
   greater tuberosity, avulsion fracture 38
   head, comminuted fracture 38
Hunter syndrome 147
Hurler's syndrome 147
hydrotherapy, elbow 96
hyperpathia 381
hyperthyroidism, frozen shoulder and 51
hypertonus, spastic 308, 309–10
hyponeurotization in spastic palsy 315–18
hypothyroidism, frozen shoulder and 51

ibuprofen 27
immobilization
   elbow stiffness after 79, 80
   fingers, joint stiffness after 232, 237
   hand, position 257, 263

interphalangeal joints 257, 260, 263
   thumb rehabilitation 300–1
   wrist
      position 200–1
      stiffness after 159, 180
impingement syndrome, shoulder 16–17, 55
   treatment 38
indomethacin 27
infection
   finger stiffness and 262
   shoulder joint 17, 63
   wrist 165, 173–5
inflammatory disorders
   shoulder 3, 4, 16–18
   wrist 165, 169–73
   see also names of specific disorders
infraspinatus muscle 10
interligamentous sulcus 137
interosseous membrane, distal radioulnar joint
      206–7
   scarring 213
   tear 213
interphalangeal (IP) joints
   anatomy 259–60
   capsular lesions 261–2
   cartilage destruction 262–3
   immobilization 263
      position 257, 260, 263
   proximal see proximal interphalangeal joint
   synovial tissue diseases 262
   thumb 277
interphalangeal joint stiffness
   aetiopathogenesis 260–1
   prevention 263
   thumb 286
irradiation, shoulder 17

Kapandji II procedure 218
Kienbck's disease 164, 165, 195
kinematics 311
kinesiology, electromyographic 310
Kinetec 8091 248
kinetics 311

leukaemia, compartment syndrome and 376, 377
Levame orthosis 302
loose bodies
   distal radioulnar joint 214
   shoulder 3
lunate, idiopathic necrosis see Kienbck's disease
lunocapitate arthrodesis 185–7
lymphocytes, wound healing 16, 20

M50 device, metacarpophalangeal joint
    rehabilitation 247
macrophages, wound healing 16, 20
Madelung's deformity 145, 211, 212
magnetic resonance imaging (MRI), shoulder 5, 35
malignancy
    compartment syndrome and 375–7
    intramuscular metastases 377
manipulation, shoulder 44–5
    contraindications 51
    frozen 50–1
    with corticosteroid injections 51
Maroteaux-Lamy syndrome 147
massage
    metacarpophalangeal joint 247, 248
    proximal interphalangeal joint 273
    shoulder 42
meniscus homologue 137
metacarpal flap, reverse flow 238
metacarpophalangeal (MP) joint
    anatomy 231–2
    arthrodesis 244
    arthrogryposis 363–4
    locked 240
    passive mobilization 248
    prostheses 244–5
    thumb 277
        capsuloplasty 343, 344
        dislocation 284–5
        stiffness 284–6
metacarpophalangeal joint stiffness
    arthroplasties 244–5
    post-traumatic 237
        causes 231–5, 247
        clinical aspects 232–3
        in extension 232–3, 237
        in flexion 233, 235
    rehabilitation 247–50
    treatment
        conservative 237
        flaps 237–40
        planning 234
        surgical 243–6
        tenolysis 239–40
methotrexate 28
midcarpal joint 135, 138
    stiffness, ankylosing spondylitis 172
    in wrist movement 140
Milwaukee shoulder 29
monocytes, wound healing 16, 20
motor neurone syndrome, upper/lower 308
motor system disorders 307–8

clinical evaluation 308–10
neurophysiological evaluation 310–13
motor unit (MU) discharge, spastic muscle 311
MP joint see metacarpophalangeal joint
mucopolysaccharidosis 147
muscle tone 308
    evaluation 309–10
        neurophysiological 310
        prolonged coma survivors 321
myoelectric upper limb exerciser (MULE) 228
myositis ossificans 78, 115, 117, 118
myostatic contracture 329, 332–3, 341, 342

naproxen 27
Neer's test 55
neurological diseases
    motor system see motor system disorders
    signs and symptoms 307
neuromuscular diseases
    elbow stiffness 77–8
    types 332–3
neuropathic joint disease 262–3
neurophysiological tests, spasticity 310
neurorehabilitation, spastic upper limb 349–54
    after prolonged coma 319–20
nitric oxide 18
non-steroidal anti-inflammatory drugs (NSAIDs)
    adverse effects 27–8
    osteoarthritis 28
    prescription guidelines 27
    rheumatoid arthritis 27

occupational therapy
    elbow 96, 123
    reflex sympathetic dystrophy 387, 388
ochronosis 262
oedema, hand 232, 237, 252–3, 258
Ollier's disease 146
orthoses
    arthrogryposis of elbow 355
    Levame 302
ossification, elbow
    capsular 80
    extracapsular tissues 79
    heterotopic 74–5, 78, 95
osteoarthritis
    distal radioulnar joint 213–14
    elbow
        primary 78
        secondary 79
    finger joints 262
    shoulder 4, 28

thumb base 299
wrist 175–6
    post-traumatic 160–4, 175–6
oxicams 27

paracetamol 27
paracrine action of cytokines 16
parkinsonism 307, 310, 312
peroxynitrite 18
phenylacetic acids 27
physiotherapy
    arthrogryposis
        elbow 355, 359
        hand and wrist 361
    distal radioulnar joint 227–8
    frozen shoulder 50
    metacarpophalangeal joint stiffness 247–8
    neurorehabilitation of spastic upper limb 352–3
    postoperative
        distal radioulnar joint 228
        elbow 88, 96
        elbow replacement arthroplasty 123
        flexor tendon repair 256
        radiocarpal joint 202
        stiff shoulder 42–3
    proximal interphalangeal joint 273
    radiocarpal joint 201–2
    reflex sympathetic dystrophy 385, 387
PIP joint see proximal interphalangeal joint
piroxicam 27
pisotriquetral joint capsule 138
platelet derived growth factor 52
polyelectromyography 310
pronator quadratus island flap 179
propionic acid derivatives 27
prostheses
    elbow 103, 113, 120
        GSB III 120–9
        Hospital for Special Surgery design 103, 104
    metacarpophalangeal joint 244–5
    proximal interphalangeal joint 270–1
    shoulder 67–8
    silastic 192, 245, 270, 295–6, 297
    thumb base 294, 295–6, 297
        partial 295
    wrist 191–2
proximal interphalangeal (PIP) joint 251
    anatomy 251–2, 259–60
    ankylosis 252
    arthrodesis 268
    arthrogryposis 363, 364
    dislocation 261–2

flexion 260–1
immobilization position 257, 260
post-coma spasticity, surgical treatment 327
prostheses 270–1
proximal interphalangeal joint stiffness
    arthrolysis 267–8
    arthroplasties 268–70
    causes 251–8, 260
        extrinsic 252, 253–7, 261
        intrinsic 261–3
    iatrogenic 257
    rehabilitation 273–5
    surgical treatment 265–72
    tenolysis 265–7
proximal row carpectomy 194–5
pseudogout see calcium pyrophosphate dihydrate
    (CPPD) crystal deposition
psoriasis, elbow joint 78
psoriatic arthritis 172, 262
pyrophosphate arthropathy, shoulder 25

rabdomyolysis, drug-induced, compartment
    syndrome and 374–5, 377
radial artery flap 179
radial club hand (radial deficiency) 143–4, 211
    treatment 144
radial forearm flaps 179, 180, 181
radiocarpal joint 197
    anatomy 135–8
    ankylosis 165, 166
        infection 174, 175
        inflammatory disorders 172
        rheumatoid arthritis 170–1
    biomechanics 138–41
    immobilization
        position 200–1
        stiffness after 159, 180
    mobilization 198, 201–2
    movement(s) 138–41, 149, 197–8
        stiffness diagnosis 152
    osteoarthritis 175–6
    prostheses 191–2
radiocarpal joint stiffness
    arthrodesis
        limited 185–9
        total 190–1
    arthroscopic arthrolysis 193–4
    causes
        extrinsic 153, 155–8
        general 169–77
        intrinsic 155, 159–66

radiocarpal joint stiffness *contd*
  congenital 143–8
  definition 149
  diagnosis 151–3
  extra-articular 153, 155–8
  flaps 179–80, 181–2
  history 149
  infection and 173–5
  inflammatory diseases and 165, 169–73
  intra-articular 155, 159–66
  pain and 151–2
  post-traumatic 149, 159–64
    chronic 160–4
    early 159–60
  preventive care 198, 200–2
  proximal row carpectomy 194–5
  rehabilitation 197–202
  scapholunate advanced collapse treatment
      185–8
  tenolysis 180–1, 182
radiocarpal ligaments 135–7, 138
  stretching 198, 199, 202
radiography
  contrast, shoulder 35
  radiocarpal stiffness 153, 162
  shoulder 5, 34–5
    frozen shoulder diagnosis 48
radiohumeral synostosis, congenital 211
radiolunate arthrodesis 189, 190
radiotherapy, frozen shoulder 51
radioulnar joint, distal see distal radioulnar joint
radioulnar synostosis, congenital 211
radius 206
  congenital abnormalities 143–4, 211
  fractures, distal radioulnar joint stiffness 212–16,
      227
  malunion
    extra-articular 159–66
    intra-articular 160, 163
recessus prescaphoideus 137
recessus prestyloideus 137
recessus pretriquetralis 137
reflex sympathetic dystrophy (RSD) 257–8, 286,
      296, 381–9
  definition 381
  management 383, 384, 385
  pathophysiology 384–7
  rehabilitation 385, 386, 387–8
reflexes 309
  neurophysiological testing 311–12
  stretch, overactive 332
rehabilitation

distal radioulnar joint 227–8
elbow
  arthroscopic arthrolysis 88
  open arthrolysis 96
  replacement arthroplasty 123
flexor tendon repair 256
metacarpophalangeal joint 247–50
proximal interphalangeal joint 273–5
radiocarpal joint 197–202
reflex sympathetic dystrophy 385, 386, 387–8
shoulder, stiff and postoperative 41–6
spastic upper limb see spasticity,
      neurorehabilitation/surgical rehabilitation
thumb 299–303
see also neurorehabilitation
replacement arthroplasty
  distal radioulnar joint 218
  elbow
    ankylosed elbows 103–29
    complications 107, 117, 128
    GSB III prosthesis 119–29
    indications 119–20
    postoperative management 123
    results 103, 107, 113–17, 118
    technique 105–7, 111–13, 123
  metacarpophalangeal joint 244–5
  proximal interphalangeal joint 270–1
  shoulder 67–70
    contraindications 69
    indications 69
    postoperative management 70
  thumb 295–6, 297
retinoic acid syndrome 376–7
rhabdomyolysis, drug-induced, compartment
      syndrome and 374–5, 377
rheumatoid arthritis
  distal radioulnar joint 216–18
  elbow 78
    replacement arthroplasty 114, 115, 119, 123–7
  finger stiffness 262
  shoulder 4, 17
    management 25–8, 29, 30
  thumb 299, 300
  wrist 165, 166, 169–71
    young people 171
rigidity 308–9, 333
  assessment, prolonged coma survivors 309
rotator cuff 10
  suprascapular nerve block 30
  tears, treatment 38
  tendonitis 4, 16
    calcific 16

Sanfilippo syndrome 147
sarcoidosis 262
Sauvé-Kapandji procedure 216, 217, 218, 221, 222,
    223, 225
    complications 224
    results 224–5
scaphoid non-union 162–3, 165
scaphoid non-union advanced collapse (SNAC)
    163, 164, 188
scaphoid-trapezium-trapezoid (STT) joint,
    osteoarthritis 175
scapholunate advanced collapse (SLAC) 160–1,
    162, 176, 185–8
scapholunate instability 162
scapulothoracic joint, mobility 41
Scheie syndrome 147
scleroderma 253–4
    finger stiffness 262
Secretan's syndrome 239
seronegative spondarthropathies, shoulder 26
sesamoid-metacarpal synsotosis 343, 344
shoulder hand syndrome 381–2
shoulder joint
    anatomy 7–13
    arthrodesis 63–6
        complications 66
        contraindications 64
        indications 63–4
        position 64
        postoperative management 66
        technique 65
    arthrogryposis 355, 357
        surgery for 357, 358
    compartment syndrome 367, 368
    destructive arthritis 29
    elderly, symptomatic disorders 30–1
    fibrosis and adhesions 15, 56
        biological molecules in 18–23
        clinical causes 15–18
    infection 17, 63
    innervation of skin 12–13
    irradiation 17
    movement(s) 3, 10
        combined 3
        sectors 41
    osteoarthritis 28
    painful arc syndrome 10, 16
    rehabilitation after surgery 41–6
    relationships to nerves and vessels 12
    rheumatoid arthritis 17
        management 25–8, 29, 30
    spastic contracture 335

    surgery for 323, 326
shoulder stiffness
    acquired 4
    assessment 33–6
        diagnostic 34
        functional 35–6
    bipolar 57
        arthroscopy 60
    bony disorders and 4
    capsular 56
        arthroscopic treatment 57–60
    causes 33
    classification 55–7
    clinical evaluation 5
    congenital 3–4
    definition 3
    extracapsular 56
    fibrosis/adhesions and 15–24
    from remote sites 4
    functional (false) 55
    inflammatory causes 3, 4, 16–18
    investigations 34–5
    neurological causes 4
    organic 56–7
    post-traumatic 4, 37–8, 57
        manipulation 44
        treatment 38–9
    postoperative 33, 34, 41–2, 57
        arthroscopy 60
        prevention 42–3
        treatment 43–5, 60
    rehabilitation 41
    replacement arthroplasty 67–70
        contraindications 69
        failed 63
        indications 69
        postoperative management 70
    transient 3
    see also frozen shoulder
silastic prostheses 192, 245, 270, 295–6, 297
skin disorders/lesions
    elbow stiffness 78
    metacarpophalangeal joint stiffness 232, 234,
        237–8, 247
    proximal interphalangeagl joint stiffness 253–4
skin flaps
    metacarpophalangeal joint treatment 237–40
    radiocarpal joint treatment 179–80, 181–2
sonography, shoulder 5
spasm 309
    assessment, prolonged coma survivors 321

spasticity
  aetiology 331
  after prolonged coma 319–30
    anaesthesiological guidelines 323
    clinical assessment 321–2
    functional assessment 322
    surgical rehabilitation 322, 323–8
  arm attitudes/movements after central lesions
      350–2
  clinical aspects 307–10
  deformities
    hand 335–7
    upper limb 335
  elbow stiffness 77–8
  extent of limb involvement 333, 335
  hyponeurotization in spastic palsy 315–18
  neuromuscular disorder types 332–3, 334
  neurophysiological evaluation 310–13
  neurorehabilitation 349–54
    after prolonged coma 319–20
  sensory impairment of hand 335
    tests 335
  surgical rehabilitation 331–48
    after prolonged coma 322, 323–8
    contraindications 332
    goals 337
    indications 337
    preoperative evaluation 331–7
    prognosis 337
    results 346–7
    techniques 338–46
  wrist stiffness 156
splints/splinting
  arthrogryposis
    elbow 355
    hand and wrist 361
  distal radioulnar joint rehabilitation 228
  elbow 85, 88, 96, 355
  fingers, wrist stiffness 180–1, 182
  metacarpophalangeal joint rehabilitation 248–9,
      250
  metacarpophalangeal joint stiffness management
      237
    postoperative 240
  proximal interphalangeal joint rehabilitation
      273–4
  reflex sympathetic dystrophy rehabilitation 387–8
  thumb rehabilitation 299, 300–3
  wrist
    arthrogryposis 361
    congenital abnormalities 144, 145
spondarthropathies, seronegative, shoulder 26

stellate ganglion block
  frozen shoulder 51
  reflex sympathetic dystrophy 385
Stener lesions 285, 286
stereognosis defects in spasticity 335
Still's disease 78, 171
stretch reflex, overactive 332
subacromial bursitis 4, 16
subacromial impingement syndrome 16–17, 55
  treatment 38
subacromial space 12, 13
subscapularis muscle 11
Suddeck syndrome 258
sulphasalazine 28
superoxide anion 18
suprascapular nerve blocks 30
  osteoarthritis 28
supraspinatus muscle 10
swan-neck deformity 256–7
  cerebral palsy 344
    surgical treatment 344–6
synovitis
  diffuse pigmented villonodular 79
  rheumatic proliferative 78
systemic lupus erythematosus
  elbow 78
  finger stiffness 262
  shoulder involvement 26

T (tendon/deep tendon) reflex 311–12
tendons
  healing 255–6
  see also extensor tendon; flexor tendon
tenoarthrolysis, total anterior 267, 268
tenodesis, wrist 151
tenolysis
  metacarpophalangeal joint 239–40
  proximal interphalangeal joint 265–7
  radiocarpal joint 180–1, 182
tenotomy
  compartment syndrome, hand 371
  spastic hand 327, 339, 342
tensor fasciae latae flaps 181
teres minor muscle 10
Thibierge-Weissenbach syndrome 78
thumb
  arthrogryposis 363–4
    thumb-in-palm deformity 363, 364
  spastic deformities 336
    adduction 336, 342
    surgery for 337, 342–4
    thumb-in-palm (adduction-flexion) 336, 337,

340, 342, 344
thumb base prostheses 294, 295–6, 297
    partial 295
thumb stiffness 277
    basal joint 289–98, 299
        aetiology 289–90
        articular surgery 290–7
        soft tissue surgery 290
    interphalangeal joint 286
    interrelated 277, 286
    metacarpophalangeal joint 284–6
    rehabilitation 299–303
    trapeziometacarpal joint 277, 278–84
    treatment 277–8
thyroid disease, frozen shoulder and 51–2
tonic vibration reflex (TVR) 312
transforming growth factor-a
    inhibition, prevention of adhesions between
        tendon and synovium 21–3
    mechanisms of action in wound healing 19–20
    role in fibrosis 18–19
trapeziectomy 290, 291, 296
trapeziometacarpal joint 277
    stiffness 277, 278–84
        extrinsic causes 279–84
        intrinsic causes 278
trauma
    compartment syndromes and 371–3
    distal radioulnar joint stiffness 212–16
    elbow stiffness 73, 74, 75, 79–80
    metacarpophalangeal joint stiffness 231–5, 237,
        247
    radiocarpal joint stiffness 149, 159–64, 175–6
    shoulder 4
        fibrosis and adhesion formation 15–16
        stiffness after 37–9, 44, 57
tremor 333
triangular fibrocartilaginous complex (TFCC) 208,
    209
trigger finger 286
trigger wrist 156
tryptophan, reflex sympathetic dystrophy 386
tuberculosis
    shoulder 17, 52
    wrist 165, 166, 174–5

ulna
    congenital abnormalities 143–4, 210, 211
    fractures, distal radioulnar joint stiffness 213–15
    matched ulna procedure (Watson) 218, 221, 222,
        223
        results 224–5
    recession 221, 223–4, 225
ulnar club hand (ulnar deficiency) 144–5, 211
    treatment 145
ulnar flap 179
ulnocarpal impaction syndrome 216
ultrasound
    metacarpophalangeal joint rehabilitation 247–8
    proximal interphalangeal joint rehabilitation 273

vagina synovialis intertubercularis 8
volar capsuloplasty 296
volar plate 251–2, 257, 259
    detachment 261
volar wounds, wrist stiffness 156
Volkmann contracture 365, 370
    perinatal 373, 374
Volkmann's disease/syndrome 79, 156, 308

wafer procedure, distal radioulnar joint 221, 223, 224
Watson procedure, distal radioulnar joint 218, 221,
    222, 223
Watson procedure, distal radioulnar joint treatment,
    results 224–5
wound healing 15
    biological molecules in 18
        transforming growth factor-a 18–23
    fractures 15–16
    soft tissue trauma 15–16
wrist
    arthrogryposis 361–3
    denervation 189–90
    spastic (flexion) contractures 336–7
        surgery for 327, 338–42
    see also radiocarpal joint
wrist stiffness
    causes 133
    see also radiocarpal stiffness; radioulnar stiffness
writer's cramp see focal dystonia

x-rays see radiography